PERIL TO THE NERVE: GLAUCOMA AND CLINICAL NEURO-OPHTHALMOLOGY

To our wives, Charlotte and Christine
To our children: Jonathan, Rachel and Jack
You make life and work easier

PERIL TO THE NERVE: GLAUCOMA AND CLINICAL NEURO-OPHTHALMOLOGY

edited by Barry J. Leader, MD and
Jonathan C. Calkwood, MD

Proceedings of the 45th Annual Symposium of the
New Orleans Academy of Ophthalmology,
New Orleans, LA, USA, April 25–28, 1996

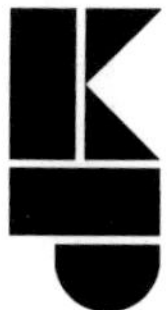

Kugler Publications / The Hague / The Netherlands

Library of Congress Cataloging-in-Publication Data

New Orleans Academy of Ophthalmology. Session (45th : 1996 : New
     Orleans, La.)
        Peril to the nerve : glaucoma and clinical neuro-ophthalmology :
     proceedings of the 45th Annual Symposium, New Orleans, LA, USA,
     April 25–28, 1996, organized by the New Orleans Academy of
     Ophthalmology; editor, glaucoma, Barry J. Leader : editor, neuro-
     ophthalmology, Jonathan C. Calkwood.
             p.   cm.
        Includes bibliographical references and index.
        ISBN 906299153X
        1. Glaucoma--Congresses.   2. Neuroophthalmology--Congresses.
     I. Leader, Barry J.   II. Calkwood, Jonathan C.   III. Title.
        [DNLM: 1. Glaucoma--therapy--congresses.   2. Optic Nerve Diseases-
     -therapy--congresses.   WW 290 N5317p   1997]
     RE871.N47   1996
     617.7'41--dc21
     DNLM/DLC
     for Library of Congress   97-13859
                                                                            CIP

ISBN 90-6299-153-X

Distributors:
For the U.S.A. and Canada:
Kugler Publications
c/o Demos Vermande, Order Department
386 Park Avenue South, Suite 201
New York, NY 10016, USA
Telefax (+212) 683 0118

For all other countries:
Kugler Publications
P.O. Box 97747
2509 GC The Hague, The Netherlands
Telefax (+31.70) 33 00 254

TABLE OF CONTENTS

Surgical treatment of glaucoma

Glaucoma: surgical challenges

NEURO-OPHTHALMOLOGY

PREFACE

Peril to the nerve

> "You don't see what you don't know".
> George Spaeth

For a half century the New Orleans Academy has been dedicated to providing an annual indepth evaluation of an important clinical topic in ophthalmology. Our symposia have always been a combination of relevant clinical thought based on outstanding knowledge and current research. In April, 1996, this tradition continued with the symposium "Peril to the Nerve" - Glaucoma and Clinical Neuro-ophthalmology. From the latest discussions of the literature to provocative round table and clinical controversy presentations, the participants discussed clinically useful topics in these fields. For four days the nearly two hundred physicians in attendance were treated to innovative thinking from speakers who were chosen for their lively approach to science and teaching.

The panelists in the glaucoma segment were a wonderful combination of acerbic wit and clinical insight. Doctors Michael Kass, Donald Minckler, Paul Palmberg, Harry Quigley, George Spaeth and Thom Zimmerman are some of the great names in this field. They enjoy teaching, are critical of each other, and like to have fun. This was a wonderful mix, which shows in their presentations.

The neuro-ophthalmology section included Doctors Ronald M. Burde, Joel S. Glazer, and Norman J. Schatz. This was a reunion of sorts for these physicians as, exactly twenty-five years previously, they appeared on the panel of the New Orleans Academy discussing neuro-ophthalmology. Although a little older, these three gentlemen used their additional wisdom and experience to make the neuro-ophthalmology section interesting and informative. Any reader needing a refresher in clinically relevant neuro-ophthalmology will find this section particularly helpful.

New Orleans has always been a fun place to visit and once a year, the New Orleans Academy makes it a fun place to learn. The more detailed presentation of each topic in this monograph expands on the oral presentations given during the symposium.

As editors, we would like to thank the president of the New Orleans Academy, Dr. William Rachal, and the executive secretary, Mrs. Emily Busby, for their tremendous help in organizing this symposium. The editorial expertise of Kugler Publications is also gratefully acknowledged. The success of this symposium, however, would not have been possible without the enthusiastic and continuing support of the ophthalmologists of New Orleans and South Louisiana who are members of the New Orleans Academy. To them we give our appreciation.

Barry J. Leader, MD
Jonathan C. Calkwood, MD

CONTRIBUTORS

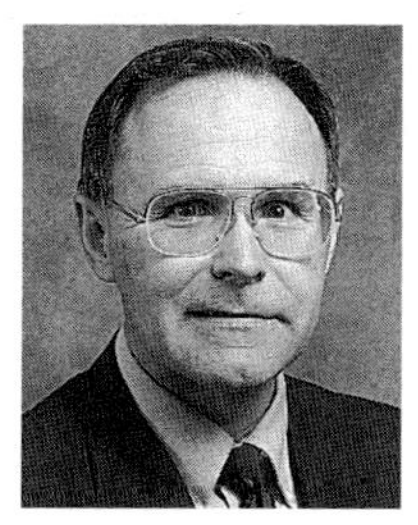

PAUL PALMBERG, MD, PhD
Professor of Ophthalmology
Bascom Palmer Eye Institute
Miami, Florida

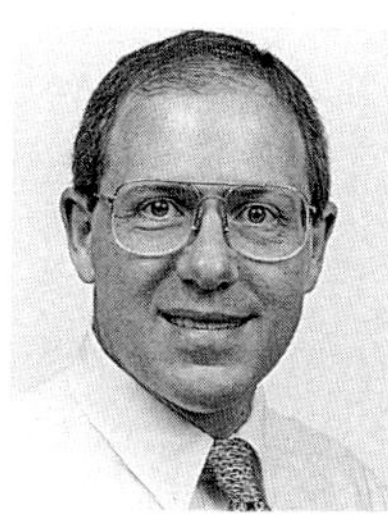

HARRY QUIGLEY, MD
A. Edward Maumenee
Professor, Ophthalmology
Baltimore, Maryland

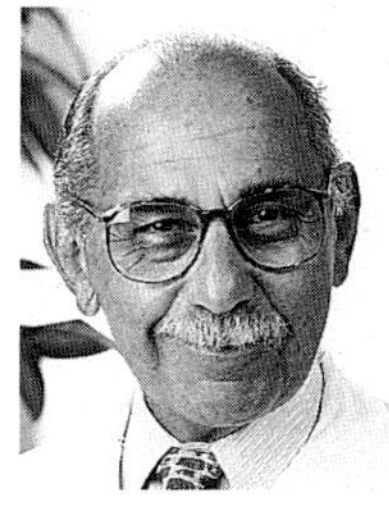

NORMAN J. SCHATZ, MD
Professor of Neuro-Ophthalmology
Mercy Neuroscience Institute
Miami, Florida

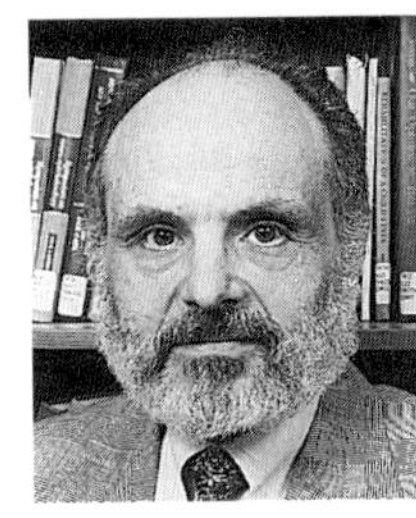

RONALD M. BURDE, MD
Professor and Chairman
Department of Ophthalmology
Montefiore Medical Ceter
Bronx, New York

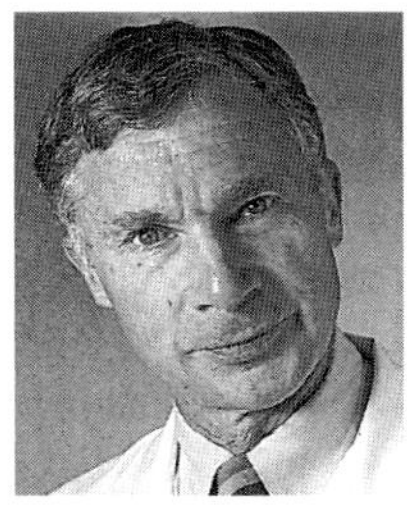

GEORGE J. SPAETH, MD
Professor of Ophthalmology
Jefferson Medical College
Director, Glaucoma Service
    Wills Eye Hospital
Philadelphia, Pennsylvania

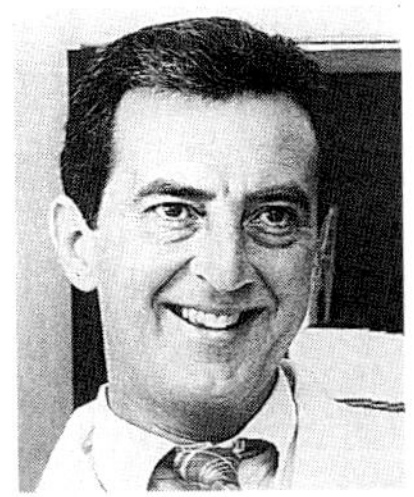

THOM J. ZIMMERMAN, MD, PhD
Professor and Chairman
Department of Ophthalmology and
    Toxicology
Kentucky Lions Research Institute
Louisville, Kentucky

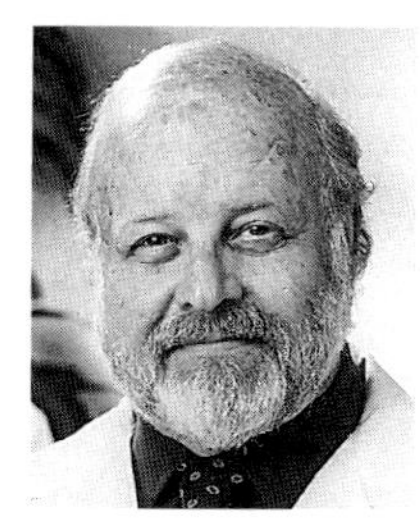

JOEL S. GLASER, MD
Professor, Neuro-Ophthalmology
Mercy Neuro-Science Institute
Bascom Palmer Eye Institute
Miami, Florida

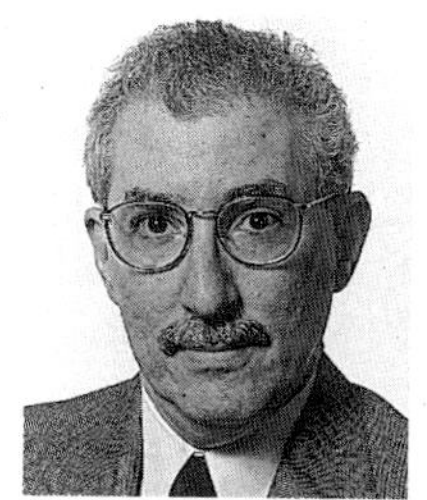

MICHAEL A. KASS, MD
Professor of Ophthalmology
    and Vice-Chairman
Department of Ophthalmology and
    Visual Sciences
Washington University Medical School
St. Louis, Missouri

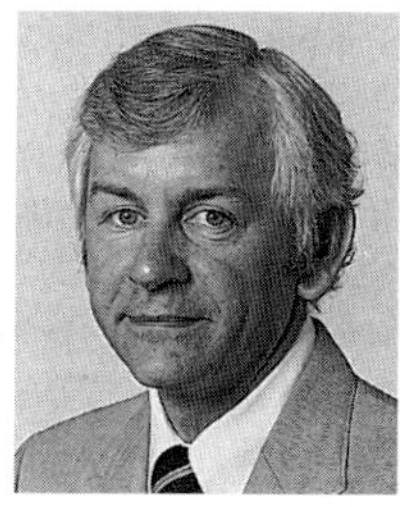

DON MINCKLER, MD
Professor of Ophthalmology
Director of Glaucoma Services
Doheny Eye Institute
University of Southern California
Los Angeles, California

GLAUCOMA

Glaucoma and the nerve

Contents

The progression of open-angle glaucoma: it isn't what you think

Harry A. Quigley

Glaucoma Service and Dana Center for Preventive Ophthalmology, Wilmer Institute, Johns Hopkins University School of Medicine, Baltimore, MD, USA

Abstract

Glaucoma is an important cause of visual disability in the United States and in the world. It is a progressive optic neuropathy related to the intraocular pressure and other risk factors. However, evidence from a variety of sources suggests that the vast majority of glaucoma patients do not go blind in their lifetime. The estimated rate at which glaucoma patients who are under therapy lose further visual function is much slower than is generally believed. As a result, the primary goal for glaucoma monitoring is to differentiate between those persons at greatest risk for visual loss and those who are going to have no significant visual loss. Only in the former are dramatic and risk-producing interventions merited. The most important problem facing glaucoma management at this time is to produce valid measures of glaucoma progression that make this separation in a cost-effective manner.

The issue

All eye care professionals are familiar with glaucoma due to its relatively high prevalence. And, most of us have encountered glaucoma patients with no remaining vision, for whom only rehabilitative services are appropriate. It is widely believed that this is a common result for glaucoma: "they're all going to go blind". I have collected a substantial amount of information over the last three years that may indicate the need to re-evaluate our expectations for the progression of glaucoma.

What factors have determined our view of glaucomatous progression?

It was not until the last 40 years that detailed observations of the actual course of glaucoma became feasible. This derived from technological developments: applanation tonometry, cameras to document alterations in the optic disc, and standardized perimetry with the Goldmann instrument. Of course, many ophthalmologists do not utilize disc photography as a means of follow-up. (I am judging this to be the case based on my viewpoint as a referral center. It would be interesting to conduct a study of actual practices in the community.) And, until the last five

Address for correspondence: Harry A. Quigley, MD, Wilmer 120, Johns Hopkins Hospital, 600 N Wolfe Street, Baltimore, MD 21287, USA

Peril to the Nerve – Glaucoma and Clinical Neuro-Ophthalmology, pp. 3–10
Proceedings of the 45th Annual Symposium of the New Orleans Academy of
Ophthalmology, New Orleans, LA, USA, April 25-28, 1996
edited by Barry J. Leader and Jonathan C. Calkwood
© 1998 Kugler Publications, The Hague/The Netherlands

years, most offices did not carry out quantitative perimetry. This has only occurred since the widespread use of the automated perimeters made by Octopus and Humphrey. Thus, we could not make a realistic estimate of glaucomatous change prior to the last three decades. Consider a person who developed glaucoma at age 40 in 1955. He or she represents the first generation of glaucoma patients whose course has been recorded by 'modern' methods. Furthermore, with the rapid expansion in the number of ophthalmologists during the last 20 years, as well as the mobility of our population, many of those now in practice have not had the opportunity to observe large numbers of glaucoma patients consistently over ten years or more. In addition, we have all learned that it is only by keeping track of progression systematically that accurate conclusions can be reached. Is it any wonder that our idea of glaucoma is in need of re-evaluation? Few observations of large numbers of persons who are representative of all glaucoma patients have been made.

The most frequent source of information about glaucoma is reports from referral centers about their patients. It is characteristic of the persons who seek care at such institutions that they are not representative of all persons with glaucoma. Often, they have had a perceived failure of therapy or complications. They are more likely to be unhappy with the result of care elsewhere, because of an outcome other than the expected one. In the Baltimore Eye Survey, we examined 5500 randomly selected persons from an urban area, half of whom were African-Americans. Among 161 persons found to have open-angle glaucoma by standard criteria, only half were already under care[1]. When the severity of glaucoma was assessed among these persons, it was quite clear that the previously diagnosed were more advanced in their stage of damage[2]. Furthermore, it is only human nature that physicians remember the worst cases (and what we perceive as our failures) much more vividly than the routine or the better results. Thus, our experience with glaucoma is affected by the fact that we care for the more severely affected persons.

In order to obtain a better estimate of the rate of blindness and visual impairment in glaucoma, I evaluated the data from the Baltimore Eye Survey and from similar population-based studies by Barbara and Ron Klein and co-workers in Wisconsin[3] and by Michelle Coffey et al. in Ireland[4]. The proportion of those in each population who were bilaterally blind averaged about 4% among white persons and 8% among African-Americans. By calculating from the prevalence of glaucoma, I estimated that there are 130,000 persons who have gone blind due to glaucoma in the US[5]. This is both a major public health problem and a personal tragedy for each affected person. But, considered in another way, this is a rather smaller proportion of those with glaucoma than would be calculated from the notion that "all glaucoma patients will go blind".

How fast does glaucoma progress?

If we wish to answer this question scientifically, a large, randomly selected group of persons with glaucoma from the US population would have to be observed for ten years or longer, using detailed automated perimetry. To learn the natural progression rate of the disease, there could be no treatment. Recognizing that this is unethical by present standards, a compromise would be to learn the 'natural history' of treated disease. For any study, the size of the sample group needs to be estimated. The question here is, how fast does measurable change occur?

Estimating the proportion who progress

It may be surprising to note that there is only a small amount of information on the progression rate of treated (or untreated) glaucoma. A small number of university centers and large practices, particularly HMOs who keep computerized databases and enforce standardized practice patterns, might provide some important clues in the future. Scott Smith, Joanne Katz and I recently studied 65,000 Humphrey visual field records at the Wilmer Glaucoma Service. We examined those followed for seven years or more whose charts could be extracted for other historical information and who had not had some other reason for change in field status. There were 200 phakic and 65 pseudophakic persons whose fields were considered informative.

The most important issue in the study was how we would decide to measure progression in automated fields. A number of potential methods for monitoring field change have been suggested, from analysis of individual points to regression of global indices. Some compare a small amount of baseline data to each individual future field (Humphrey glaucoma change probability). Recent software has been implemented to perform regression analysis on points, indices and even (with some customizing) on clusters of points (Octopus/Peridata or Dicon/Fieldview). There are several glaucoma clinical trials now ongoing that had to decide on methods to define field progression. As these trials begin to examine their data, it is clear that their methods have serious limitations. For example, the progression criteria used in the Glaucoma Laser Trial were found to be contradicted by subsequent fields in 50% of those originally called progressive. The Low Tension Glaucoma Study has had to revise its progression criteria dramatically after discovering that many of those originally thought to have progressed were simply undergoing long-term fluctuation. Clearly, it is vital to develop widely accepted, valid analytic tools for monitoring field progression that would be applicable to clinical trials and the broader population of glaucoma patients.

In seeking to develop such methods, there is no dearth of ideas for analytic strategies, but the availability of suitable databases for hypothesis testing is quite limited. Among clinical trials, only the Glaucoma Laser Trial has five-year field data and its sample size is quite modest. The Low Tension Glaucoma Study has fewer than 300 persons enrolled and these are possibly distinct in that all have normal intraocular pressures. The other trials will not have long-term data for several years and their populations might be considered to be lacking in generalizability. The Ocular Hypertension Treatment Study only includes persons with initially normal fields. The Collaborative Glaucoma Treatment Study only has newly diagnosed persons. The Advanced Glaucoma Intervention Study includes only those failing on medical therapy, all of whom undergo a surgical procedure as part of the trial. None of these represents data from the medically treated glaucoma patient in the mainstream of those being followed with mild and moderate field loss.

For our study, we tried many different methods for measuring progression. I will state here only the conclusion of a paper[6]. Comparing the trend for change by linear regression analysis had the most to offer, and in doing so, we grouped points into clusters, much as is done in the Glaucoma Hemifield Test of the Humphrey instrument. Using this technique, we found that only about 20% of the eyes worsened during follow-up. This progression rate of 3% per year of glaucoma eyes seemed lower than is generally believed to be true, especially since two-thirds of the group consisted of referred glaucoma patients and one-third African-Americans served by a resident clinic. Could it be that this is a reasonable estimate?

Modelling the course of glaucoma

In order to put this progression rate in perspective with the blindness rate that we have already presented, it is necessary to know at what age the glaucoma patient will develop disease and for how many years the disease will be present before the person's death. Then, the worsening rate from initial damage could be multiplied by the number of affected years. In carrying out such calculations a number of assumptions need to be made. First, we must deal with a heterogeneous group of glaucoma patients as if they behaved in some consistent fashion. The progression must be assumed to start at a relatively small degree of damage and to progress in a monotonic fashion over time, rather than episodically. The damage rate is assumed to be similar in early and in later disease. These are clearly not always the case, but for the purpose of dealing with large numbers of persons, the average behavior may be modelled quite accurately by these assumptions. Furthermore, we need a model of glaucoma that is based on large amounts of data. I have constructed such a model, using the prevalence of glaucoma provided in over 111 studies[7]. The model system[6] uses the fact that glaucoma is a disease in which the prevalence (number in a group with disease at one point in time) can be used to calculate the incidence (number of new cases over time in a group). I started a theoretical group of 30-year-olds (white and black separately) in the model and applied the incidence rate of glaucoma and the mortality rate of US Census data. In this way, we can calculate the number of those who would develop glaucoma in the group and how long the average person has the disease. The average white person is estimated to have glaucoma for only 12.8 years from initial field loss to death, while the comparable figure for blacks is 16.3 years. This points to what may be the major difference between black and white persons with glaucoma – blacks are exposed to disease for 25% longer. For whites, at a worsening rate of 3% per year, 38% would be expected to become worse (though not blind) in their lifetime exposure to glaucoma.

Progression estimates from cross-sectional prevalence and age

I have taken another approach to estimating the progression rate in glaucoma through the use of modelling[2]. We tested the visual field of the 161 glaucoma subjects in the Baltimore Eye Survey with detailed static and kinetic perimetry on the Goldmann perimeter (automated perimetry was not available at the outset of the study). I categorized each of these fields on a nine-level severity scale and compared the level of field damage in each person to other attributes of each person, including age, race, gender, intraocular pressure, treatment, and cup/disc ratio. The severity of visual field damage was significantly associated with age and intraocular pressure. Reasoning that we could use age as a surrogate for duration of disease, I estimated the individual rate of deterioration. For both black and white glaucoma subjects, the rate was a deterioration of two field grading levels per decade.

At this rate, the average person with initial field loss in one eye at age 40 would worsen by eight levels by age 80. This is equivalent to becoming legally blind in one eye and developing an initial field defect in the second eye. An average person who developed first field loss at age 60 would not be legally blind in either eye in the typical lifetime of a person in the US. If the estimates of the average duration of disease that I presented above are correct, the typical worsening in the typical patient is not very substantial.

Previous reports on progression rate

It is interesting to survey the available literature on glaucoma progression rates for comparison. One prospective study followed 42 untreated persons to estimate the natural history of glaucoma in those with normal pressure levels[8]. Forty-four percent of subjects satisfied the chosen criterion (4 dB deterioration in mean defect on Octopus perimetry). While half the subjects progressed in four years, the use of a simple 'all-or-none' criterion of worsening does not allow a progression rate to be estimated. And, this crossing of a criterion was shown by the Glaucoma Laser Trial to overcall progression.

All published studies of progression in glaucoma with history of pressure above normal levels involve persons who were treated to lower intraocular pressure, either medically or surgically. Five studies that I reviewed had multilevel Goldmann or other perimeter scales to judge progression which can be extrapolated to give data that are comparable to my study[9-13]. Their estimated rate of visual field loss was one to two units in ten years, similar to my estimate. Three other studies used linear regression of automated perimetric data to judge progression rates[14-16], but they had short follow-up times (two to four years). From 25% to 50% of patients worsened. Thirteen other studies used 'all or none', categorical criteria (worse or stable)[17-29]. When the worsening rate is estimated, 8% of eyes deteriorated per year. One report estimated rates of glaucoma progression by comparing age and prevalent field findings (similar to my modelling)[31]. Several different progression rate estimates were given, and it is difficult to compare their data to my own. In addition, they studied a clinic-based group, not persons selected randomly, potentially overstating progression rate.

In summary, the literature suggests that half of those with glaucoma do not measurably deteriorate in a five-year period, even when 'worsening' means crossing a single categorical threshold. Studies that give a graded level of damage to estimate the progression rate seem to agree with our estimate.

What effect does treatment have on progression?

As described above, we have no satisfactory information on progression rates in large numbers of untreated persons who already have visual field loss from glaucoma (I assume here that the only treatment is lowering of pressure). Others in this symposium will describe the rate at which therapy influences the development of initial visual field loss. However, the rate of first damage in suspects may be different from the progression rate in those who have already shown their susceptibility by having damage. And, the therapeutic effect may be different as well. With respect to those already injured, the clinical trials now being conducted will develop information only on the value of one treatment compared to another: *e.g.*, drops *versus* surgery, or laser *versus* surgery. The only exception is a trial in Sweden, where early field loss eyes are being randomized to therapy or no treatment.

Based on the presently available information, which I will not summarize here, there is no question that some beneficial effect occurs from pressure lowering. It is more a question of how much benefit and how much that benefit outweighs the negative features of therapy. These include not only side-effects that are transient, but also significant (hopefully infrequent) events such as loss of vision from surgery or death from the effects of beta-blocking eyedrops. For the sake of the present discussion, let us estimate that the standard pressure lowering reduces the progression rate by 50%. That is the best estimate from the studies that Kass[32] and

Epstein[33] and their colleagues reported.

Treatment only has an effect if it is actually applied to the person affected. From the population studies cited above, only half of those with open-angle glaucoma are presently diagnosed and under care. The majority of those who are being treated are receiving eyedrop therapy alone. Dr. Kass and his colleagues have elegantly shown us that the average patient takes only 80% of the prescribed drops[34]. Thus, we could multiply the treatment effect times the compliance rate, suggesting that therapy might mitigate the progression rate by 80% times 50%, or 40%. If we wish to analyze from a public health perspective, therapy is only being applied to one half of those with the disease; hence, its overall present effect would be half of 40% or 20%. Thus, the progression rate we calculated from age and field severity data of the Baltimore Eye Survey (a population-based sample) is likely to represent the true progression rate minus a treatment effect that slows it by 20%. Our conclusion that glaucoma progresses rather more slowly than was previously suspected is, then, not likely to be much different even when treatment is factored into the equation.

What is the effect of field loss on quality of life?

While it may not be directly related to the subject of progression, it is important to consider how dysfunctional the person with glaucoma becomes with the development of field loss. The fact that few persons detect their own field loss until it is rather advanced must be meaningful. Questionnaires that measure how much their vision problems bother them have been developed. These should be applied to glaucoma patients with various levels of field loss. In this way, we can obtain a better idea of the true personal and social cost of progression in glaucoma.

Conclusion: So glaucoma isn't that bad?

It would not be correct to conclude that glaucoma is a benign public health problem and that we have been overtreating it. As the second most prevalent cause of blindness worldwide, glaucoma clearly blinds as many as seven million persons among the world's peoples. The data presented here suggest that the rate at which glaucoma progresses, on average, may be slower than conventional wisdom has it. Our past ideas have derived in part from the ascertainment bias of the more severely affected presenting for care and from inadequate technology to monitor progression. Since there clearly are persons whose vision will be taken by glaucoma, it is our challenge to develop better means to identify as efficiently as possible those persons who will be severely affected and to treat them aggressively by whatever means is validated by appropriate clinical studies. I suggest that those who are affected early in their lives are more likely to be damaged eventually. At the same time, the remainder of the glaucoma population should not be subjected to needlessly dangerous treatments and procedures that are not merited by the risk level of their disorder.The clinical management of glaucomatous eyes should include careful and repeated confirmation of progression by automated visual field testing prior to initiation or change in therapy.

References

1. Tielsch JM, Sommer A, Katz J, Royall RM, Quigley HA, Javitt J: Racial variations in the prevalence of primary open angle glaucoma: the Baltimore Eye Survey. JAMA 266:369-374, 1991
2. Quigley HA, Tielsch JM, Katz J, Sommer A: The rate of progression in open-angle glaucoma. Am J Ophthalmol 122:355-363, 1996
3. Klein BEK, Klein R, Sponsel WE, Franke T, Cantor LB, Martone J et al: Prevalence of glaucoma: the Beaver Dam Eye Study. Ophthalmology 99:1499-1504, 1992
4. Coffey M, Reidy A, Wormald R, Xian WX, Wright L, Courtney P: Prevalence of glaucoma in the west of Ireland. Br J Ophthalmol 77:17-21, 1993
5. Quigley HA, Vitale S: Models of glaucoma prevalence and incidence in the United States. Invest Ophthalmol Vis Sci 38:83-91, 1997
6. Smith SD, Katz J, Quigley HA: Analysis of progressive change in automated visual fields in glaucoma. Invest Ophthalmol Vis Sci 37:1419-1428, 1996
7. Quigley HA: The number of people with glaucoma worldwide. Br J Ophthalmol 80:389-393, 1996
8. Shirai H, Sakuma T, Sogano S, Kitazawa Y: Visual field change and risk factors for progression of visual field damage in low tension glaucoma. Acta Soc Ophthalmol Jpn 96:352-358, 1992
9. Berggren L, Widengard I: Visual impairment of open angle glaucomas at first presentation and after a five to ten year follow-up. Uppsala J Med Sci 97:251-260, 1992
10. Jay JL, Allan D: The benefit of early trabeculectomy versus conventional management in primary open angle glaucoma relative to severity of disease. Eye 3:528-535, 1989
11. Olivius E, Thorburn W: Prognosis of glaucoma simplex and glaucoma capsulare: a comparative study. Acta Ophthalmol (Kbh) 56:921-934, 1978
12. Pohjanpelto P: Long-term prognosis of visual field in glaucoma simplex and glaucoma capsular. Acta Ophthalmol (Kbh) 63:418-423, 1985
13. Popovic V, Sjostrand J: Long term following trabeculectomy: II. Visual field survival. Acta Ophthalmol (Kbh) 69:305-399, 1991
14. O'Brien C, Schwartz B, Takamoto T, Wu DC: Intraocular pressure and the rate of visual field loss in chronic open-angle glaucoma. Am J Ophthalmol 111:491-500, 1991
15. Noureddin BN, Poinoosawmy D, Fitzke FW, Hitchings RA: Regression analysis of visual field progression in low tension glaucoma. Br J Ophthalmol 75:493-495, 1991
16. Vogel R, Crick RP, Mill KB, Reynolds PM, Sass W, Clineschmidt CM: Effect of timolol versus pilocarpine on visual field progression in patients with primary open-angle glaucoma. Ophthalmology 99:1505-1511, 1992
17. Chumbley LC, Brubaker RF. Low-tension glaucoma. Am J Ophthalmol 81:761-767, 1976
18. Mao LK, Stewart WC, Shields MB: Correlation between intraocular pressure control and progressive glaucomatous damage in primary open-angle glaucoma. Am J Ophthalmol 111:51-55, 1991
19. Harbin TS, Podos SM, Kolker AE, Becker B: Visual field progression in open-angle glaucoma patients presenting with monocular field loss. Trans Am Acad Ophthalmol Otol 81:253-257, 1976
20. Werner EB, Drance SM, Schulzer M: Trabeculectomy and the progression of glaucomatous visual field loss. Arch Ophthalmol 95:1374-1377, 1977
21. Kolker AE: Visual prognosis in advanced glaucoma: a comparison of medical and surgical therapy for retention of vision in 101 eyes with advanced glaucoma. Trans Am Ophthalmol Soc 75:539-555, 1977
22. Hart WM Jr, Becker B: The onset and evolution of glaucomatous visual field defect. Ophthalmology 89:268-279, 1982
23. Mikelberg FS, Schulzer M, Drance SM, Lau W: The rate of progression of scotomas in glaucoma. Am J Ophthalmol 101:1-6, 1986
24. Leydhecker W, Gramer E: Long term studies of visual field changes by means of computerized perimetry (Octopus 201) in eyes with glaucomatous field defects after normalization of the intraocular pressure. Int Ophthalmol 13:113-117, 1989
25. Araie M, Sekine M, Suzuki Y, Koseki N: Factors contributing to the progression of visual field damage in eyes with normal-tension glaucoma. Ophthalmology 101:1440-1444, 1994
26. Gliklich RE, Steinmann WC, Spaeth GL: Visual field change in low-tension glaucoma over a five-year follow-up. Ophthalmology 96:316-320, 1989
27. Shirakashi M, Iwata K, Sawaguchi S, Abe H, Nanba K: Intraocular pressure-dependent progression of visual field loss in advanced primary open-angle glaucoma: 15 year follow-up. Ophthalmologica 207:1-5, 1993
28. Kidd MN, O'Connor M: Progression of field loss after trabeculectomy: a five-year follow-up. Br J Ophthalmol 69:827-831, 1985
29. De Natale R, Glaab-Schrems E, Krieglstein GK: The prognosis of glaucoma investigated with computerized perimetry. Doc Ophthalmol 58:385-392, 1984

30. Glaucoma Laser Trial Research Group: The Glaucoma Laser Trial (GLT): 6. Treatment group differences in visual field changes. Am J Ophthalmol 120:10-22, 1995
31. Jay J, Murdoch JR: The rate of visual field loss in untreated primary open angle glaucoma. Br J Ophthalmol 77:176-178, 1993
32. Kass MA, Gordon MO, Hoff MR, Parkinson JM, Kolker AE, Hart WM, Becker B: Topical timolol administration reduces the incidence of glaucomatous damage in ocular hypertensive individuals. Arch Ophthalmol 107:1590-1598, 1989
33. Epstein DL, Krug JH, Hertzmark E, Remis LL, Edelstein DJ: A long-term clinical trial of timolol therapy versus no treatment in the management of glaucoma suspects. Ophthalmology 96:1460-1468, 1989
34. Kass MA, Gordon M, Morley RE, Meltzer DW, Goldberg JJ: Compliance with topical timolol treatment. Am J Ophthalmol 103:188-193, 1987

The pathophysiology of visual field injury in glaucoma

Correlating anatomy and tissue alterations with clinical field analysis

Don Minckler

Department of Ophthalmology, University of Southern California School of Medicine, Los Angeles, CA, USA

Visual field examination remains a mainstay of the clinical management of glaucoma, especially in mild to moderately severe disease. In the early stages of glaucomatous optic nerve injury, visual field examination as normally performed is actually far less likely than careful disc examination to reliably detect early nerve injury. Perimetry has its most efficacious application in the moderately damaged glaucoma eye, where expansion or increasing density of a visual field defect is most likely to be measurable. In the advanced stages of glaucoma, perimetry becomes decreasingly useful as a method of assessing progression. This is especially true in eyes with compromised central vision, because fixation and reliability deteriorate.

Anatomy of the anterior visual pathway

The normal human optic nerve contains approximately 1.2 million axons projecting from retinal ganglion cells to the lateral geniculate body[1]. The distribution of ganglion cells varies with retinal location, being maximal in number and layers in the perifoveal (macular) region[2]. Excepting a minor population of 'displaced' ganglion cells with uncertain function in the middle nuclear layer, retinal ganglion cells reside in the inner nuclear layer[2-4]. The human retina is 'convergent' with numerous photoreceptors projecting to fewer middle nuclear cells which in turn project to fewer ganglion cells[1]. Only in the central retina does the relationship between photoreceptors and ganglion cells approach one to one[3].

Anatomical modifications in the fovea, which subserve high resolution central vision, necessitate that axons from temporal portions of the retina project around those from more nasal locations. Peripheral axons from temporal regions remain deep in the retinal nerve fiber layer and project into peripheral portions of the optic nerve (Figs. 1 to 4)[1,5,6]. Ganglion cells from peripapillary locations project through those from peripheral regions and assume a relatively central location in

Address for correspondence: Professor Don S. Minckler, MD, Department of Ophthalmology, University of Southern California School of Medicine, Doheny Eye Institute, 1450 San Pablo Street, Los Angeles, CA 90033-4666, USA

Peril to the Nerve – Glaucoma and Clinical Neuro-Ophthalmology, pp. 11–19
Proceedings of the 45th Annual Symposium of the New Orleans Academy of
Ophthalmology, New Orleans, LA, USA, April 25-28, 1996
edited by Barry J. Leader and Jonathan C. Calkwood
© 1998 Kugler Publications, The Hague/The Netherlands

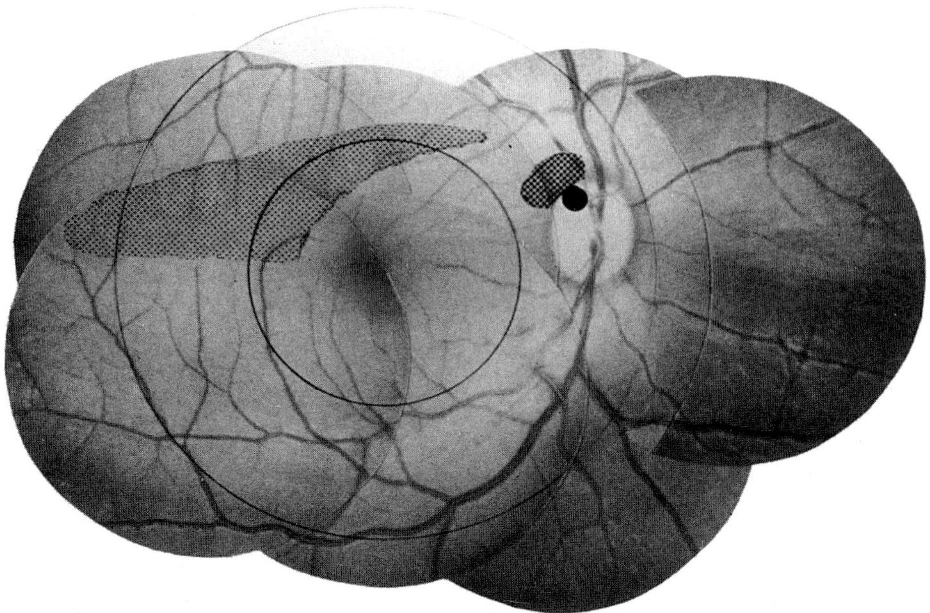

Fig. 1. Montage fundus photograph of rhesus monkey eye after direct disc injection (black circle) of horseradish peroxidase (HRP) 24 hours before sacrifice and histologic examination. Reconstruction by light microscopy permitted construction of a geographic display of ganglion cells (cross-hatched area) with cytoplasmic labeling by retrograde axonal transport of HRP from the injection site. HRP appears as golden brown granules in cytoplasmic lysosomes of ganglion cells after appropriate cytochemical reactions (Fig. 2). Cross-hatched peripapillary area represents location of ganglion cells labeled by 'passive diffusion' of HRP from the injection site. Circles represent 10° and 20°, respectively, of visual angle around the fovea, including the 'Bjerrum' region of the retina. (Reproduced from Minckler[6], by courtesy of the *Archives of Ophthalmology* [Fig. 2].)

the optic nerve. Axons from temporal regions respect both a horizontal and vertical raphe temporally, providing the anatomical basis for distinguishing 'neurological' from 'glaucomatous' visual field injury[1].

Retinal ganglion cell axons 'arborize' within the nerve fiber layer as they stream to the optic nerve head, providing for lateral dispersion of axons from any single location (Figs. 5 to 7)[7]. Axons 'meander' within individual bundles both in the retinal nerve fiber layer and as they traverse the nerve head (Figs. 6 and 7). This dispersion presumably provides some protection from total loss of function due to severe injury to any small region of the retina. Anatomical dispersion and functional overlap of ganglion cell domains in the retina may partially explain the difficulties commonly encountered with intertest fluctuation and inconsistent reproducibility of scotomas. The boundaries of early glaucomatous perimetric scotomas are very likely to be ill defined and variable based on the anatomical dispersion of axons as they ascend to the disc. Besides the distribution of projecting retinal ganglion cell axons, other factors including patient fatigue and inconsistent fixation contribute to intertest and intratest fluctuation in an individual's visual field performance.

Large diameter axons, which may be selectively vulnerable to pressure-induced injury, occur with increased frequency in the inferior nerve fiber layer arcades correlating with the tendency for initial visual field defects to occur superiorly[1,8].

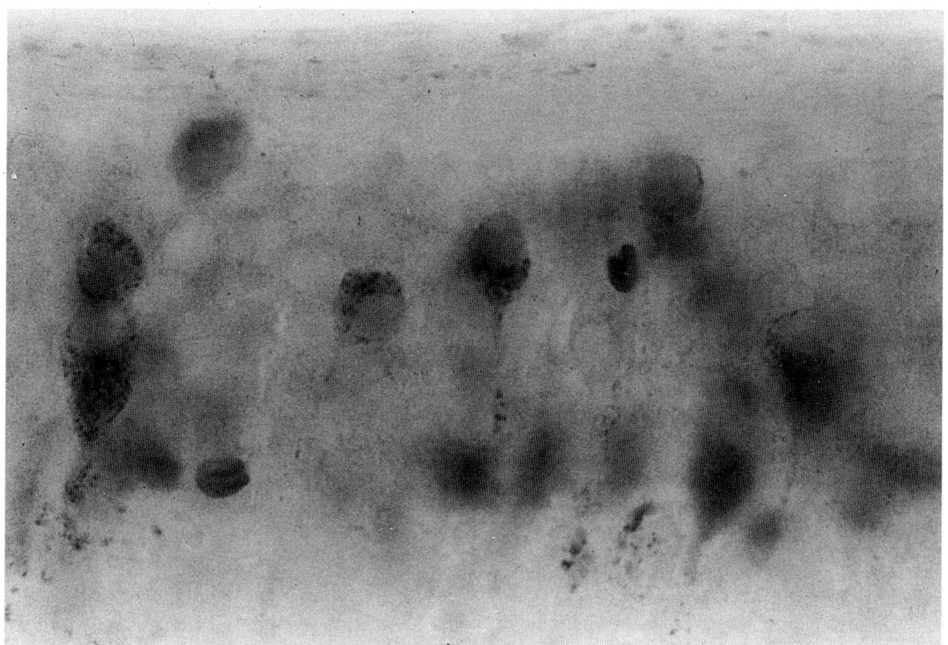

Fig. 2. Ganglion cells near the fovea in monkey retina labeled by retrograde axonal transport of HRP following a disc injection. Examination of serially sectioned or flat mounted retinas after disc injections of HRP in several eyes clarified the topographic relationship between the disc injection site and the region of labeling of retinal ganglion cells, summarized in Figures 3 and 4. (HRP reacted, x 80 µm section, x 787.)

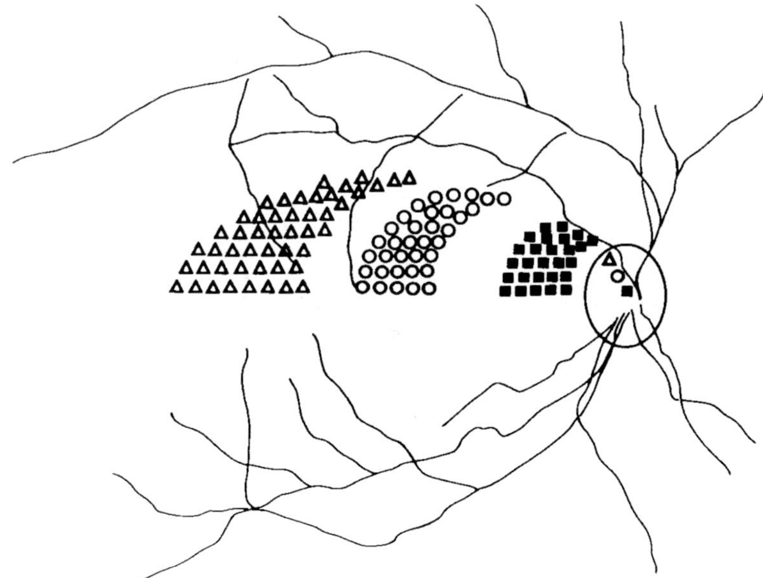

Fig. 3. Symbols on the disc correspond to the location of disc injections of HRP. Matching symbols in the retina correspond to the locations of HRP labeled ganglion cells which resulted from injection of the three disc locations. The clinical implication is that the location of a field defect can be used to localize disc (laminar) injury to axonal bundles. (Reproduced from Minckler[6], by courtesy of the *Archives of Ophthalmology* [Fig. 10].)

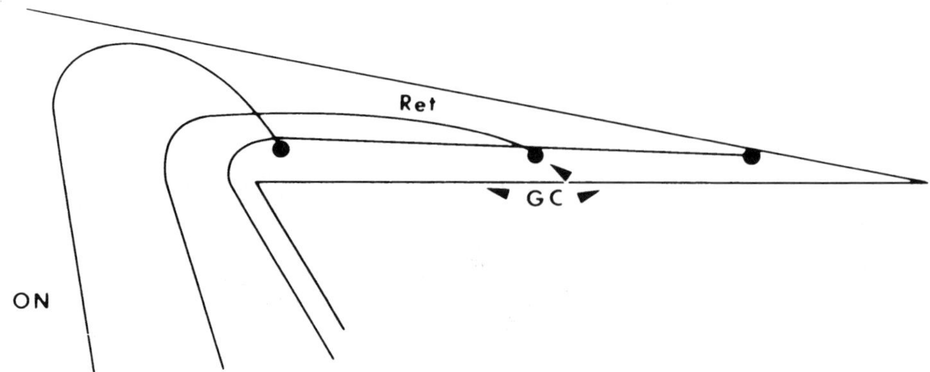

Fig. 4. Diagrammatic representation of anteroposterior organization of axons determined by analysis of multiple HRP injections in different monkey optic discs. Light microscopic analysis of peripapillary axon labeling revealed 'filled' ganglion cells, whose axons could be followed in thick section preparations. (Reproduced from Minckler[6], by courtesy of the *Archives of Ophthalmology* [Fig. 9].)

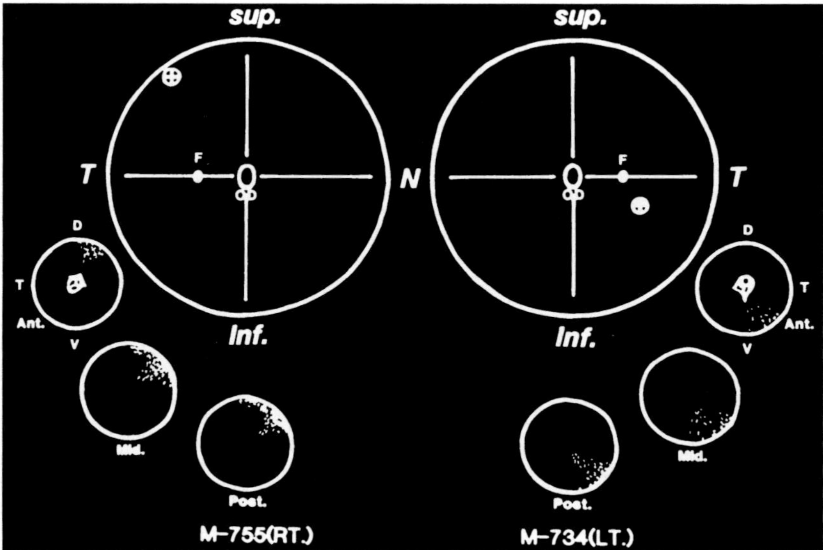

Fig. 5. Diagrammatic representation of location of 100 μm Argon laser retinal burns in right and left eyes of one rhesus monkey and corresponding location of degenerating axons subsequently demonstrated in cross-section displays of the optic nerve heads. The projecting axons from ganglion cells in the tiny area of the burn have been dispersed over the entire quadrant of the nerve (arborization) by the time they reach the lamina. (Reproduced from Ryu and Minckler[7], by courtesy of *Proceedings of the Japanese Academy (Series B)*.)

Fig. 6. Flat mount display of HRP labeled bundles of nerve fibers near the disc in a rhesus monkey following direct disc injection of HRP. Interchange of axon bundles is obvious between collections of bundles. (HRP reacted, original magnification x 160.)

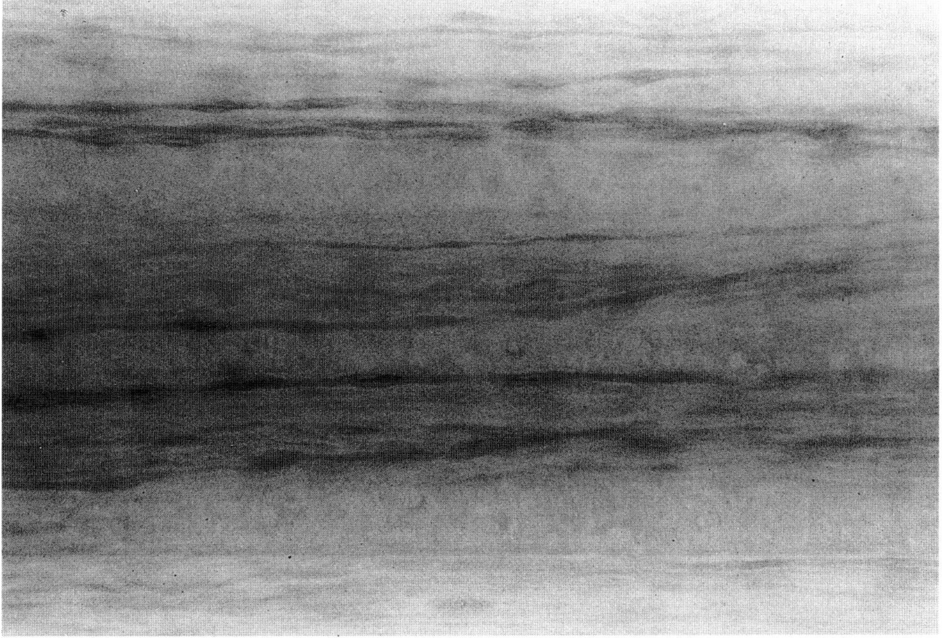

Fig. 7. Higher magnification of bundles of axons demonstrating 'meandering' of individual axons (beaded structures) within the bundle. (HRP reacted, original magnification x 400.)

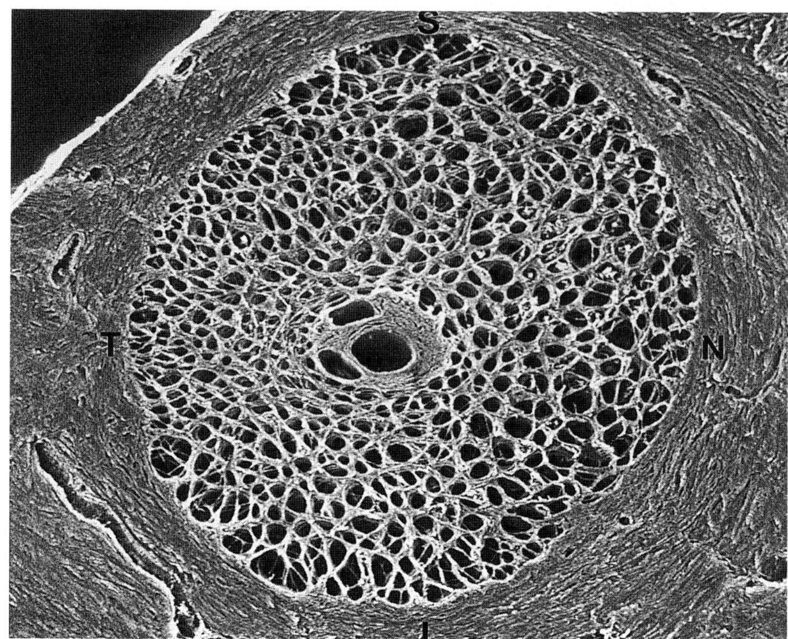

Fig. 8. Scanning electronmicrograph of dissection and digestion preparation of normal human optic nerve obtained at autopsy. The section includes the lamina cribrosa and is nearly perpendicular to the axis of the nerve. The central retinal vein has bifurcated and identifies the temporal (T) portion of the pore system. Superior (S), nasal (N) and inferior (I) are also indicated. Temporal pores (T) are smaller and appear to have more substantial surround by collagen beams than other areas. (SEM original magnification x 75.)

Controversy about axon damage in glaucoma

Controversy persists about the mechanism of axon injury in glaucoma. Historically, concepts about glaucomatous optic nerve injury have been very much oversimplified and generally categorized as either 'mechanical' or 'vascular[1]. There is however agreement that the anatomical site of initial injury in experimental studies and clinicopathological correlations in humans is in the laminar portion of the optic nerve head[1].

Vascular mechanisms, most elaborately proposed by Hayreh, have suggested that increased intraocular pressure (IOP) impairs blood flow to the optic nerve head and that optic nerve injury in glaucoma is fundamentally a form of ischemic injury[9]. Over the last several decades, numerous experimental and anatomical studies have not clearly established the role of ischemia in the pathogenesis of optic nerve injury. Limitations of past methodology and the remarkable ability of the optic nerve to autoregulate blood flow may have confused interpretation of past experimental findings. Newer imaging techniques, especially color Doppler studies, may clarify some of these issues. They may identify at least some sub-types of human glaucoma in which vascular disease plays an important role. Newer laboratory studies, especially those investigating the autoregulation of blood flow by capillary endothelium are also likely to provide new insight into the role of ischemia in glaucomatous optic nerve injury[10].

The mechanical concept of injury to the optic nerve in glaucoma has been rein-

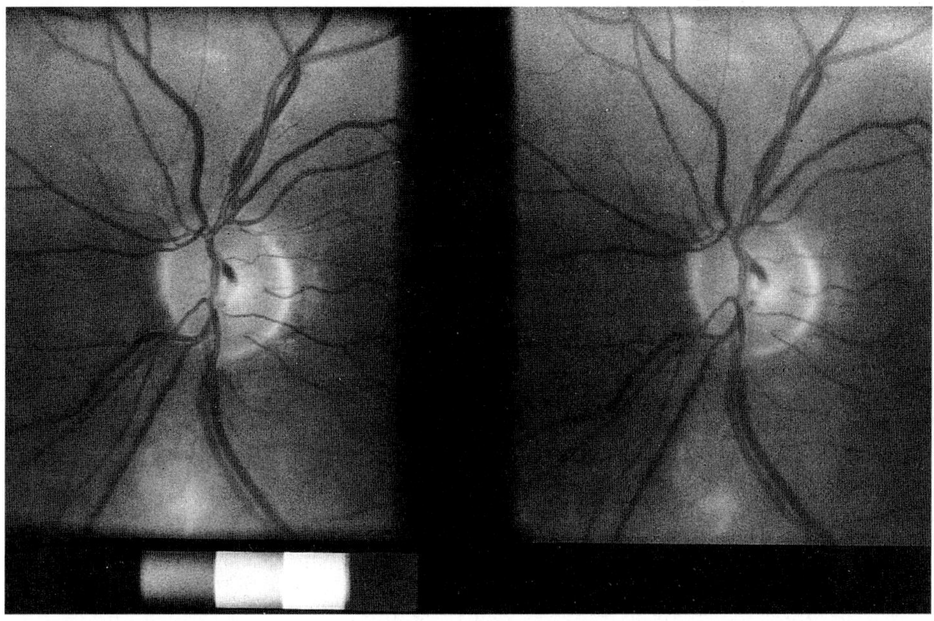

A.

B.

Fig. 9A. Split-field stereo disc photograph and visual field from left eye of a patient with long-standing modest elevation of IOP, not previously recognized to have pressure-induced disc injury. Visual field examination (*Fig. 9B*) suggested an early paracentral scotoma. Careful stereo disc examination did reveal compression of the mid portion of the disc in the inferior temporal quadrant. Disc compression is occurring in a location predicted from HRP injection studies. (Stereo view can be obtained by using low power plus lenses and convergence.)

forced by the recognition that either elevating or decreasing IOP blocks axonal transport in the lamina cribrosa[4]. Blockage of both orthograde and retrograde axonal transport correlates with morphological 'constriction' of axons impacted by distortion of the glial-collagen boundaries of axonal canals. Anatomical features of the lamina cribrosa may have relevance to the patterns of optic nerve injury in glaucoma. The apparent vulnerability of the arcuate bundles correlates with a relative paucity of collagenous support for large axonal bundle pores at the superior and inferior poles. Laminar pores carrying the macular fibers on the temporal side of the nerve have relatively greater support by surrounding collagen bundles perhaps partially explaining their relative 'resistance' to glaucomatous injury (Fig. 8).

Axonal transport, seemingly a 'basic science' issue, is actually a clinically observable phenomenon with either direct or indirect ophthalmoscopy. Disc swelling, whether ocular or central nervous system in origin, is a manifestation of obstruction of axonal transport in the nerve head[11]. Enlargement of the optic disc characterizes several ophthalmologic disorders including papilledema from increased intracranial pressure, anterior optic neuritis, postoperative disc swelling associated with hypotony, acute angle-closure glaucoma, and decompressive retinopathy following filtering surgery[12]. The filling in (normalization) of an enlarged cup following lowering of IOP in babies or young adults is also a consequence of obstruction of axonal transport at the lamina. Enhancement of nerve fiber bundle defects following filtering surgery is also probably a reflection of orthograde axonal transport obstruction in the lamina with backup into the surrounding retina[4]. Cotton-wool spots including 'cytoid bodies' are additionally a manifestation of axonal transport obstruction with axonal enlargement in the retinal nerve fiber layer.

Typical, chronic open-angle glaucoma produces slowly progressive optic nerve and visual field damage, requiring years from onset to end-stage injury. Such slowly progressive injury seems unlikely to be the result of a vascular occlusion but chronic vascular disease might aggravate whatever other mechanisms are active. Rarely, visual field defects demonstrate an abrupt deterioration or 'stair step change'. A sudden worsening of a visual field defect field would be consistent with an infarction or 'ischemic' mechanism of injury. We may eventually be able more accurately to categorize optic discs as to their vulnerability to specific types of visual field damage in glaucoma by assessing anatomic features visible ophthalmoscopically (Fig. 9).

Several anatomical, genetic and physiologic 'risk factors' may modify the clinical course and accelerate or predispose to visual field injury in glaucoma. Advanced age, myopia, and black race are probably the most 'accepted' factors thought to increase the risk of visual field damage in glaucoma. Other less clearly established risk factors include associated systemic disorders such as hypertension and diabetes. Anatomical and local tissue features which may increase the risk of visual field loss in glaucoma include optic nerve head drusen, peripapillary pigment epithelial atrophy, pre-existing large cup to disc ratio, and degeneration or defects in collagen or elastic tissue components of the lamina cribrosa[1].

References

1. Varma R, Minckler DS: Pathology of the optic nerve. In: Ritch R, Shields MB, Krupin T (eds) The Glaucomas, pp 139-175. St Louis, MO: CV Mosby 1995
2. Van Buren JN: Retinal Ganglion Cell Layer. Springfield, IL: Charles C Thomas 1993

3. Bunt AH, Minckler DS: Displaced ganglion cells in the retina of the monkey. Invest Ophthalmol Vis Sci 16:95-98, 1977
4. Minckler DS, Milam AH: Optic nerve axonal transport. In: Tasman W, Jaeger EA (eds) Duane's Foundations of Clinical Ophthalmology, ch 27. Philadelphia, PA: JB Lippincott 1994
5. Bunt AH, Minckler DS: Foveal sparing: new anatomical evidence for bilateral representation of the central retina. Arch Ophthalmol 95:1445-1447, 1977
6. Minckler DS: The organization of nerve fiber bundles in the primate optic nerve head. Arch Ophthalmol 98:1630-1636, 1980
7. Ryu DT, Minckler DS: The retinal nerve fibers in the primate optic nerve head. Proc Jpn Acad (Series B):328-331, 1983
8. Minckler DS, Ogden T: Primate arcuate nerve fiber bundle anatomy. In: Greve EL, Heijl A (eds) Seventh International Visual Field Symposium, Amsterdam, September 1986, pp 605-612. Dordrecht, NL: Martinus Nijhoff/Dr W Junk Publishers 1987
9. Hayreh SS: The pathogenesis of optic nerve lesions in glaucoma. Trans Am Acad Ophthalmol Otolaryngol 81:OP 197, 1976
10. Haefliger IO, Anderson DR: Blood flow regulation in the optic nerve head. In: Ritch R, Shields MB, Krupin T (eds) The Glaucomas, pp 189-197. St Louis, MO: CV Mosby 1995
11. Minckler DS, Bunt AH: Axoplasmic transport in ocular hypotony and papilledema in the monkey. Arch Ophthalmol 95:1430-1436, 1977
12. Fechtner RD, Minckler DS, Weinreb RN, Frangei G, Jampol LM: Complications of glaucoma surgery: ocular decompression retinopathy. Arch Ophthalmol 110:965-968, 1992
13. McLeod D, Marshall J, Kohner Em, Bird AC: The role of axoplasmic transport in the pathogenesis of retinal cotton-wool spots. Br J Ophthalmol 61:177, 1977

The clinical impact of new optic nerve imaging techniques

Harry A. Quigley

Glaucoma Service and Dana Center for Preventive Ophthalmology, Wilmer Institute, Johns Hopkins University School of Medicine, Baltimore, MD, USA

Abstract

In order to monitor glaucoma for the development of initial damage or for progressive worsening, it is important to assess the physical state of the retinal ganglion cells and their axons. This complements visual function testing. There have been an unprecedented number of new approaches suggested in order to monitor the optic nerve structure. None of these has reached the point of proven clinical impact. However, analysis of the various methods shows what might be features of the ideal system. These are: comfort for the patient, low acquisition and maintenance cost, rapid analysis per eye, high reproducibility and high validity.

What do we want to examine?

To monitor damage in glaucoma, we wish to quantify the loss of retinal ganglion cells. There is no evidence for loss of other retinal cells in primary open-angle glaucoma[1]. The loss of ganglion cells was first monitored by examination of the optic disc, where all ganglion cell fibers exit the eye. Their bulk makes up the rim of the disc. Thinning of the rim, as well as its typical excavation in glaucoma[2], are useful screening and clinical signs of disease. Hoyt and co-workers initially pointed to the value of examining the peripapillary nerve fiber layer[3], where loss of ganglion cells may also be detected. This examination is highly predictive of progressive glaucoma damage[4], and can be taught as either a clinical technique or by evaluation of photographs[5]. Finally, it is conceivable that the loss of ganglion cell bodies could be detected, particularly in areas of the retina in which they make up a substantial proportion of the retinal thickness, or if a means could be devised to measure their loss specifically.

Standard clinical methods

The preferred practice patterns for glaucoma and glaucoma suspects of the American Academy of Ophthalmology indicate that documentation of the status of the optic disc is the appropriate method to follow structural loss. This can be done either by estimation of the cup/disc ratio, by drawing the disc and its configura-

Address for correspondence: Harry A. Quigley, MD, Wilmer 120, Johns Hopkins Hospital, 600 N Wolfe Street, Baltimore, MD 21287, USA

Peril to the Nerve – Glaucoma and Clinical Neuro-Ophthalmology, pp. 21–27
Proceedings of the 45th Annual Symposium of the New Orleans Academy of
Ophthalmology, New Orleans, LA, USA, April 25-28, 1996
edited by Barry J. Leader and Jonathan C. Calkwood
© *1998 Kugler Publications, The Hague/The Netherlands*

tion, or by performing color stereophotographs. It is fair to say that the vast majority of glaucoma patients in the US are followed by these techniques.

Despite the widespread use of such methods, they may be relatively insensitive. I believe that most of us would agree that, for long-term monitoring, a drawing is unlikely to be as sensitive as a clear stereophotograph of a disc. Thus, I will consider here the value of photography. For example, I performed a study[6] with a group of persons who had developed initial glaucoma field loss during follow-up. Each had undergone annual color stereophotography and nerve fiber layer photography for at least five years prior to developing damage. These converters to field loss were matched with an equal number of suspects who did not develop field loss (at least during the follow-up period) and all pictures were examined in masked fashion. The idea was to determine whether disc examination would separate the progressing eyes from the stable ones.

The conditions should certainly have been ideal: cooperative patients with generally clear media, experienced photographers, and a glaucoma specialist able to compare serial stereophotographs. Despite this, only one out of five of the progressing glaucoma eyes was singled out as changed. While the actual measured cup/disc ratio did slightly enlarge in the progressive group on average, the changes were so small that a clinician observing the discs would not be alerted often enough.

This result was challenged by some of my colleagues who were sure that if they assessed the disc pictures using their favorite methods they would surely be able to do better than I. One such system simultaneously compares two pairs of stereophotographic pairs through one eyepiece[7]. With that system and the same photographs, 40% of the progressives had 'changed' – but an equally substantial proportion of the stable eyes were read as changed as well (my original readings found that fewer than 5% of the stable ones changed). Hence, the specificity of the method (at least for this set of pictures) was insufficient. Another system for evaluating change in disc photographs produces the appearance of motion in areas of compared discs where change has occurred[8]. With this system and my pictures, a number of the photographs could not be evaluated, as there are certain conditions that must be fulfilled before adequate examination is possible. Among the 'readable' pictures, there was no greater sensitivity and specificity than I had achieved.

I conclude that annual stereophotographs can detect some progressive glaucoma eyes, but that the sensitivity of this method is far from adequate. In the study to which I refer, it was early glaucoma damage that was monitored. The average cup/disc ratio for the progressive eyes was between 0.5 and 0.6. This should be the cup size that allows best determination of structural change. When the rim is narrow, the detection of further loss is much more difficult. Thus, I do not believe that my conclusion would have been any different if more advanced glaucoma cases had been included. In fact, I suspect it would be even more difficult to detect change.

Nerve fiber layer examination

In the same eyes that were evaluated in the study described above, the reading of nerve fiber layer photographs detected 50% of the progressive eyes (2.5 times more than the disc examination). Since I have spent considerable time developing this reading system, I should point out that others have found that it is not better than optic disc evaluation. Caprioli and co-workers have compared disc and nerve fiber layer examinations (by methods that are not given in enough detail for me to compare their methods to my own)[9]. They found that the techniques were both about the same in information value. However, even if this is accurate, note that my study found that even the nerve fiber layer examination did not identify half of the progressive eyes.

It is clear that there is additive information in the peripapillary area to that available within the disc rim. However, the examination of either area by human observers needs improvement.

Optical methods of analysis

Measuring disc features by hand

A variety of methods have been designed in order to derive more information from optic disc and nerve fiber layer photography. These can be summarized by the incorporation of two features into standard photography: *quantification* and *enhancement of topographical imaging*. A number of persons have used what might be called home-made systems of quantification. I placed a piece of film with a micrometer scale on it over my stereoviewer in my progression study to measure the diameter of the disc and cup horizontally and vertically. In this way, the neural rim area can be estimated. Drance and colleagues[10] and Jonas *et al.*[11] have used such systems with their own variations. While these add useful information, they are quite time-consuming for standard clinical practice. In some clinical trials and epidemiologic studies, investigators have used transparent overlays to estimate the size of the disc and cup compared to standard, marked circles[12]. Again, these methods are more useful for research than in practice. To be of wider usefulness, such techniques must be performed automatically by machines, converting the photographic information into digital form for reprocessing automatically.

Topcon Imagenet system

One of the first and now the longest-lasting systems for this purpose is the Topcon Imagenet system. It is essentially a fundus camera in which two images of the optic disc are obtained at fixed angle to each other, simultaneously through the pupil. However, instead of film, two television cameras collect the images and these are reprocessed. The generation of topographical information occurs by comparison of the relative brightnesses of the same areas in the two images. The second feature, namely enhancement of imaging, was added as a projected light and dark pattern into the eye, that improves the instrument's ability to determine the position of the surface of the disc and peripapillary retina. One important feature of any system is how the machine decides what position in the image is to be called the zero point for reference to all the other heights. For this system, zero was (for a number of years) the height of the surface of the retina at the disc rim. More recently, software alterations have moved reference zero to the nasal and temporal retina. This is very important, as the surface of the disc rim changes with glaucomatous atrophy; essentially, the surface subsides. Any system that uses the rim position as zero will understate the change in topography in glaucoma, perhaps missing it altogether.

A number of studies have compared the Imagenet system to human evaluations. Our recent studies asked the specific question: which is better at detecting changes in the disc configuration, humans reading stereophotographs or the machine? This is the classical John Henry, the steel-driving man against the steam pile-driver paradigm. Claude Burgoyne tested this in a series of monkey eyes in which the pressure was artificially raised and lowered and the machine read digital images, while humans read color stereophotographs of the same eyes[13]. It was not even close – the Imagenet was clearly better than human observers at detecting small changes. In part, this is because it is so easy for the machine to acquire a large number of stereo observations and to average the findings statistically (in the cited study, eight images were averaged at each time point by the machine). Humans would take a long time to evaluate eight stereopairs at each point and still would not come up with the answer.

However, the Topcon system requires a human observer to mark the disc perimeter with a series of points. This is not only time-consuming, but the subsequent analysis time is not trivial. It is probably more time than the clinician has on a busy patient day, thus moving the availability of the data to the end of the day. Or, technical persons could perform these steps, but the variability in the method increases substantially if different observers perform the human steps.

Furthermore, the Imagenet retains several of the other disadvantages of fundus photography – it requires a well-dilated pupil, clear media, and it produces very bright flashes to acquire the pictures (patients remember the brightness of fundus photography long after their last set of images). Nonetheless, the Imagenet and some other similar systems that have been described are practical, available, and have been proven to be better than human disc analysis alone.

Glaucoma-Scope

This system also combines the principles of optical imaging, quantitative analysis, and enhancement. It projects a series of horizontal lines over the disc and digitally collects the non-stereo image produced by a dim red illuminating light source (there is no alternative of using a camera-back as in the Topcon if the operator wishes to use color film as an alternative). The deflection of the projected lines provides the information needed to read the position of the surface of the disc, cup and peripapillary retina. The reference zero position is read from parallel zones outside the disc in the nasal and temporal retina, avoiding the problem described above.

The analysis of images still requires that an observer must mark positions along the disc rim, retaining the disadvantages described above for the Topcon machine. Analysis times are falling with faster computers, but still represent a barrier to be overcome.

This machine has no bright flashes and can image through pupils smaller than required by a stereocamera. Its red light is able to penetrate cataract better than white light, flash cameras. And, its cost is lower than most of the other systems described here. Software development (in which I have participated) has shown that analysis of the peripapillary height of the retina can be used to estimate the nerve fiber layer thickness. This approach has allowed reasonable estimates of the total number of nerve fibers in an eye (validated by histological comparisons in monkeys)[14].

In addition, the Glaucoma-Scope can detect with equal precision to that of the Imagenet system the type of small deflections in the disc and cup that occur in monkey eyes after alterations in eye pressure. The sensitivity of this instrument in this paradigm is at least equivalent to that of the Imagenet.

Retinal thickness analyzer

Among optical imaging systems, one other device deserves mention, as it utilizes visible light to detect the structures in the eye. Zeimer and colleagues projected a slit beam into the eye and detected the position of the vitreoretinal interface and the retinal pigment epithelium in the image. By essentially subtracting the two from each other, and taking into account the angle at which imaging is performed, the thickness of the retina can be estimated. The method has been recently applied to the evaluation of glaucoma in an interesting manner. The technique is most reproducible for imaging in the retina surrounding the macula. It might superficially be thought that this is irrelevant to glaucoma, since the prejudice is that the perifoveal ganglion cells are immune to glaucoma damage.

However, initial studies have suggested that glaucoma eyes with asymmetric damage are easily detected with the technique. This appears to result from the fact that a substantial minority of the retinal thickness in the perifovea is occupied by the cell bodies of ganglion cells, and the fact that many ganglion cells in this area are lost in glaucoma by the time significant visual field loss occurs[15].

Scanning laser ophthalmoscopy

An entirely new technology entered glaucoma analysis when laser energy was used to image the disc and retina. In addition to using coherent light, these systems combined confocal optics, a method in which the light energy is selected from a particular level of the reflected image and the data that are received from either anterior or posterior to that position are ignored. As a result, a dissection of any tissue of appropriate optical clarity can be conducted. The system produces 32 images at planes through the tissue that begins with some designated position. In fact, the system has no flashes, since a red laser light is used and imaging is performed through small pupils (in fact, dilating the pupil is a disadvantage).

There are two commercial instruments at this time, the LDT and the Heidelberg, which have been evaluated in modest numbers of glaucoma patients and appear to provide interesting information[16]. Their most significant problem appears to be that the reference zero point has not been adequately determined. This bothersome issue may severely limit the usefulness of the entire system. If a solution to the problem cannot be found, the progressive change in glaucoma cannot be considered to be measurable. The advantage of being able to image within the tissue (by confocal optics) ironically becomes the disadvantage that we cannot be assured that change detection is based on an invariant reference zero.

Further issues with this methodology relate to which software methods will turn out to be the most useful ones. The traditional cup/disc ratio will almost certainly give way to other, more specific features of glaucoma damage that are detected with these instruments.

Among the most important practical issues is the high cost and service expense of these systems. If they represent a substantial improvement in glaucoma management, then either the cost must somehow be absorbed, or it must be decreased through some aspect of volume assessment or decrease in unit cost.

Optical coherence tomography

A promising new imaging system has been proposed to determine the thickness of retinal components surrounding the disc[17]. This system is, as yet, a prototype without a commercial product. It appears to be able to image the retinal thickness, and, perhaps to differentiate between the thickness of the nerve fiber layer and the remainder of the retina. This, in itself, is an important feature, but there are questions at present for future research about the instrument's ability to define important parameters. No studies have been conducted to determine the practicality or the validity of this system to measure glaucoma change. Neither is the degree of operator input to the generation of images known at present.

Nerve fiber analyzer

This is the only instrument that may be able to measure the actual nerve fiber layer thickness, using the principle that the nerve fibers change the polarization of light that passes through them[18]. It promises to detect the specific loss of retinal ganglion cells (as opposed to the use of surrogates such as the position of the vitreoretinal interface, or the total retinal thickness). The instrument has all the advantages of laser imaging, including no flashes, no need for a large pupil, and imaging through moderate cataract. It is presently undergoing extensive changes in software and imaging systems. The cost is presently at the higher end of the machines that are being considered here.

References

1. Kendell KR, Quigley HA, Kerrigan LA, Pease ME, Quigley EN: Primary open-angle glaucoma is not associated with photoreceptor loss. Invest Ophthalmol Vis Sci 36:200-205, 1995.
2. Quigley HA, Addicks EM, Green WR, Maumenee AE: Optic nerve damage in human glaucoma. II. The site of injury and susceptibility to damage. Arch Ophthalmol 99:635-649, 1981
3. Hoyt WF, Frisen L, Newman NM: Fundoscopy of nerve fiber layer defects in glaucoma. Invest Ophthalmol 12:814-829, 1973
4. Sommer A, Katz J, Quigley HA, Miller NR, Robin AL, Richter, RC, Witt KA: Clinically detectable nerve fiber atrophy precedes the onset of glaucomatous field loss. Arch Ophthalmol 109:77-83, 1991
5. Quigley HA: Diagnosing Early Glaucoma with Nerve Fiber Layer Examination. New York:Igaku-Shoin Publ 1995
6. Quigley HA, Katz J, Derick RJ, Gilbert D, Sommer A: An evaluation of optic disc and nerve fiber layer examinations in monitoring progression of early glaucoma damage. Ophthalmology 99:19-28, 1992
7. Dehm EJ, Wilensky JT, Hillman DS, Lindenmuth KA, Viana MAG: Optic disc evaluation using the Deltascope versus +10 diopter lenses. Invest Ophthalmol Vis Sci (ARVO Abstracts) 35(Suppl):1349, 1994
8. Heijl A, Bengtsson B: Diagnosis of early glaucoma with flicker comparisons of serial disc photographs. Invest Ophthalmol Vis Sci 30:2376-2384, 1989
9. O'Connor DJ, Zeyen T, Caprioli J: Comparisons of methods to detect glaucomatous optic nerve damage. Ophthalmology 100:1498-1503, 1993
10. Balazsi AG, Drance SM, Schulzer M, Douglas GR: Neuroretinal rim area in suspected glaucoma and early chronic open-angle glaucoma: correlation with parameters of visual function. Arch Ophthalmol 102:1011-1014, 1984
11. Jonas JB, Gusek GC, Naumann GO: Optic disc morphometry in chronic primary open-angle glaucoma. II. Correlation of the intrapapillary morphometric data to visual field indices. Graefes Arch Clin Exp Ophthalmol 226:531-538, 1988
12. Klein BE, Moss SE, Magli YL, Klein R, Johnson JC, Roth H: Optic disc cupping as clinically estimated from photographs. Ophthalmology 94:1481-1483, 1987
13. Burgoyne CF, Varma R, Quigley HA: Comparison of clinician judgment with digitized image analysis in the detection of induced optic disk change in monkey eyes. Am J Ophthalmol 120:176-183, 1995
14. Quigley HA, Pease ME: Change in the optic disc and nerve fiber layer measured with the Glaucoma-Scope in monkey eyes. J Glaucoma 5:106-116, 1996

15. Glovinsky Y, Quigley HA, Pease ME: Foveal ganglion cell loss is size dependent in experimental glaucoma. Invest Ophthalmol Vis Sci 34:395-400, 1993
16. Weinreb RN: Diagnosing and monitoring glaucoma with confocal scanning laser ophthalmoscopy. J Glaucoma 4:225-227, 1995
17. Schuman JS, Hee MR, Puliafito CA, Wong C, Pedut-Kloizman T, Lin CP, Hertzmark E, Izatt JA, Swanson EA, Fujimoto JG: Quantification of nerve fiber layer thickness in normal and glaucomatous eyes using optical coherence tomography. Arch Ophthalmol 113:586-596, 1995
18. Weinreb RN, Dreher AW, Coleman A, Quigley HA, Shaw B, Reiter K: Histopathologic validation of Fourier-ellipsometry measurements of retinal nerve fiber layer thickness. Arch Ophthalmol 108:557-560, 1990

Glaucoma management dilemmas

Contents

Ocular hypertension: does treatment work?

Michael A. Kass

Department of Ophthalmology & Visual Sciences, Washington University School of Medicine, St. Louis, MO, USA

Introduction

Glaucoma is a common cause of blindness in the United States and other industrialized countries. One study suggests that two million people in the United States have glaucoma and that 80,000 of these individuals are legally blind from the disease[1]. Glaucoma is the leading cause of blindness in African Americans. In the Baltimore Eye Survey, the prevalence of glaucoma in African Americans was four to five times higher than in whites[2]. Elevated intraocular pressure (IOP) is one of the major risk factors for open-angle glaucoma. It is estimated that three to six million people in the United States have elevated IOP without glaucomatous damage that is detectable using current clinical tests. Armaly reported that 1.2% of individuals in their thirties and 10.5% of people in their seventies had IOPs of 23 mmHg or greater[3]. In the Baltimore Eye Survey, 6.6% of those tested had pressures of 21 mmHg or greater in one or both eyes[2]. Up to now, there has been no consensus on how to manage this large group of people. Various experts have recommended treating all people with increased IOP, treating none of them until they develop damage and finally treating those thought to be at greatest risk of developing glaucoma. In order to select the correct approach for this common condition, we need to answer at least four major questions about ocular hypertension including the following:

1. What is the incidence of primary open-angle glaucoma among ocular hypertensive individuals?
2. Which ocular hypertensive subjects are most likely to develop open-angle glaucoma, *i.e.*, what are the risk factors for glaucoma in this group?
3. Can we predict accurately which ocular hypertensive individuals will develop open-angle glaucoma?
4. Does treatment to lower IOP alter the prognosis of ocular hypertensive subjects?

Address for correspondence: Michael A. Kass, MD, Department of Ophthalmology & Visual Sciences, Washington University School of Medicine, St. Louis, MO 314-362-5713, USA

Peril to the Nerve – Glaucoma and Clinical Neuro-Ophthalmology, pp. 31–38
Proceedings of the 45th Annual Symposium of the New Orleans Academy of Ophthalmology, New Orleans, LA, USA, April 25-28, 1996
edited by Barry J. Leader and Jonathan C. Calkwood
© 1998 Kugler Publications, The Hague/The Netherlands

Table 1. Long-term follow-up of untreated ocular hypertensive subjects

Authors	IOP (mmHg)	Follow-up (years)	No. of patients	Percent developing open-angle glaucoma
Sorensen *et al.*[4]	≥20	15	55	7.4
Linner[5]	22-26	10	92	0.0
Walker[6]	≥21	10	109	10.1
Hovding and Aasved[7]	≥21	20	29	27.6
Lundberg *et al.*[8]		20	41	34.1

What is the incidence of open-angle glaucoma in ocular hypertensive subjects?

Many studies indicate that between 0.5% and 1% of ocular hypertensive subjects develop glaucoma per year. This relationship appears to hold true even after follow-up periods as long as 10 to 20 years (Table 1)[4-8]. From these data, two observations can be made, 1. the conversion rate to glaucoma does not appear to rise precipitously with time and 2. there is no period of time after which an ocular hypertensive individual is safe from developing open-angle glaucoma.

Despite the uniformity of these data, the published studies have a number of limitations including the following:

1. Most of these prospective studies classified patients on the basis of a single IOP measurement recorded during screening. Thus it is possible that some of the patients were misclassified.
2. Most of the studies utilized out-dated visual field testing strategies.
3. Most of the studies excluded the optic disc as a potential endpoint and this has an impact on the incidence of glaucoma.

In contrast to the reports above, three recent studies on the development of glaucomatous visual field loss in ocular hypertensive subjects found conversion rates of 3.4-3.9% per year[9-11]. The patients in these three studies were recruited from university practices as opposed to population-based samples and also had higher IOPs at study inception.

What are the risk factors for open-angle glaucoma in ocular hypertensive subjects?

It is clear that no factor taken by itself is a good predictor of the development of glaucoma. This is perhaps best exemplified by elevated IOP. Although elevated IOP is a major risk factor for the development of open-angle glaucoma, in most studies one-third to one-half of newly diagnosed glaucoma patients have normal IOPs upon initial screening[3,12,13]. In addition, as indicated earlier, only a minority of individuals with elevated IOP eventually develop open-angle glaucoma[4-8]. Finally, ocular hypertension is eight to ten times more prevalent in the population than open-angle glaucoma[3,12,13].

In order to refine our predictions, we need to turn to multivariate models. In the multivariate analyses done to date, the major risk factors for developing open-angle glaucoma in the ocular hypertensive population are the level of IOP, the appearance of the optic disc (or nerve fiber layer), increasing age and family history

Table 2. Risk factors for the development of open-angle glaucoma

	Drance et al.[14,15]	Kitazawa[16]	Hart et al.[17]	Armaly et al.[18]	Wilson et al.[19]
Elevated IOP	+	+	+	+	n/a
Optic disc abnormality	+	+	+	+	n/a
Increasing age	n/a	+	+	+	n/a
Family history glaucoma	+	+	+	n/a	+
Abnormal tonography	n/a	+	-	+	n/a
Vascular disease	+	+	-	-	+

Table 3. Risk factors and predictions about the development of glaucoma[20]

Coefficient of risk by quartiles	Developed open-angle glaucoma
0.00-0.24 (lowest)	3/143 (2.2%)
0.25-0.49	3/41 (7.3%)
0.50-0.74	6/53 (15.1%)
0.75-1.00 (highest)	7/26 (26.9%)

of glaucoma (Table 2)[14-19]. Some studies have also implicated systemic vascular disease, decreased outflow facility, African American heritage and myopia as risk factors.

How can one predict which ocular hypertensive individuals will develop open-angle glaucoma?

If we apply the risk factors given above, how accurate are our estimates of risk? Hart and co-workers[17] did a retrospective study developing estimates of risk in a group of ocular hypertensive patients. On the basis of their modeling they would have identified correctly 97% of those who developed glaucoma and 80% of those who did not[17]. Drance and co-workers made predictions in a group of ocular hypertensive subjects. After an eight- to ten-year follow-up, they determined that their predictions had been correct in approximately 80% of the subjects[14,15]. Kolker and co-workers utilized the model developed by Hart *et al.*[17], and predicted risk in 243 ocular hypertensive subjects on the basis of IOP, age, family history of glaucoma and vertical cup/disc ratio by contour[20]. Kolker and co-workers found that the incidence of open-angle glaucoma was directly related to the assessment of risk at baseline (Table 3).

Does treatment affect the prognosis of ocular hypertension?

The final question posed was does reduction of IOP delay or prevent the onset of glaucomatous damage? For the answer to this question, we might first turn to animal studies. While there are a number of animal models of ocular hypertension, there is no published information indicating that lowering IOP in these animals protects them from developing glaucoma.

There are a number of published studies on reducing IOP in ocular hyperten-

Table 4. Medical treatment in ocular hypertension (modified from Kass[29])

Investigator	Sample size	Treatment	Developed visual field loss	Comments
Graham[24]	201	Pilocarpine 1% and/or epinephrine 1%	One person developed visual field loss	Low rate of conversion to glaucoma; non-randomized treatment assignment; short follow-up; < 50% of patients used eye-drops regularly; very small IOP differential between treated and untreated individuals
Norskov[25]	110	Not specified	0/68 untreated people; 3/42 treated people	Retrospective design; non-randomized treatment assignment; low rate of conversion to glaucoma
Levene[26]	59	2% pilocarpine or phospholine iodide 0.125%	3/59 untreated eyes; 5/59 treated eyes	Low rate of conversion to glaucoma; small sample size; little pressure differential between treated and untreated eyes
David *et al.*[27]	61	Pilocarpine 2%-4%. epinephrine, carbonic anhydrase inhibitors	3/67 untreated eyes; 9/50 treated eyes	Variable follow-up; non-randomized treatment assignment with eyes at greatest risk receiving medication
Chisholm *et al.*[28]	101	Not specified;	Unclear;	Difficult to interpret
Schulzer *et al.*[11]	143	timolol 0.25%-0.5%	13/73 untreated people; 15/70 treated people	High rate of conversion to glaucoma; treatment limited to a single drug
Becker and Morton[21]	50	Epinephrine 2%	7/50 untreated eyes; 2/50 treated eyes	Small sample size; variable follow-up due to side-effects; treatment limited to a single drug
Shin *et al.*[22]	19	Epinephrine 1-2%	6/19 untreated eyes; 0/19 treated eyes	Small sample size; unresponsive patients dropped from trial; treatment limited to a single drug

Table 4. Cont'd

Investigator	Sample size	Treatment	Developed visual field loss	Comments
Kitazawa[23]	52	Timolol 0.25%-0.5%	2/24 untreated people; 1/30 treated people	Small sample size; low conversion rate to glaucoma; short follow- up; treatment limited to a single drug
Epstein *et al.*[9]	107	Timolol 0.25%-0.5%	7/54 untreated people; 4/53 treated people	Treatment limited to a single drug
Kass *et al.*[10]	62	Timolol 0.25%-0.5%	10/62 untreated eyes; 4/62 treated eyes ·	Small sample size; treatment limited to a single drug

sive individuals using various medications. Unfortunately, these are almost equally divided between those that find ocular hypertensive therapy to be effective[9,10,21-23] in protecting ocular hypertensive individuals and those that find that treatment is not effective (Table 4)[11,24-28]. Furthermore, most of these studies are limited by factors such as small sample size, limited ethnic and racial representation, short duration of follow-up, non-randomized treatment assignment, insensitive techniques for detecting glaucomatous damage and limitation to a single drug for lowering IOP.

In a recent study by Schwartz and co-workers, 37 ocular hypertensive patients were randomly assigned to topical timolol treatment or placebo. The timolol-treated patients had lower IOPs and an improvement in the appearance of the optic disc and nerve fiber layer. None of the patients in the study developed visual field loss[30,31].

Ocular Hypertension Treatment Study

The Ocular Hypertension Treatment Study (OHTS) is now under way and is attempting to answer the question of the efficacy of medical reduction of IOP in ocular hypertension. OHTS is a long-term, randomized, multi-center, clinical trial. At this time, more than 1500 ocular hypertensive subjects judged to be at moderate risk for developing open-angle glaucoma have been randomized to either medical treatment or close observation. The investigators in the study are free to choose from all commercially available topical anti-glaucoma medications. The eligibility and exclusion criteria for the study are given in Table 5. Subjects are examined every six months with automated threshold visual fields and yearly with stereoscopic optic disc photographs. We believe that after a few years we will be able to definitively answer the question of whether lowering IOP by medical means protects these individuals. In addition, we should be able to refine the models of risk using this national sample. The OHTS also includes ancillary studies on blue on yellow perimetry and scanning laser ophthalmoscopy of the optic disc. These new tests may redefine early changes (damage) in glaucoma.

To a clinician faced with a patient in the office, the OHTS offers some hope for the future but no definitive guidance now. Until the study is completed, clinicians

ond, the diagnosis of OAG has now been generally agreed to consist of optic nerve damage typified by visual field loss and excavation of the optic nerve head. Studies must not only examine persons selected at random from a population, but they must also utilize examination techniques that include field testing and/or optic disc evaluation.

ACG has been thought of as a symptomatic disorder of acute attacks. As a result, many surveys of glaucoma had assumed that it was satisfactory to determine the type of glaucoma by initial screening with tonometry and occasionally with field testing, than to determine the type of glaucoma after the fact by having an expert perform gonioscopy. More recent studies have shown that the differentiation of OAG and ACG requires gonioscopy at screening.

In 1995, there were two summary articles reviewing the number and distribution of persons with glaucoma in the world. Thylefors and Negrel[1] utilized a broad range of blindness prevalence surveys that were conducted in many countries. These have the advantage of rapid, low cost assessment, since a population may be screened using only a visual acuity chart. The small minority of those who are blind are then examined in detail by an expert, in an attempt to determine what the cause of the blindness might be. With data generated largely from such blindness prevalence surveys, it was estimated that nearly six million persons in the world are blind from glaucoma. The approach of the blindness prevalence survey may understate the number with glaucoma, since most persons with the disease are not blind, and would pass the initial screening, never coming to definitive examination.

The ideal approach to enumerating those with glaucoma is a disease prevalence survey, in which a large, randomly selected population is studied, and in which every person is subjected to sufficient testing to determine the presence or absence of the type of glaucoma that is present. This requires that as many persons as possible must undergo visual field testing[2], as well as gonioscopy, tonometry, and optic disc examination. Clearly, the expense and logistics of such studies are formidable, yet there have been a number of studies in the last ten years in Europe, Australia, and North America that satisfy these criteria. I recently summarized[3] a substantial group of data on the various types of glaucoma around the world that allow us to confirm some of the past notions of glaucoma prevalence and raise some questions about what is important in practical management.

In my evaluation of available prevalence data, glaucoma is the second most frequent cause of blindness in the world after cataract, affecting at least as many persons as does trachoma, and far exceeding diabetes, macular degeneration, onchocerciasis, and xerophthalmia. Over 66 million persons were estimated to be affected and as many as one in ten of these is legally blind in both eyes.

While there are adequate survey data on Europeans and those of European derivation, and even substantial data on those of African origin (albeit in studies carried out in the Caribbean and the US), there is a paucity of information among those living in Latin America, the Near and Middle East, and particularly among the half of the world living in China, India, and the remainder of Asia. Nonetheless, with the best estimates possible, it is likely that half of those with glaucoma in the world have ACG. Furthermore, the vast majority of those with glaucoma are both undiagnosed and untreated. Even in developed countries, at least half of those with glaucoma are unrecognized. The obvious challenge is to devise effective screening and treatment programs.

Glaucoma among European-derived persons

Among those of European ancestry, OAG is at least ten times more common than ACG. Throughout this discussion, I will use designations such as European-derived, African-derived, Chinese, etc. It is not trivial to decide how to assign ethnic labels such as these to areas of the world with diverse populations. In general, I have taken the simple expedient of assuming that persons living in a European country are similar, or I have used the method of the Baltimore Eye Survey, in which persons were asked to categorize themselves as either white or black. See Quigley[3] for a fuller discussion of this issue related to the prevalence estimates used here. The frequency of both OAG and ACG is quite low prior to age 50 and rises exponentially with advancing age. As a result, the average person with glaucoma in this group is affected for only about 12.8 years, from the point of initial visual field loss to death. This latter figure was derived from a model incorporating estimated incidence (number of new cases per year per 100,000 persons) and mortality data from the US Census Bureau[4]. Naturally, those (uncommon) persons whose glaucoma begins in middle life have disease much longer than a decade, but there are many others who develop it in the last five years of life, producing the average of 12.8 years.

Interestingly, those with ACG frequently do not fit what some clinicians think of as its 'typical' case history. Those who have suffered either a symptomatic acute attack or even intermittent acute symptoms are a minority (perhaps only 20%) of the total with a pupillary block mechanism. The remainder have chronic ACG, with peripheral anterior synechiae, and optic disc and visual field abnormalities. This suggests that screening for ACG may be performed most efficiently by a combination of searching for the anatomical configurations of the anterior chamber that predispose to this condition, together with the same disc/field methods that are most efficient for OAG detection.

Glaucoma among Asian persons

While Asians make up a substantial proportion of the world's population, it is sad that only few effective prevalence studies have been conducted among them. Those studies that have been performed suffer from a variety of problems, even after difficulties in translation have been solved[3,5]. Nonetheless, it is reasonable to conclude that the prevalence of ACG is greater than that of OAG in most Asian groups. At the same time, the rate of OAG is similar to that in Europeans. This means that the burden of ACG is additive, not a 'substitution'. Hence, Asians have a greater total proportion of their population affected by glaucoma than do Europeans. Among those in China, the estimated ratio of ACG to OAG may be as great as three to one.

Given the obvious importance of ACG among Asians, screening for this disorder takes on major significance, yet no rapid, inexpensive, effective method has been developed. With respect to ocular biometry, recent screening indicates that hand-held ultrasonographic methods may be of use. Our recent studies in collaboration with Por T. Hung and co-workers in Taiwan suggest that the high frequency of ACG among Chinese persons does not derive from a difference in ocular dimensions between all Asians and European or African persons. In fact, in terms of most ocular measurements (chamber depth, axial length, etc.), a population-based evaluation among samples of these three groups showed no significant differences[6]. To be sure, those who are diagnosed by gonioscopy as having ACG do have significantly smaller eyes and shallower anterior chambers. The difference between Asians and others seems to be that there are more of those with smaller eyes and ocular dimensions (and who develop ACG), but not that all Asians have smaller eyes. This is, of course, a happy result for screening, since if all Asians had smaller eyes, the sorting out of those with ACG would be that much harder. On the other hand, since a large proportion of those with ACG may have already suffered disc and field damage, the effective screening methods to detect nerve injury (as in OAG) may be appropriate.

It is tempting to speculate that extensive application of laser iridotomy might have a major impact on ACG among Asians. Certainly those who have not yet suffered pupillary block and appositional closure (with attendant meshwork damage) might benefit. Even if some synechiae or meshwork trauma had occurred, iridotomy would prevent more injury to the outflow channels. But, for those with established pressure difficulties, it will require more than iridotomy to help. And, this may be a substantial proportion. Further, it has been suggested that Asians seem to retain the capability to close the angle even after iridotomy – a plateau iris-like behavior. In recent clinical examinations of nearly 50 ACG patients in Taiwan, I was unable to confirm this. However, it is clear that clinical trials of iridotomy with extended follow-up are needed to assess the potential role of iridotomy.

The knowledge of ACG and OAG rates among Asian persons is assuming greater importance for US eye care professionals, since the immigration of persons from the Far East has increased substantially in recent decades.

Glaucoma among Latin American and Middle Eastern persons

There is simply no evidence other than clinically based observations upon which to base firm estimates for rates of ACG and OAG in these two groups. There is no reason to suppose that the rate of OAG is very different from that of European or Asian persons. In fact, with the exception of African people, OAG prevalence may prove to be broadly constant. It is not surprising that ophthalmologists in Latin America and the Middle East frequently cite a 'high' rate of ACG. Since those with this condition are more likely to be symptomatic and to present for care, our experience may be colored with more of them than is typical in the population at large, the phenomenon known as ascertainment bias. This same bias has been shown to have played a role in our concepts of severity of OAG and in associations between diabetes and OAG. The Baltimore Eye survey data indicate that only a small minority of those with OAG will go blind in their lifetime. Yet, many ophthalmologists seem to express the fear that "all these glaucoma patients are going blind". Perhaps our clinical experience is loaded with more advanced examples than are typical in an unselected population. In fact, our data show that the severity of glaucoma among those in the care system is significantly worse than among the undiagnosed[7].

It is interesting to speculate that the portion of those living in North, Central and South America whose ethnicity is related to persons who migrated across the land bridge from Mongolia about 20,000 years ago may share ocular features with their progenitors. Since one of the highest rates of ACG in the world is in north China, it may be that some retention of this tendency is characteristic of these persons.

As with Asian persons, the increasing proportion of the American population who are of Hispanic and Arabic heritage leads to the conclusion that much further study is needed of the prevalence of glaucoma among them to guide public policy.

Glaucoma among African-derived persons

Large studies of those of African descent in St. Lucia, East Baltimore (Maryland), and Barbados have now confirmed that these persons have a substantially higher risk of OAG than any other ethnic group. The fact that this tendency has been retained among African-Americans and African-Caribbean populations is strong support for genetic determinant(s). Some genetic traits that are highly prevalent among African persons seem to have modest beneficial effects despite their clinically negative features. This is true of sickle cell anemia, a genetic trait that has persisted despite its symptoms, and in spite of potential evolutionary pressure for its elimination, since it affects those of child-bearing age. The theory has been proposed that sickle cell disease has persisted because it confers protection against an even greater disease, malaria, which is a severe problem in much of Africa.

Why has OAG been genetically conserved among Africans? Certainly it has minimal influence on reproductive capability. In fact, throughout much of human history, the life expectancy was probably too short for a substantial proportion to develop the disease. Hence, there may be little selective pressure for its elimination. It is interesting to suggest that there may be an, as yet, undiscovered protective feature of OAG that functions to preserve its high prevalence, like sickle cell disease. The only ocular condition that affects the internal eye of persons in Africa that is uncommon elsewhere is onchocerciasis. Perhaps studies of the effect of glaucoma on this disorder would be illuminating.

The prevalence of ACG among Africans appears to be even lower than among Europeans.

Comparison of OAG susceptibility among African- and European-derived persons

The comparison of known similarities and differences between these two groups in their susceptibility to OAG may provide insight into the pathogenesis of the disease. First, in both groups the disorder increases in prevalence with age. The incidence is substantially higher especially between ages 30 and 50 among African-Americans. Among European-derived persons, the age-prevalence relation is quantitatively lower than in black persons, but increases with a steeper slope with age. This can be expressed as the average length of disease in a mathematical model. The average African-American has the disease for 25% longer than the average white American. Even if all other factors of susceptibility, treatment, and compliance were identical, this single fact would produce a less favorable outcome for blacks. In fact, their age-adjusted prevalence of OAG is four times higher and the rate of blindness is six times that of whites[8] in the United States.

Since the most consistent risk factor after age for OAG is the level of intraocular pressure (IOP), it is interesting that the Baltimore Eye Survey data do not indicate that African-Americans have statistically higher IOP than white Americans[9]. As discussed above with respect to ACG in Asians, not all African-derived persons have higher pressures than European-derived persons, but those who have a higher IOP are more common among African-Americans.

George L. Spaeth, MD: May we ask a couple of questions first?

Dr. Minckler: Of course.

Dr. Spaeth: Why did you use 5-FU and why did you get a flat chamber?

Dr. Minckler: I think we chose 5-FU because he was having his first surgery and other than guessing that he might have a lot of inflammation based on his long history of multiple drug use, I had no reason to think that he would have the level of inflammatory reaction that he did have.

Dr. Spaeth: Why did he get a flat chamber?

Dr. Minckler: He probably got a flat chamber because we used 5-FU and I guess the justification for an antimetabolite was that I wanted a low pressure postoperatively.

Dr. Spaeth: Why, since you had corneal endothelial disease and the cataract already?

Dr. Minckler: I thought his advanced nerve injury justified a low target pressure.

Harry A. Quigley, MD: I wanted to know what you thought his target pressure was, *i.e.,* you may have started seeing him after he had been seeing someone else for awhile. Did you have an idea of what his untreated eye pressure was to give you an idea of where his damage started? These pictures show somebody who is well along the process toward being one of my 5% blind. So, do you know what his pressure was?

Dr. Minckler: No.

Dr. Quigley: You told us that you wanted to set a low target, I understand that.

Dr. Minckler: The highest pressures he admitted to were in the 30 to 35 range, as I recall.

Dr. Quigley: If you say to some patients what is the highest pressure you were ever told, they can fairly reliably say, oh, yeah, the day the doctor told me about it he said it was 37. Of course, you would love to know what it was on two or three occasions before the person was under treatment to give you a feeling for where the damage really happens.

Dr. Minckler: All we knew was that the diagnosis had preceded our first examination by about three years.

Dr. Quigley: My experience has been too, to answer George's question, when you have a flat chamber and you shoot Healon into the anterior chamber at the slit-lamp, if there is no conjunctival wound leak the Healon will probably hold. If you shoot Healon in and it has gone by the next morning and you put it in that day and it has gone by the next morning, it is exiting through the conjunctiva, and even though you cannot detect the conjunctival wound leak because there is no aqueous around, when you go to the OR you will see everything leaking like a sieve up there.

Dr. Minckler: He did not have a wound leak externally.

Dr. Quigley: I mean at the incision line.

Dr. Minckler: I am not sure I am getting at George's basic question here the way he wants. The reason he got shallow chamber might be because the ciliary body was under-performing and he developed an effusion which was relatively anterior, and the entire lens/iris diaphragm certainly moved forward.

Dr. Spaeth: There are some patients you kind of get a feeling for. The way you presented it, it sounds as though you felt this patient was going to be trouble from the start.

Dr. Minckler: I could have guessed that based on his personality alone.

Dr. Spaeth: In that sort of situation, what responsibility do you have to him and to yourself to suggest to this guy that his eye problems are a small part of his real problem? Maybe he should get himself a little straightened out emotionally and then come back to see you. He is putting you in a position where he is really setting you up for this sort of situation.

Dr. Minckler: In summary, you could characterize his approach as, "I want this fixed and I do not want any responsibility for managing it. And it has to turn out well."

Thom J. Zimmerman, MD, PhD: Don, I think you ought to present this case to every patient that shows up like that. We in fact will go through the possibilities that can happen and I will sit down and go through a compliance thing and put the ball in his court. I say, look pal, how much longer do you want to see, and we know all the words to say and stuff. But you have new medicines coming down the line that were not far off. I would have really beaten him into compliance. This was almost a predictable future in a way.

Paul Palmberg, MD: Thom, I usually agree with you, but I do not think I would here because I do not think you can change people's personalities very much. A person like this gets to be 64 years old and they are really not going to change, so *you* have to find something that will save *them*. Just a couple of reflections. One, no flat chamber is due to 5-fluorouracil or mitomycin. They are all scleral flap construction problems or something else. You cannot get a flat chamber from the use of an antimetabolite. I think I had one out of 750 with 5-FU. I have had one out of 1100 with mitomycin. I do think once you have used 5-FU or mitomycin, you are much more likely to have to go back and fix that scleral flap than to be able to ride through with Healon or a contact lens or Simmons shell. Those kinds of things we used to depend on to get us out of our trouble do not work when you have used antimetabolites. I was a little surprised that it persisted because you probably stopped giving the 5-FU fairly early and you had the opportunity to back out.

Dr. Minckler: We did. We were concerned about his cornea, of course, and we generally desist with 5-FU if we have problems with shallow or flat chambers.

Dr. Palmberg: In trying to decide what to do at this point, a lot of it has to do with what kind of a wound it was and the location you used for the first surgery. Can you tell us what your scleral flap was like?

Dr. Minckler: Important point. I feel rather strongly that the first filter should be superior nasally if possible. I generally make about a 3 x 2 trapezoidal-shaped flap, a miniflap. I like the idea of keeping the initial incision in one quadrant to protect as much territory as possible for future surgery. That issue relates to where one might want to do the cataract surgery. And in fact, I will make a plea that, at least in glaucoma patients or ocular hypertensives who may become glaucoma patients and need cataract surgery, consideration be given to using a temporal approach for the simple reason that it spares both upper quadrants.

Dr. Spaeth: One last question before we get to what you wanted, what do you think this cornea was really like? Is this a patient who is going to end up with a graft in six months?

Dr. Minckler: My presumption at the beginning was that he was at high risk for corneal trouble down the road. So the best method of proceeding includes protecting the cornea at every option. That concerned me terribly because of all the problems.

Michael A. Kass, MD: Quick answer then to your question. I think this patient ought to have phacoemulsification done wherever you think you can get at it most easily. Forget about the previous trab, it is not going to work. Combine it with a penetrating keratoplasty and put in a tube shunt procedure at the same time.

Dr. Minckler: In other words, the tube shunt would be the glaucoma control procedure of choice at this point and you would put it in the anterior chamber.

Dr. Spaeth: If you thought there was an element of aqueous misdirection in this procedure, then you might conceivably want to combine that cataract extraction with a vitrectomy at the same time, and put the tube back in the posterior chamber.

Dr. Kass: You said you did pachymetry here. What were the results?

Dr. Minckler: The cornea team said it was still within the range of normal, but barely.

Dr. Kass: Did you do a specular count as well?

Dr. Minckler: Actually, yes we did. The central cells looked terrible, very irregular.

Dr. Kass: I think that is decision one, are you going to just do a cataract or are you going to combine with a PKP?

Dr. Minckler: In case you do not mention it, I want you to rate the likelihood that this plastic surgeon, who by the way does microsurgery on fingers and hands specifically, is going to wind up able to function after a PK.

Dr. Kass: You did not give him all these conditions. If you just do the cataract and in three to six months he needs a PKP, he will not thank you because he has bullous keratopathy and it renders him essentially monocular and throws off his depth perception. You are left to deal with what you have here. And if you think that even a skilfully done next procedure is likely to tip him over into bullous keratopathy within a year or so, then I think you have made the decision to do a combined PKP with the cataract. I must say, with due respect to Dr. Spaeth, that I would not do a tube, but that I would probably do a mitomycin filter with this and I would use lots of releasable or laserable sutures and viscoelastics. Lots of people have published papers saying that having a flat chamber does not matter after a filter. I do not believe that. I think it does matter. I think it very much increases inflammation and works against the procedure. So I would try very hard to avoid this. I would recommend that he have a combined PKP cataract or phaco along with a mitomycin filter and take enormous steps, even putting in extra sutures that you could zap one at a time or release one at a time, to try to keep him from being flat again.

Dr. Minckler: Do you think the flattening or recurrence of choroidal effusion is more likely having had the recent experience, or less; is there any way to predict that?

Dr. Kass: My gut instinct is that it is, but I do not have any real proof of that.

Dr. Palmberg: I think it means you would like to keep the early postoperative pressure at 15 or more so that you do not get into a cycle of choroidals and having done it once, sure he is more likely to do it again. I would do a phaco/mito, but I think unless that cornea really has gone, I would just do that. I would work very, very deep with plenty of Healon. If the cornea is borderline, once it gets a proper flow of aqueous and once there is no inflammation in the eye any more, most of those will actually turn out pretty well.

Dr. Minckler: In defense of the approach you are suggesting, I do recall that his cornea, in spite of the obvious central problems, remained crystal clear, even when the lens was right up against it. There never was any obvious decompensation of the cornea.

Dr. Quigley: For all the surgeons here who are going to do this phacoemulsification and who are not going to take the cornea off, would they like to tell the audience how they are going to get the posterior synechiae off the lens and do the capsulotomy?

Dr. Minckler: Good point.

Dr. Spaeth: With regard to Mike's point, those sutures are not going to be that easy to laser postoperatively. That is going to be a red eye. You are going to have trouble seeing them. These are the ones when you go take him to the laser and all of a sudden you have a hole right through the conjunctiva and you say a four letter word.

Dr. Minckler: By the way, just a little anecdote, he was travelling because he was a prominent person in the plastic surgery society. I had arranged for him to have some 5-FU shots after the last procedure, in a distant city, and the first time he got a 360-degree subconjunctival hemorrhage. The eye looked like a tomato when he came back. Any other thoughts about how to proceed, have we covered pretty much everybody's thoughts here?

Here in fact is what we did. Under local anesthesia, which was with anesthetic irrigation into the peribulbar space with a blunt cannula, which by the way I think is a good way to get prolonged retrobulbar anesthesia in complicated cases. We did in fact put a glaucoma drain implant upper temporally. The retina-vitreous person who was helping me with this did a pars plana vitrectomy/lensectomy. We put the tube in through the pars plana to keep it away from the anterior segment, and we actually put the implant into the sulcus on top of the anterior lens capsule which was left intact through that point, to spare the corneal endothelium as much as possible and to make it safer to put the implant in after the vitrectomy. He did a capsulotomy by reinserting the vitrector at the end of the procedure to remove what in effect was the anterior capsule behind the lens, which worked out rather well. We did what we call a 'rip cord' suture to temporarily occlude the drain which is simply a side tie arrangement so that you can pull the suture out at the slit-lamp a week or two later. We did that at about nine days out through a little snip in the conjunctiva. The problem is you do not know what the pressure is going to do immediately. There are a variety of tricks that have been suggested in terms of how to manage a temporary ligature, but we chose the rip cord. We had resumed Trusopt in the operated eye after surgery to help us with pressure control temporarily. This actually worked out reasonably well. The last question I should ask everybody is what to do about the opposite eye. In the interim, latanaprost has become available through a compassionate access program. As far as I know, it is not associated with aggravation of asthma. Remember, he is unable to use beta blockers and actually his pressure on the other side has been remarkably better controlled since we instituted that drug and discontinued his pilocarpine. Finally, at least as proof that we may temporarily have done the right thing, his cornea has actually remained relatively stable, his vision is excellent, and he has gone back to work, although not entirely happy with his vision.

Dr. Spaeth: Trusopt does not usually work too well in those patients with corneal endothelial changes because they get corneal edema with it.

Dr. Minckler: Trusopt?

Dr. Spaeth: Yes. So it would be nice to get him off on something else if you can.

Dr. Minckler: We have him on Latanaprost now. Actually, we have stopped the Trusopt.

Dr. Palmberg: Obviously, the cleverness of what you did was to avoid trauma to the endothelium, and it has turned out very well so far.

Dr. Minckler: The proof of the pudding as they say is in the pie, but just because it turned out does not mean that we did the right thing.

Dr. Palmberg: That is actually the comment I wanted to make. I have observed that when tubes are put in the pars plana in people with an intraocular lens present and a capsule present, frequently the corneas do not do well, especially in transplanted patients. I had the feeling that the fluid was going from their posterior chamber out the tube and never getting to the anterior chamber. There was not much flow through the anterior chamber. So, in those patients...actually, I liked having tubes in the anterior chamber but obviously here it did not make any difference. But I have seen several corneas go bad in that circumstance and I kind of wonder, as a long-term strategy for lots of patients, whether it is a good idea to have a tube in the pars plana in an eye that is not unicameral. If it is a unicameral eye, you are going to get nice, and more circulation. But I have seen corneas go bad.

Dr. Minckler: I guess off the top of my head my impression would be that a tube in the anterior chamber is in fact the worst long-term problem you get into with drain tubes because of corneal decompensation.

Grand Rounds I

Topics: ganglion cell loss and visual fields, disc hemorrhages, cell suicide (apoptosis), ocular hypertension dilemmas

Moderator: Kenneth Haik

Kenneth Haik, MD: *First, Dr. Quigley, you seem to be very excited about the future of nerve fiber analyzers. Do you have a financial interest in the companies that are doing it?*

Harry A. Quigley, MD: No, I have no financial interest in Laser Diagnostic Technologies. Heidelberg Instruments does not even talk to me, so I have no interest whatever. I do get royalties from the book I sell on examination of the nerve fiber layer and those royalties are being donated to the Hoffberger Program for the Prevention of Blindness in East Baltimore, Maryland.

Dr. Haik: *What is the percentage of ganglion cell loss necessary before the loss can be detected with threshold automated perimetry versus the loss related to Goldmann perimetry?*

Dr. Quigley: The question was how much damage.

Dr. Haik: *How much damage do you have before you can have a loss as detected by automated perimetry?*

Dr. Quigley: It is important to know where the numbers come from when you answer a question. There is a paper that I published about people who had automated perimeter testing who had donated their eyes. In one case, a patient of mine unfortunately committed suicide, and those eyes were studied. So three eyes have been studied that had had automated perimetry and the ganglion cell number was counted. That gives you an idea that the estimates could have very broad variability. There are several things you can conclude from looking at the numbers if you are willing to accept that. The first is that it is intuitively obvious that we will never catch the first ganglion cell disappearing because there is a lot of reserve in the visual system. So, the number is definitely going to be that more than zero ganglion cells have to be lost. The second is that human data provide you with some outside estimates. That is, if you are talking about 5 dB lost at a location or 10 dB lost at a location in automated perimetry, I can give you estimates about that. You have to take account of the fact that it is different in the central part of the field compared to the peripheral part of the field. The data were very clear on that. And the reason for that is you have so many more ganglion cells in the center of the field than you do in the periphery. So, in the center of the field, to lose 5 dB, you had to have lost more than half the ganglion cells living in that area. In the peri-

Peril to the Nerve – Glaucoma and Clinical Neuro-Ophthalmology, pp. 55–59
Proceedings of the 45th Annual Symposium of the New Orleans Academy of
Ophthalmology, New Orleans, LA, USA, April 25-28, 1996
edited by Barry J. Leader and Jonathan C. Calkwood
© 1998 Kugler Publications, The Hague/The Netherlands

phery, to lose 5 dB it was less than half, but it was in the range of 30 or 40%. The numbers I am giving you are not good enough. As a result, since that report, we have collected 60 eyes, 40 of which are useable and 20 of which have been counted so far. These are additional persons who had Humphrey perimetry, in whom the retina and the optic nerve are amenable to counting. That will be reported before the end of another 12 months.

Dr. Haik: *Another question for you was on the first talk you mentioned blindness due to glaucoma. The question is, how do you define that blindness? Is it by visual acuity alone or by visual field loss?*

Dr. Quigley: All the reports that I was talking about today are blindness by visual acuity, and the things I showed you today are all using the United States definition, which is 20/200 or worse. In general, the reports you will read that I have written will also include worse than 3/60, which is the World Health Organization rules. We took a look at the data from Baltimore as to whether, if you took account of people who had only a two central island, how much would that increase the blindness rate? In other words, they still had 20/25 vision, but they had these terribly constricted fields, and it does not dramatically change the rates of bilateral blindness to do that. So, it is probably not terribly important to answer.

Dr. Haik: *Dr. Minckler, what is the pathophysiology of the disc hemorrhage in glaucoma and is it pathognomonic?*

Don Minckler, MD: I do not think that anything is absolutely pathognomonic. My impression about what disc hemorrhages mean in the ordinary course of ongoing nerve injury is that they probably occur when small vessels are stretched beyond their limits; as the disc is collapsing, those little vessels that are coming over the corner of the edge of the disc there basically get stretched and break. My inclination has been to interpret that as evidence of ongoing tissue collapse, but not necessarily as evidence of a cause-and-effect sort of relationship. If you use fluorescein angiography to look at what is going on in the vasculature of the disc, disc hemorrhages continue to occur or changes in the vasculature continue to occur long after the field defect is stabilized. We have certainly had cases where disc hemorrhages occurred after the area of the field corresponding to this portion of the disc where the hemorrhage occurred was basically not reacting at all to targets. And the other way around. We have had hemorrhages occur in portions of the disc that correspond to the best part of the field as well as the worst part of the field, subsequent to recognizing that the patient already had major damage and a big field defect. Approximately ten years ago, Stephen Drance and many others got very interested in disc hemorrhages, especially with regard to low-tension glaucoma. I guess my suggestion would be that, while all that may be true, again what you are probably seeing is the consequences of rupture of these small vessels as the tissue is collapsing. So I think it is a bad sign. I am not so sure how seriously to take it with regard to management decisions. Although, all other things being equal and you also have a disc hemorrhage, it probably means that there is ongoing tissue collapse and you expect progression of the injury. I am sure other people on the panel might have some strong feelings about these issues.

Dr. Haik: *Are there any other comments? Dr. Spaeth?*

George L. Spaeth, MD: I agree with you entirely Don. The one thing I think is interesting to add are the ongoing studies in The Netherlands which have shown a very good correlation between progression of the disease and the presence or absence of disc hemorrhages. When the disc hemorrhages continue, the disease continues to get worse and when they stop, it seems to be slowing down. Which comes first, the chicken or the egg, is another question. But there certainly does seem to be a relationship between the occurrence of disc hemorrhage and progressive glaucomatous damage.

Dr. Minckler: Just an aside related to a specific patient, a retired ophthalmologist. He had a variation of Gaucher's disease with sort of perpetual low platelet counts. He had the most horrendous disc hemorrhages I had ever seen. There were sort of cycles of these things. I could never correlate them with his field problems. His fields actually remained relatively stable in spite of these massive peripapillary and disc hemorrhages that would occur periodically.

Dr. Spaeth: One last thought along those lines. You can correlate the presence of disc hemorrhages with the later occurrence of acquired pit of the optic nerve. There are a couple of patients who have been followed. We published one of them in whom the nerve was pretty normal, there was a disc hemorrhage; following the disc hemorrhage exactly in the same area of the development of acquired pit of the optic nerve. But I agree entirely with Don, they are not well correlated with the presence or absence of visual field defects. And I do not think of them as a sign of an ischemic process.

Dr. Minckler: Could I ask Harry a question before I forget, related to his talk? Apoptosis, have you carried out studies or are there studies related to the appearance of these characteristic cells in normal aging?

Dr. Quigley: Yes, what was on our poster at ARVO a couple of days ago was looking at the rate at which you find apoptotic cells in normal control human eyes, controlled human eyes from persons who had diabetes mellitus, and persons who had a history of glaucoma. The diabetics had a few more than the controls, but there were cells dying in the controls. When you look at the rate in the controls, it was one per 100,000 per day. If you calculate the number, it comes close to the rate of aging loss of ganglion cells, so that kind of fitted. It was 1/15 as fast as the glaucoma eyes were losing ganglion cells, approximately. The glaucoma eyes, interestingly, had a higher rate in the more severe cases. That is, in glaucoma eyes that had fewer remaining axons in the optic nerve, which may mean that that was why they were more severe. We saw definite apoptosis in control eyes.

Dr. Minckler: I like the concept that, perhaps in this disease or the pressure-related thing that we call glaucoma, sometimes, the cell body may not be recognizing or recognizing and doing the wrong thing in response to an injury in the lamina.

Dr. Haik: *Dr. Kass, there is a question for you. How would you treat a 65-year-old white individual with an intraocular pressure of 32 in the right eye, 27 in the left? There has been no visual field loss over a two-year period, open angles and a cup to disc ratio of 0.5 on the right and 0.4 on the left.*

Michael A. Kass, MD: Obviously, you have some choices here. If you have followed this patient for a long time and they have not gotten any worse, you may choose to continue to follow them, depending on their general health and what you think their life expectancy and all would be. If I saw this patient new, so far what I would call the only major risk factor is the pressure of 32 on a single reading here. We did not say anything about family history. This is a white person. So, there are some other factors missing here that you might choose to consider. If this patient routinely ran pressures of 30 or above, I probably would give them a trial on simple medical treatment and see how they respond.

Dr. Haik: *There is a follow-up question. You talked about not being overly aggressive in patients with ocular hypertension, so if you have a patient with a pressure of 28 and you elect to treat them, what is your target pressure in that instance? What happens if you do not achieve your target pressure with simple medications?*

Dr. Kass: In an ocular hypertensive, I would assume you would be looking for a 20 or 25% decrease in intraocular pressure. I do not think there is much reason to treat somebody and lower their pressure by a millimeter of mercury, not in this situation. So I think, if you had somebody who had a pressure of 26, you are probably looking for perhaps a 5-mm fall. If you can obtain that by simple means, and by simple means I would say try a beta blocker, assuming that the patient's health will allow it and see what you get. If you find that you cannot achieve this by simple means, in a patient like this, then I would say back off and see what happens. The odds are still in this patient's favor that they would do well for a long period of time, and you always have the option of intervening more aggressively at a later time.

Dr. Haik: *Dr. Minckler?*

Dr. Minckler: Just a comment. My most dramatic example of an ocular hypertensive, I guess we would call it, was a fellow in his 40s who maintained pressures between 50 and 60 mmHg in both eyes for three years before we elected to operate on him finally because one disc actually started having reproducible compression. He still did not have a field defect. The reason we followed him for so long was because he either did not respond at all to anything we gave him or could not tolerate it systemically. I think he also basically refused any aggressive intervention until we convinced him that his nerve was actually changing. In retrospect, I was glad we had procrastinated because both surgeries, that is, the first and the second eye, were subsequently complicated by any number of problems.

Dr. Kass: I do not remember if Paul Palmberg actually remembers this lady during residency or fellowship. She used to see Dr. Becker, and she would run pressures routinely in the 60s and 70s. She had no damage that we could detect at that time by Goldmann perimetry. There were normal optic nerves. When you treated her, she would drop to maybe 45 or 50 with epinephrine or whatever we had available at that time. She was followed for many years by Dr. Becker and I think died with very good vision.

Dr. Quigley: I just wanted to add a couple of comments. If I remember rightly, the cup to disc ratio was 0.5 and 0.4?

Dr. Kass: Correct.

Dr. Quigley: If this was a physician who examined the nerve fiber layer, and if it was different between the two eyes so there was nerve fiber layer atrophy in the 0.5 eye that matched with the asymmetry, I would personally be much more likely to say to that patient, I think you have early structural damage. We still can avoid treating you if you do not want to, but I would probably do a therapeutic trial more often in that sort of setting than I would otherwise. Nerve fiber layer asymmetry is a pretty good predictor that the person has about a three times higher rate than anybody else of being the one who is going to get the field loss in the future.

Dr. Haik: *One last question on the relationship between exercise, aerobic exercise, and ocular hypertension and anything to do with the control of open-angle glaucoma? Any comments?*

Dr. Kass: There is some evidence, mostly from Van Buskirk's group, that if you get people on a chronic exercise program, it has a modest positive effect on being able to reduce intraocular pressure. I tell this to people because people always ask if there is anything I can do. I figure this is something they can do, and even if the effect on intraocular pressure is negligible, probably the other effects on their body are worthwhile. It gives them something that they can do and makes them feel less helpless. So I use this suggestion quite a bit.

Dr. Spaeth: I agree with Mike entirely. And I think it is not just a placebo effect. From your program, Mike, Ivan Goldberg some years ago did a lovely study on the effect of being sedentary on the progression of low-tension glaucoma. He correlated progressive damage in patients who were sedentary at a much higher rate than in those who were more prone to exercise. So, I think there is theoretical and good data out there to suggest that exercise is good for people with glaucoma long term.

The treatment of normal-tension glaucoma

Michael A. Kass

Department of Ophthalmology & Visual Sciences, Washington University School of Medicine, St. Louis, MO, USA

Introduction

The diagnosis of normal-tension glaucoma is made when a patient has glaucomatous-type cupping and visual field loss, intraocular pressure (IOP) in the normal range, open angles and the absence of any other disease causing visual loss. A synonym is low-tension glaucoma, but this term is a misnomer because IOP is rarely low in this condition.

Normal-tension glaucoma has perplexed ophthalmologists for more than a hundred years. It challenges the time-honored causal relationship between elevated IOP and glaucomatous damage. Normal-tension glaucoma also challenges our therapeutic approach to glaucoma because it is unclear whether lowering IOP helps to stabilize this condition. A substantial portion of this article is devoted to a review of the therapeutic options for normal-tension glaucoma.

Clinical features

The clinical features of normal-tension glaucoma resemble primary open-angle glaucoma. Typically, the pressure in normal-tension glaucoma is in the mid to high normal range (*i.e.*, 15 to 21 mmHg)[1,2]. Some investigators have used 21 mmHg as the cut-off between normal-tension glaucoma and primary open-angle glaucoma, while others have used 22 or even 24 mmHg. Clearly, all these boundary choices are arbitrary. Patients with normal-tension glaucoma have been noted to have wider diurnal and postural fluctuations of IOP than normal individuals[3-6].

Some authorities believe that normal-tension glaucoma and primary open-angle glaucoma have identical visual field and optic disc changes, whereas others believe there are notable differences between the findings of the two conditions. Some researchers have reported that visual field defects are denser, steeper, more focal or localized, and closer to fixation in normal-tension glaucoma than open-angle glaucoma[7-17]. The opposite hemifield is also more likely to be normal in normal-tension glaucoma[18,19]. However, other researchers have not confirmed these differences[20-22]. Similarly, some authorities believe that the optic discs are more

Address for correspondence: Michael A. Kass, MD, Department of Ophthalmology & Visual Sciences, Washington University School of Medicine, St. Louis, MO 314-362-5713, USA

Peril to the Nerve – Glaucoma and Clinical Neuro-Ophthalmology, pp. 61–72
Proceedings of the 45th Annual Symposium of the New Orleans Academy of
Ophthalmology, New Orleans, LA, USA, April 25-28, 1996
edited by Barry J. Leader and Jonathan C. Calkwood
© *1998 Kugler Publications, The Hague/The Netherlands*

cupped, have more focal and diffuse loss of the rim and have more peripapillary atrophy than is noted in primary open-angle glaucoma[23-32].

There are two reports that the optic discs are larger in patients with normal-tension glaucoma[33,34]. However, others have not confirmed these differences between normal-tension glaucoma and open-angle glaucoma[35-38]. Optic disc hemorrhages are more common in normal-tension glaucoma, with some patients experiencing multiple episodes[35,39-41]. Hoyng *et al.* reported 41.6% of patients with normal-tension glaucoma had one or more episodes of disc hemorrhage[39]. To some extent, the differences described between normal-tension glaucoma and open-angle glaucoma may reflect the different stages at which the two conditions are detected. Most cases of primary open-angle glaucoma are detected because of elevated IOP whereas most cases of normal-tension glaucoma are detected because of optic disc cupping. Since it is easier to detect a suspicious IOP than a suspicious optic disc, cases of normal-tension glaucoma are usually diagnosed at a later stage of the disease process. When eyes with normal-tension glaucoma and primary open-angle glaucoma are matched for the degree of cupping, the pattern of visual field loss is identical. Similarly, when eyes with normal-tension glaucoma and primary open-angle glaucoma are matched for the degree of visual field loss, the cupping is identical[42]. Even if we accept some of these differences between normal-tension glaucoma and open-angle glaucoma, they do not imply a difference in pathogenesis or of therapeutic options.

Patients with normal-tension glaucoma often demonstrate abnormalities on fluorescein angiography including diffuse and focal hypofluorescence of the disc and abnormal transit time[43-49]. These abnormalities are also seen in open-angle glaucoma.

It is estimated that one-third of the patients who present with cupping of the optic disc and visual field loss have normal IOP when first measured[50-53]. Many of these patients continue to have normal pressures throughout repeated examinations including diurnal measurements. It is thought that low-tension glaucoma constitutes 5-15% of the cases of open-angle glaucoma in caucasian populations. In the Baltimore Eye Survey, 16.7% of glaucomatous individuals never had a recorded IOP exceeding 21 mmHg[54]. Shiose has reported a high prevalence of normal-tension glaucoma in Japan[55].

Approximately 50% of the cases referred with the diagnosis of normal-tension glaucoma do not appear to progress as assessed by kinetic perimetry over long periods of follow-up[56-59]. Some investigators believe higher rates of progression are detected with computerized visual fields[60,61]. However, in the Low-Tension Glaucoma Study, which utilizes computerized visual field tests, only about 1% of the patients demonstrate reproducible progression per year[62]. Using data from that study, Schulzer has demonstrated that basing conclusions on two visual fields yields false positive answers about progression 57% of the time. He recommends increasing the number of field tests to three or four before determining whether progression has occurred. Risk factors for progressive visual loss in normal-tension glaucoma include a large cup/disc ratio, a high ratio of peripapillary atrophy to disc area and higher levels of IOP[63-66].

Typically, normal-tension glaucoma is seen in older individuals with patients presenting in the sixth and seventh decades of life[47,67]. Some investigators have reported normal-tension glaucoma to be more common in women and myopic individuals[47,67], but others have not confirmed these associations[50]. Although there have been a few descriptions of families with normal-tension glaucoma[25,28], most cases appear to be sporadic.

Orgal and Flammer have reported that 60% of patients with normal-tension glaucoma have perilimbal conjunctival aneurysms, compared to 20% of open-angle glaucoma patients and 13% of normal individuals[68].

Differential diagnosis

Many conditions can produce an atrophic appearance of the optic disc with accompanying visual field loss despite IOP in the normal range (Table 1). It is impor-

Table 1. Differential diagnosis of normal-tension glaucoma (modified from Hoskins and Kass[69])

1. Glaucoma
    a. Elevated IOP not detected
        1. undetected wide diurnal variation
        2. low scleral rigidity
        3. systemic medication
        4. elevation in supine position only
    b. Glaucoma in remission
        1. past corticosteroid administration
        2. pigmentary glaucoma
        3. associated with past uveitis or trauma
        4. glaucomatocyclitic crisis
        5. burned-out primary open-angle glaucoma
        6. angle closure
2. Optic nerve disorders
    a. Congenital optic nerve conditions
        1. pits
        2. colobomas
        3. tilted discs
    b. Ischemic optic neuropathy
        1. arteritic
        2. non-arteritic
    c. Compressive lesions
        1. tumors
        2. aneurysms
        3. cysts
        4. chiasmatic arachnoiditis
    d. Drusen
    e. Demyelinating diseases
    f. Inflammatory diseases
    g. Hereditary optic atrophy
    h. Toxic drugs or chemicals
3. Ocular disorders
    a. Myopia
    b. Retinal degeneration
    c. Myelinated nerve fibers
    d. Branch vascular occlusions
    e. Choroidal nevus or melanoma
    f. Choroidal rupture
    g. Retinoschisis
    h. Chorioretinal disease or scars
4. Systemic vascular conditions
    a. Anemia
    b. Carotid artery obstruction
    c. Acute blood loss
    d. Arrhythmia
    e. Hypotensive episodes
5. Miscellaneous: hysteria

tant to distinguish these conditions because some of them may very well be progressive (*i.e.*, open-angle glaucoma) and some are likely to be stable (*i.e.*, a coloboma of the optic disc).

The most common conditions in the differential diagnosis of normal-tension glaucoma are the following:

1. Open-angle glaucoma
IOP readings in the office may be misleading because of diurnal variation, low scleral rigidity or systemic medications that reduce pressure. Some patients demonstrate elevated IOP only in the morning or only in the supine position[4-6]. Patients referred for normal-tension glaucoma may need to be reclassified after diurnal or postural pressure readings[5,6]. Glaucoma may also have been present in the past, but now the patient is in remission (*i.e.*, angle-closure glaucoma or pigmentary glaucoma).
2. Congenital defects of the optic disc, including pits, colobomas and tilted discs.
3. Ischemic optic neuropathy.
4. Compressive lesions of the optic nerve.
5. Retinal diseases including branch vascular occlusions.

Work-up

The most important part of the work-up of a patient with normal-tension glaucoma is a careful history. This includes questions about past and present health, previous elevations of IOP and treatment, ocular trauma and inflammation, and exposure to toxins. It is especially important to ask about corticosteroid administration to the eye, to the skin or systemically. Patients must be queried about hemodynamic crises including blood loss, arrhythmia, transfusions and hypotensive episodes.

The eye examination should include measurements of IOP at different times of day and evening. Measurements should be taken in the sitting and supine positions. Palpation and auscultation of the carotid arteries may indicate obstructive disease. The results of the history and physical examination may suggest that some patients should receive a general medical work-up, a neurological examination, serological tests for syphilis, ophthalmodynamometry, measurements of hematocrit and hemoglobin levels, antinuclear antibodies or imaging of the carotid arteries or the brain and orbits. If the history and physical examination are unremarkable, routine imaging studies of the brain and orbits are rarely useful.

Pathogenesis

There has been great controversy about the pathogenesis of normal-tension glaucoma. Some authorities believe normal-tension glaucoma is a variant of primary open-angle glaucoma in which the optic disc demonstrates greater vulnerability to the effects of IOP[35]. This could occur because the lamina cribosa is weak or maldeveloped in some fashion[70-72]. Quigley and co-workers reported that the lamina cribosa of patients with normal-tension glaucoma has less connective tissue and larger pores than the lamina of patients with open-angle glaucoma[70,71]. Some authorities have noted an association between the level of IOP and damage in normal-tension glaucoma[65,73-76]. However, others have failed to confirm this association[77].

Another school of thought proposes that normal-tension glaucoma and primary open-angle glaucoma have different etiologies and that normal-tension glaucoma is primarily a vascular or an immune disease[23,59]. As proof of this hypothesis, some authors cite differences in the visual field and the optic disc appearance of the two conditions (see previous section on 'Clinical features'). Patients with normal-tension glaucoma have been noted to have a higher prevalence of a variety of vascular problems, including hemodynamic crises, hypercoagulability, abnormal ophthalmodynamometry, hypertension, hypotension, increased blood viscosity, elevated blood cholesterol and lipids, carotid artery disease, coronary artery disease, migraine and vasospasm[35,78-89]. However, other studies have found no difference in the prevalences of vascular disorders in normal-tension glaucoma and primary open-angle glaucoma[3,90,91]. Using color-Doppler analysis, fluorescein angiography or measurements of ocular pulsatile blood flow, some investigators find decreased flow and/or increased resistance in the orbital and ocular vessels in normal-tension glaucoma[92-99].

Other investigators have noted an increased incidence of immune disorders in patients with normal-tension glaucoma[100]. Wax and co-workers have reported an increased prevalence of autoantibodies to a variety of antigens including rhodopsin in the sera of patients with normal-tension glaucoma[101,102].

Even if vascular diseases or immune abnormalities occur more frequently in normal-tension glaucoma, it does not necessarily imply that there is a different pathogenesis of normal-tension glaucoma and open-angle glaucoma. A vascular disease or an immune disorder could reduce optic nerve resistance to either pressure-induced damage or some other type of damage.

Discussing the etiology of normal-tension glaucoma naturally raises the issue of the etiology of open-angle glaucoma. A number of investigators have now postulated that open-angle glaucoma is an optic neuropathy that may or may not be associated with increased IOP[103-105]. In many patients, it appears that IOP plays a significant or even the major role. Normal-tension glaucoma may not differ from open-angle glaucoma in this regard. However, in other patients alternative causes for the optic nerve degeneration such as vascular or immune phenomena may be more important. Thus it is likely that some patients with normal-tension glaucoma (and open-angle glaucoma) will be helped greatly by reducing IOP, others will be helped a little, and others may not be helped at all.

Treatment

The treatment of normal-tension glaucoma has been even more controversial than the pathogenesis. Patients with a stable form of the disease require no treatment. This is especially true if the patient appears to have optic neuropathy related to a previous hemodynamic episode. Progression of the disease is unlikely unless the patient has another episode of hypotension or blood loss.

In patients with normal-tension glaucoma, diseases such as anemia, arrhythmia, hypotension, hypertension, or congestive heart failure should be treated to improve their general health and to improve circulation to the eye. In patients with progressive normal-tension glaucoma most clinicians have advocated reducing IOP even though firm evidence to support this approach is lacking.

Medical treatment

Some authorities have questioned whether it is even possible to lower pressure in normal-tension glaucoma short of performing filtering surgery[64]. In the Normal Tension Glaucoma Study the investigators attempted to reduce IOP by 30% in patients randomized to treatment. They were able to achieve this goal in 27% of the patients by pilocarpine alone, in 7% of the patients by argon laser trabeculoplasty alone, in 23% of the patients by pilocarpine and argon laser trabeculoplasty and in 43% of the patients by filtering surgery[106]. Thus, it is clear that substantial reductions of IOP can be obtained by standard approaches.

A number of investigators have attempted to treat normal-tension glaucoma by reducing IOP with standard medications[28,35,47]. At this point, it is impossible to say whether such treatment is successful in stabilizing the condition for reducing the rate of progression. If medical treatment is to be employed it is important to do diurnal IOP measurements to assess the response to therapy.

Some authorities have questioned whether epinephrine and the beta blockers, particularly the non-selective beta blockers are contraindicated in normal-tension glaucoma because they might affect perfusion to the eye. Harris and co-workers utilized color-Doppler imaging of orbital vessels in patients with normal-tension glaucoma. They found that timolol significantly reduced IOP but had no effect on peak systolic and/or diastolic velocity or resistive index in any of the vessels studied. In contrast, the betaxolol was less successful in reducing IOP but decreased resistive index and increased end diastolic velocity in the vessels studied. This was a one-month study so no long-term effects in visual function could be detected[107]. In other studies the beta blockers have been more successful than pilocarpine in lowering IOP[108]. Other investigators have utilized drugs such as bunazosin, an α_1-adrenergic blocker, or prostaglandin analogs to reduce IOP in normal-tension glaucoma[109,110]. Unfortunately, none of the standard or new therapeutic agents has been evaluated in a controlled study for a sufficient period of time in order to assess efficacy in protecting the visual field.

Because of the association of normal-tension glaucoma and vasospasm some investigators have utilized calcium channel blockers[111,112]. Netland and co-workers noted that patients with normal-tension glaucoma who were coincidentally taking calcium channel blockers for other conditions had less progression than other patients not taking these agents[111]. Gaspar and co-workers utilized nifedipine in a mixed group of patients with visual field loss. They noted that the patients treated with the calcium channel blockers had an improvement of the visual fields which was not noted in patients who did not receive these agents. The younger the patients and the healthier the optic discs, the greater the improvement in the visual fields[112].

In a similar fashion, one group of investigators has attempted to treat normal-tension glaucoma with seratonin blockers particularly naftidrofuryl, a specific S2 inhibitor. The treated patients showed an increase in visual acuity and a better preservation of visual field over six months of follow-up[113,114].

Finally, one group attempted to study the effect of magnesium, a 'physiological' calcium channel blocker, on normal-tension glaucoma. All of the patients in this study had normal-tension glaucoma with cold-induced vasospasm of the fingers. After four weeks of treatment the four normal-tension glaucoma patients in the study had improvement of their visual fields[115].

Argon laser trabeculoplasty has been reported to lower IOP in normal-tension glaucoma[103,116,117]. However, no long-term studies are available on the efficacy of laser surgery in maintaining visual function.

Some clinicians believe that reductions of IOP to low-normal or even sub-normal levels are necessary to stabilize progressive normal-tension glaucoma. This is best achieved through filtering surgery either with full-thickness procedures or with guarded procedures employing antimetabolite agents[117-119]. Hitchings and co-workers have reported that they did a trabeculectomy in one eye of 18 patients with progressive normal-tension glaucoma. The fellow eye was followed without treatment for two to seven years. IOP was reduced by more than 31% in the eyes that received surgery and less than 1% in the fellow eyes. Beginning two years postoperatively, the visual function tests began to diverge with the surgically treated eyes appearing to have better preservation of vision[118]. Similar results have been reported by other investigators[117,119]. Yamamoto and co-workers performed trabeculectomy with mitomycin C in 42 eyes of 29 patients who had progressive normal-tension glaucoma. This procedure reduced IOP from the mean preoperative level of 13.9 mmHg to a mean postoperative level of 7.9 mmHg. The visual field deteriorated in only two of the eyes postoperatively. However, cataract progressed in eight eyes and hypotonous maculopathy developed in 11 eyes. The authors note that the postoperative IOP level approaches hypotony in this situation and that filtering surgery is associated with a high rate of complications[121]. Other clinicians have reported that filtering surgery is not helpful in normal-tension glaucoma[11,59,72,122]. One group attempted optic nerve sheath decompression for low-tension glaucoma but the results were disappointing[123].

If we accept the hypothesis that normal-tension glaucoma has a variety of causes it is likely that no one therapeutic approach will be successful in each case. Unfortunately, we have been forced to use the same approach for all patients with the diagnosis. At present, we are unable to distinguish subclasses of patients with normal-tension glaucoma. If we were able to distinguish subclasses we might be able to determine which agent or approach would be most likely to help which patient.

It is clear that no therapeutic approach has proven to be successful in normal-tension glaucoma. In part, this relates to the small retrospective studies that have been performed. It is hoped that the Normal Tension Glaucoma Study will definitively determine the impact of reducing IOP. A plea is made for additional randomized prospective trials to assess other approaches including calcium channel blockers, serotonin antagonists, and other agents. Until such information is available, the author will continue to reduce IOP in patients with progressive normal-tension glaucoma. If medical and laser therapy do not reduce IOP by 30%, a trabeculectomy will be performed with mitomycin C in one eye. The decision about the fellow eye is made depending on the response of the first eye to surgery and the patient's preference.

Acknowledgments

Supported in part by an unrestricted grant from Prevent Blindness America, New York, NY, USA.

References

1. Best W: Glaucoma ohne Hochdruk. Klin Monatsbl Augenheilkd 159:280-286, 1971
2. Leighton DA, Phillips CI: Systemic blood pressure in open-angle glaucoma, low tension glaucoma and the normal eye. Br J Ophthalmol 56:447-453,1972
3. Hatsuda TA: Low-tension glaucoma. Folia Ophthalmol Jpn 28:244-251,1977
4. De Vivero C, O'Brien C, Lanigan L, Hitchings R: Diurnal intraocular pressure variation in low-tension glaucoma. Eye 8:521-523,1994
5. Yamagami J, Araie M, Aihara M, Yamamoto S: Diurnal variation in intraocular pressure of normal-tension glaucoma eyes. Ophthalmology 100:643-650, 1993
6. Sogano S, Yamamoto T, Kitazawa Y: IOP change over time in normal-tension glaucoma. Nippon Ganka Gakkai Zasshi – Acta Soc Ophthalmol Jpn 97:65-70, 1993
7. Caprioli J, Spaeth GL: Comparison of visual field defects in the low-tension glaucomas with those in the high-tension glaucomas. Am J Ophthalmol 97:730-737, 1984
8. Harrington DO: Pathogenisis of the glaucomatous visual field defects: individual variations in pressure sensitivity. In: Newell FW (ed) Conference on Glaucoma; Transactions of the Fifth Josiah Macy Conference. New York, NY: Josiah Macy Foundation 1960
9. Lyle DJ: Arteriosclerotic optic atrophy. Proc Soc Med 50:937-940, 1957
10. Primrose J: Clinical review of glaucomatous discs. In: Cant JS (ed) The Optic Nerve. St. Louis, MO: The CV Mosby Co, 1972
11. Sourdille GP: Champ visuel rétréci et possibilités opératoires dans le glaucome. Bull Soc Ophtalmol Fr 2:361-366, 1956
12. Takada M, Araie M, Suzuki Y, Koseki N, Yamagami J: The central visual field defects in low-tension glaucoma. A comparison of the central visual field defects in low-tension glaucoma with those in primary open angle glaucoma. Nippon Ganka Gakkai Zasshi – Acta Soc Ophthalmol Jpn 97:1320-1324, 1993
13. King D, Drance SM, Douglas G, Schulzer M, Wijsman K: Comparison of visual field defects in normal-tension glaucoma and high-tension glaucoma. Am J Ophthalmol 101:204-207, 1986
14. Yamagami J, Araie M, Suzuki Y, Shirato S, Koseki N: A comparative study of visual field damage in low-tension and primary open-angle glaucoma. Nippon Ganka Gakkai Zasshi – Acta Soc Ophthalmol Jpn 97:383-389, 1993
15. Lachenmayr BJ, Drance SM, Chauhan BC, House PH, Lalani S: Diffuse and localized glaucomatous visual field changes in light sense, flicker and visual acuity perimetry. Evidence of pressure damage. Fortschr Ophthalmol 88:530-537, 1991
16. Samuelson TW, Spaeth GL: Focal and diffuse visual field defects: their relationship to intraocular pressure. Ophthalmic Surg 24:519-525, 1993
17. Arai M, Yamagami J, Suziki Y: Visual field defects in normal-tension and high-tension glaucoma. Ophthalmology 100:1808-1814, 1993
18. Drance SM, Douglas GR, Airaksinen PJ, Schulzer M, Hitchings RA: Diffuse field loss in chronic open angle glaucoma and low tension glaucoma. Am J Ophthalmol 104:577-580, 1987
19. Chauhan B, Drance SM: The influence of intraocular pressure on visual field damage in patients with normal tension and high tension glaucoma. Invest Ophthalmol Vis Sci 97:2367-2372, 1990
20. Drance SM: The visual field of low tension glaucoma and shock-induced optic neuropathy. Arch Ophthalmol 95:1359-1361, 1977
21. Mosquera JM: El pseudo-glaucoma: caudro clinica y problemas terapeuticos. Arch Oftalmol (B. Aires) 33:245-248, 1959
22. Motolko M, Drance SM, Douglas GR: Visual field defects in low-tension glaucoma: comparison of defects in low-tension glaucoma and chronic open-angle glaucoma. Arch Ophthalmol 100:1074-1077,1982
23. Caprioli J, Spaeth GL: Comparison of the optic nerve head in high- and low-tension glaucoma. Arch Ophthalmol 103:1145-1149, 1985
24. Chervin M: Glaucoma por hipersecretion, glaucoma sin hipertension, pseudoglaucoma. Arch Oftalmol (B. Aires) 42:187-202, 1967.
25. Knapp E: Glaukom ohne Hochdruck bei Mutter und Tochter. Klin Monatsbl Augenheilkd 153:669-673, 1968.
26. Kuhl W: Glaukom ohne Hochdruck und Tonographietest. Ophthalmologica 163:245-253, 1971
27. Paufique L, Barut C, Bonnet M, Voinot MJ: A propos du glaucome à basse tension. Bull Soc Ophtalmol Fr 64:464-470, 1964
28. Sandvig K: Pseudoglaucoma of autosomal dominant inheritance: a report of 3 families. Acta Ophthalmol (Kbh) 39:33-37, 1961
29. Tomita G, Yamada T, Matsubara K, Kitazawa Y: Glaucoma-like disc without increased intra-ocular pressure or visual field loss and early stage normal-tension glaucoma disc. Nippon Ganka

Gakkai Zasshi – Acta Soc Ophthalmol Jpn 97:225-231, 1993
30. Yamagami J, Araie M, Shirato S: A comparative study of optic nerve head in low- and high-tension glaucomas. Graefes Arch Clin Exp Ophthalmol 230:446-450, 1992
31. Huang LN, Zhou WB: Comparison of optic disc damages and fluorescein filling defect of the disc between low tension and primary open angle glaucoma. Chung-Hua Yen Ko Tsa Chih (Chinese J Ophthalmol) 28:209-213, 1992
32. Buus DR, Anderson DR: Peripapillary crescents and halos in normal-tension glaucoma and ocular hypertension. Ophthalmology 96:16-19, 1989
33. Jonas JB: Size of glaucomatous optic discs. Germ J Ophthalmol 1:41-44, 1992
34. Burk, RO, Rohrschneider K, Noack H, Volcker HE: Are large optic nerve heads susceptible to glaucomatous damage at normal intraocular pressure? A three-dimensional study by laser scanning tomography. Graefes Arch Clin Exp Ophthalmol 230:552-560, 1992
35. Drance SM, Sweeney VP, Morgan RW, Feldman F: Studies of factors involved in the production of low tension glaucoma. Arch Ophthalmol 89:457-465,1973
36. Ourgard HG, Etienne R: L'Exploration Fonctionelle de l'Oeil Glaucomateux. Paris: Masson, 1961
37. Harrington DO: The visual fields, 4th Edn. St. Louis, MO: The CV Mosby Co 1976
38. Winstanley J: Discussion on low-tension glaucoma. Proc R Soc Med 52:433-437, 1959
39. Hoyng PFJ, DeJong H, Oosting H, Stilma J: Platelet aggregation, disc haemorrhage and progressive loss of visual fields in glaucoma. Int Ophthalmol 16:65-73, 1992
40. Gloster J: Incidence of optic disc haemorrhages in chronic simple glaucoma and ocular hypertension. Br J Ophthalmol 65:452-456, 1981
41. Kitazawa Y, Shirato S, Yamamoto T: Optic disc haemorrhage in low-tension glaucoma. Ophthalmology 93:853-857, 1986
42. King D, Drance SM, Douglas G, Schulzer M, Wijsman K: Comparison of visual field defects in normal-tension glaucoma and high-tension glaucoma. Am J Ophthalmol 101:204-207, 1986
43. Begg IS, Drance SM, Goldmann H: Fluorescein angiography in the evaluation of focal circulatory ischaemia of the optic nerve head in relation to the arcuate scotoma in glaucoma. Can J Ophthalmol 7:68-74, 1972
44. Hitchings RA, Spaeth GL: Fluorescein angiography in chronic simple glaucoma and low-tension glaucoma. Br J Ophthalmol 61:126-132, 1977
45. Inoue Y, Inoue T, Shishida Y: Fluorescein angiography of the optic disc in low-tension glaucoma. Folia Ophthalmol Jpn 26:1400-1410, 1975
46. Laatikainen L: Fluorescein angiographic studies of the peripapillary and perilimbal regions in simple, capsular and low tension glaucoma. Acta Ophthalmol (Kbh) 111:3-83, 1971
47. Levene RZ: Low tension glaucoma: a critical review and new material. Surv Ophthalmol 24:621-664, 1980
48. Spaeth GL: Fluorescein angiography: its contribution towards understanding the mechanisms of visual loss in glaucoma. Trans Am Ophthalmol Soc 73:491-553, 1976
49. Spaeth GL: The Pathogenesis of Nerve Damage in Glaucoma: Contributions of Fluorescein Angiography. New York, NY: Grune & Stratton, Inc 1977
50. Hollows FC, Graham PA: Intraocular pressure, glaucoma and glaucoma suspects in a defined population. Br J Ophthalmol 50:570-586, 1966
51. Bankes JLK, Perkins ES, Tsolakis S, Wright JE: Bedford glaucoma survey. Br Med J 1:791-796, 1968
52. Wallace J, Lovell HG: Glaucoma and intraocular pressure in Jamaica. Am J Ophthalmol 67:93-100, 1969
53. Perkins ES: The Bedford glaucoma survey. I. Longterm followup of borderline cases. Br J Ophthalmol 57:179-185, 1973
54. Sommer A, Tielsch JM, Katz J, et al: Relationship between intraocular pressure and primary open angle glaucoma among white and black americans The Baltimore Eye Survey. Arch Ophthalmol 109:1090-1095, 1991
55. Shiose Y: Prevalence and clinical aspects of low tension glaucoma. Acta XXIV Int Congr Ophthalmol 1:587-591, 1983
56. Drance SM: Some factors in the production of low tension glaucoma. Br J Ophthalmol 56:229-242, 1972
57. Drance SM, Morgan RW, Sweeney VP: Shock-induced optic neuropathy: a cause of nonprogressive glaucoma. N Engl J Med 288:392-395, 1973
58. Anderton SA, Coakes RC, Poinoosawmy S, Clarke P, Hitchings RA: The nature of visual loss in low tension glaucoma. In: Heijl A, Greve E (eds) 6th International Visual Fields Symposium, Santa Margharita Ligure 1984, pp 383-387. The Hague: Junk 1985
59. Chumbley LC, Brubaker RF: Low tension glaucoma. Am J Ophthalmol 81:761-763, 1976
60. Nourreddin B, Poinoosawmy D, Fitzke F, Hitchings RA: Regression analysis of visual field progression in low tension glaucoma Br J Ophthalmol 74:493-495, 1991

61. Glicklich RE, Steinman WC, Spaeth GL: Visual change in low tension glaucoma over a five year follow up. Ophthalmology 96:316-320, 1986
62. Schulzer M: Errors in the diagnosis of visual field progression in normal tension glaucoma. Ophthalmology 101:1589-1594, 1994
63. Araie M, Sekine M, Suzuki Y, Koseki H: Factors contributing to the progression of visual field damage in eyes with normal tension glaucoma. Ophthalmology 101: 1440-1444, 1994
64. Geijssen CH: Studies on Normal Tension Glaucoma. Amsterdam: Kugler Publications 1991
65. Cartwright MJ, Anderson DR: Correlation between asymmetric damage with asymmetric intraocular presure in normal tension glaucoma. Arch Ophthalmol 106:898-900, 1988
66. Crichton A, Drance SM, Douglas G, Schulzer M: Unequal IOPs and its relation to asymmetric visual field defects in low tension glaucoma. Ophthalmology 96:1313-1314, 1989
67. Sjøgren H: A study of pseudoglaucoma. Acta Ophthalmol (Kbh) 24: 239-243, 1946
68. Orgal S, Flammer J: Perilimbal aneurysms of conjunctival vessels in glaucoma patients. Germ J Ophthalmol 4:94-96, 1995
69. Hoskins HD, Kass MA: Diagnosis and Therapy of the Glaucomas. St. Louis, MO: CV Mosby 1989
70. Quigley HA, Addicks EM: Reginal differences in the structure of the laminar cribosa and their relation to optic nerve damage. Arch Ophthalmol 99:137-142, 1981
71. Tengroth B, Amitzboll T: Changes in the content and composition of collagen in the glaucomatous eye. Basis for a new hypothesis for the genesis of chronic open-angle glaucoma – a preliminary report. Acta Ophthalmol (Kbh) 62:999-1010, 1984
72. Quigley HA, Green WK: The histology of human glaucoma cupping and optic nerve damage: clinicopathologic correlation in 21 eyes. Ophthalmology 86:1803-1830, 1979
73. Haefliger IO, Hitchings RA: Relationship between asymmetry of visual field defects and intraocular pressure difference in an untreated normal (low) tension glaucoma population. Acta Ophthalmol (Kbh) 68:564-567, 1990
74. Shirai H, Sakuma T, Sogano S, Kitazawa Y: Visual field change and risk factors for progression of visual field damage in low tension glaucoma. Nippon Ganka Gakkai Zashi – Acta Soc Ophthalmol Jpn 96:352-358, 1992
75. Weber J, Koll W, Krieglstein GK: Intraocular pressure and visual field decay in chronic glaucoma. Germ J Ophthalmol 2:165-169, 1993
76. Yoshikawa K, Inoue T, Inoue Y: Normal tension glaucoma: the value of predictive tests. Acta Ophthalmol (Kbh) 71:463-470, 1993
77. Orgul S, Flammer J: Interocular visual-field and intraocular-pressure asymmetries in normal-tension glaucoma. Eur J Ophthalmol 4:199-201, 1994
78. Morax V: Glaucome simple au atrophie avec excavation. Ann Ocul (Paris) 153:25-37, 1916
79. Thiel R: Glaukom ohne Hochdruck. Ber Dtsch Ophthalmol Gesellsch 48:133-139, 1930
80. Gafter F, Goldmann H: Experimentelle Untersuchungen über den Zusammenhang von Augendrucksteigerung und Gesichtsfeldschädigung. Ophthalmologica 130:357-361, 1955
81. Winder AF: Circulating lipoprotein and blood glucose levels in association with low-tension and chronic simple glaucoma. Br J Ophthalmol 61:641-645, 1977
82. Winder A, Patterson G, Miller SJH: Biochemical abnormalities associated with ocular hypertension and low tension glaucoma. Trans Ophthalmol Soc UK 94:518-524, 1974
83. Goldberg I, Hollows FC, Kass MA, Becker B: Systemic factors in patients with low-tension glaucoma. Br J Ophthalmol 65:56-62, 1981
84. Corbett JJ, Phelps CD, Eslinger P, Montague PR: The neurologic evaluation of patients with low-tension glaucoma. Invest Ophthalmol Vis Sci 26:1101-1104, 1985
85. Graham SL, Drance SM, Sijsman K, Douglas GR, Mikelberg FS: Ambulatory blood pressure monitoring in glaucoma. The nocturnal dip. Ophthalmology 102:61-69, 1995
86. Kaiser HJ, Flammer J, Burckhardt D: Silent myocardial ischemia in glaucoma patients. Ophthalmologica 207:6-7, 1993
87. Kaiser HJ, Flammer J, Graf T, Stumpfig D: Systemic blood pressure in glaucoma patients. Graefes Arch Clin Exp Ophthalmol 231:677-680,1993
88. Hayreh SS, Zimmerman MB, Podhajsky P, Alward WL: Nocturnal arterial hypotension and its role in optic nerve head and ocular ischemic disorders. Am J Ophthalmol 117:603-624, 1994
89. Gasser P, Flammer J: Blood-cell velocity in the nailfold capillaries of patients with normal-tension and high-tension glaucoma. Am J Ophthalmol 111:585-588, 1991
90. Duke-Elder S: Fundamental concepts in glaucoma. Arch Ophthalmol 42:538-544,1949
91. Joist JH, Lichtenfeld P, Mandell AI, Kolker AE: Platelet function, blood coagulability and fibrinolysis in patients with low tension glaucoma. Arch Ophthalmol 94:1893-1895,1976
92. Nagata A, Mishima H, Choshi K, Shimada S, Furumoto Y: Fluorescein fundus angiography of optic nerve head in primary open angle glaucoma and low tension glaucoma. Nippon Ganka Gakkai Zasshi – Acta Soc Ophthalmol Jpn 96:1423-1428, 1992

93. Harris A, Sergott RC, Spaeth GL, Katz JL, Shoemaker JA, Martin BJ: Color Doppler analysis of ocular vessel blood velocity in normal-tension glaucoma. Am J Ophthalmol 118:642-649, 1994
94. Ravalico G, Pastori G, Toffoli G, Croce M: Visual and blood flow responses in low-tension glaucoma. Surv Ophthalmol 8:173-176, 1994
95. Abe H, Hasegawa S, Takagi M, Usui T, Shirakashi M, Iwata K: Fluorescein angiographic findings regarding the optic disc in cases of low-tension glaucoma and the chronic stage of anterior ischemic optic neuropathy. Nippon Ganga Gakkai Zasshi – Acta Soc Ophthalmol Jpn 97(10): 1225-1230, 1993
96. Rojanapongpun P, Drance SM, Morrison BJ: Ophthalmic artery flow velocity in glaucomatous and normal subjects. Br J Ophthalmol 77:25-29, 1993
97. Yamazaki Y, Hayamizu F: Analysis of ophthalmic arterial flow by color Doppler imaging in glaucomatous eyes. Nippon Ganga Gakkai Zasshi – Acta Soc Ophthalmol Jpn 98:1115-1120, 1994
98. Rankin SJ, Walman BE, Buckley AR, Drance SM: Color Doppler imaging and spectral analysis of the optic nerve vasculature in glaucoma. Am J Ophthalmol 119:685-693, 1995
99. Butt Z, McKillop G, O'Brien C, Allan P, Aspinall P: Measurement of ocular blood flow velocity using colour Doppler imaging in low tension glaucoma. Eye 9:29-33, 1995
100. Cartwright MJ, Grajewski AL, Friedberg ML et al: Immune-related disease and normal-tension glaucoma. Arch Ophthalmol 110:500-502, 1992
101. Wax MB, Barrett DA, Pestronk A: Increased incidence of paraproteinemia and auto antibodies in patients with normal pressure glaucoma. Am J Ophthalmol 117:561-568, 1994
102. Romano C, Barrett DA, Li Z, Pestronk A, Wax MB: Ant. Rhodopsin antibodies in sera from patients with normal-pressure glaucoma. Invest Ophthalmol Vis Sci 36:1968-1974, 1995
103. Anderson DR: Glaucoma: the damage caused by pressure. XLVI Edward Jackson Memorial Lecture. Am J Ophthalmol 108:485-495, 1989
104. Van Buskirk EM, Cioffi GA: Glaucomatous optic neuropathy. Am J Ophthalmol 113:447-452, 1992
105. Drance SM: Bowman Lecture: glaucoma changing concepts. Eye 6:337-345, 1992
106. Schulzer M: The intraocular pressure reduction in normal-tension glaucoma patients. The Normal Tension Glaucoma Study Group. Ophthalmology 99:1468-1470, 1992
107. Harris A, Spaeth GL, Sergott RC, Katz LJ, Cantor LB, Martin BJ: Retrobulbar arterial hemodynamic effects of betaxolol and timolol in normal-tension glaucoma. Am J Ophthalmol 120:168-175, 1995
108. Nyman K: Intraocular pressure reduction with topically administered pilocarpine, timolol and betaxolol in normal tension glaucoma. Acta Ophthalmol (Kbh) 71:686-690, 1993
109. Fujimore C, Yamabayaski S, Hosoda M, Hosaha O, Makino F, Henme T, Toukahara S, Ueno R: The clinical evaluation of VF-021, a new prostaglandin related compound, in low tension glaucoma patients. Nippon Ganka Gakkai Zasshi – Acta Soc Ophthalmol Jpn 97:1231-1235, 1993
110. Azuma I: Progress in medical treatment for glaucoma. Nippon Ganka Gakkai Zasshi – Acta Soc Ophthalmol Jpn 97:1353-1369, 1993
111. Netland PA, Chaturvedi N, Dreyer EB: Calcium channel blockers in the management of low-tension glaucoma and open-angle glaucoma. Am J Ophthalmol 115:608-613, 1993
112. Gaspar AZ, Flammer J, Hendrickson P: Influence of nifedipine on the visual fields of patients with optic nerve-head disease. Eur J Ophthalmol 4:24-28, 1994
113. Mermoud A, Faggioni R: Treatment of normal pressure glaucoma with a serotonin S2 receptor antagonist, naftidrofuryl (praxilen). Klin Monatsbl Augenheilkd 198:332-334, 1991
114. Mermoud A, Faggione R, Van Melle GD: Double-blind study in the treatment of normal tension glaucoma with naftidrofuryl. Ophthalmologica 201:145-151, 1990
115. Gasper AZ, Gasser P, Flammer J: The influence of magnesium on visual field and peripheral vasospasm in glaucoma. Ophthalmologica 209:11-13, 1995
116. Schwartz AL, Perman KI, Whitten M: Argon laser trabeculoplasty in progressive low-tension glaucoma. Ann Ophthalmol 16:560-566, 1984
117. Abedin S, Simmons RJ, Grant WM: Progressive low-tension glaucoma: treatment to stop glaucomatous cupping and field loss when they progress despite normal intraocular pressure. Ophthalmology 89:1-6, 1982
118. Hitchings RA, Wu J, Pianissemi D, McNaught A: Surgery for normal tension glaucoma. Br J Ophthalmol 79:402-406, 1995
119. Szymanski A, Brozyna-Zylka B, Sobiery A, Otrzonsek D: Surgical treatment of low pressure glaucoma. Klin Oczna 94:294-296, 1992
120. DeJong D, Greve EL, Hoyng PEJ, Geijssen C: Results of filtering procedure in low tension glaucoma. Int Ophthalmol 13:131-138, 1989

121. Yamomoto T, Ichien M, Suesmori-Matsuskita H, Kitazawa Y: Trabeculectomy for normal-tension glaucoma. Nippon Ganka Gakkai Zasshi – Acta Soc Ophthalmol Jpn 98:579-583, 1994
122. Bloomfield S: The results of surgery in low tension glaucoma. Am J Ophthalmol 36:1067-1070, 1953
123. Wax MB, Barrett DA, Hart WM Jr, Custer PL: Optic nerve sheath decompression for glaucomatous optic neuropathy with normal intraocular pressure. Arch Ophthalmol 111:1219-1228, 1993

Medical management of glaucoma

Thom J. Zimmerman and Robert D. Fechtner

Department of Ophthalmology and Visual Sciences, University of Louisville, Louisville, KY, USA

Introduction

The patient in front of you has primary open-angle glaucoma. You have determined this by appropriate visual field testing, examining the optic nerve head, and measuring the intraocular pressure (IOP). On several occasions, the pressure has been in the low 30s. The patient has a positive family history of glaucoma. You are convinced this patient has primary open-angle glaucoma and is at risk of further visual field loss. You have decided to take measures to lower the IOP.

The main factors in choosing the correct medical agent are pointed out by a ratio called the 'therapeutic index'. The therapeutic index (TI) is that ratio with the desired effect as the numerator and all other effects of the agent as the denominator (TI = desired effect/all others). This denominator can also be called side-effects. This concept of the therapeutic index is useful for patient medication decisions. The idea is to consider TI by learning everything about the patient and appropriate drugs and to find the best marriage of drug for this particular patient. In this process one gets a thorough medical history as we were taught to do in medical school and internship. Listing all the patient's current medications, allergies, present and past medical conditions, previous surgeries, and family history is the minimum information needed. Obtaining information regarding lifestyle, basic feelings and sentiments about their problem, will be useful in establishing compliance with medical therapy.

A good time to consider compliance and related problems is prior to beginning therapy. As stated many times in this chapter, if we are going to commit a patient to lifelong therapy, it is our responsibility to make sure the patient understands, accepts, and complies.

Let us look at the compliance issues a little more closely. By way of review, glaucoma is usually asymptomatic. In fact, in early glaucoma the only noticeable symptoms may be those related to the medication! The patient notices no improvement with the lifetime medication commitment, and only if we are 100% successful does he get no worse. Then there is the matter of cost, side-effects, and drug interactions with medical therapy. We have always imagined it very difficult for a patient to come in for an examination, be told that he has glaucoma, and then be

Address for correspondence: Thom J. Zimmerman, MD, University of Louisville, Department of Ophthalmology and Visual Sciences, 301 E. Muhammad Ali Boulevard, Louisville, KY 40202, USA

Peril to the Nerve – Glaucoma and Clinical Neuro-Ophthalmology, pp. 73–85
Proceedings of the 45th Annual Symposium of the New Orleans Academy of
Ophthalmology, New Orleans, LA, USA, April 25-28, 1996
edited by Barry J. Leader and Jonathan C. Calkwood
© 1998 Kugler Publications, The Hague/The Netherlands

given a lifetime sentence from which there are no weekends off, vacations, or holidays. Treatment is not going to make him any better, it is just going to keep him from getting worse.

Education can help most of these patients understand their problem. We must design and tailor this education for the particular patient. Some patients can take the entire course of education in the first visit and be fine for a lifetime. Most patients need to have a little bit on this visit, a little bit more on the next visit with continuing education. We are never free from providing reinforcement.

After initially educating the patient about the disease and the consequences, the groundwork is set for explaining that there will be frequent follow-ups and that diagnostic testing will be needed. A discussion of cost of care should be started.

We must work with the patients on follow-up visits by continuing to explain the disease and the possible consequences, and by trying to simplify their treatment regimes and minimize their inconvenience. Predicting and discussing likely side-effects will not only decrease calls to your office, but will also instill confidence and help your patients deal with and overcome the problems. Some patients might benefit from the use of compliance aids, pamphlets, or other literature in order better to understand the disease, the treatment goals, and the need for frequent follow-up and testing. All of this can significantly improve compliance.

Before we initiate treatment with the selected agent, there are several other considerations that are part of our routine. For many people we consider a *one-eyed trial*. This allows us to judge exactly how much efficacy we are obtaining, and allows us to ascertain systemic or local side-effects that may have occurred with only half the usual amount of medication on board. We also teach, stress, and reinforce nasolacrimal occlusion with eye drop application[1]. Our routine is to ask patients to use whatever agent we select for one week in one eye only and then to return for further education, reinforcement and to tailor the drop application to their lifestyle. Unless there is a contraindication, we would then ask the patient to treat both eyes and return after one week. Much of the education, reinforcing, checking efficacy and side-effects are repeated.

If the pressure is at the target level or below, the patient is asked to return in approximately three months for follow-up examination. This one-eyed trial process is very useful for both education and reinforcing benefits of care early in the relationship with the patient. Not only do we do one-eyed trials when initiating therapy on most patients, but we often repeat these yearly in order to make sure that we have not lost the effect of a drug due to tolerance. This allows us to stop a drug that has lost its effect and replace it with another.

One of the things we see frequently is people on multiple drugs without all these drugs having satisfactory efficacy. In glaucoma care when the pressure goes up we typically add another medication. If that pressure has gone up because of tolerance of one of the drugs already on board, then we have allowed the continuation of a medication that no longer gives the efficacy we wish, but does continue to expose this patient to the possible side-effects of this drug and the possible drug interactions with other systemic or topical medications. Many patients develop tolerance to adrenergic drugs over time and it is important to stop them, instead of just adding another drug when the pressure goes up. If a drug is not doing what we want it to do (in this case, lowering IOP) then the therapeutic index is zero. Stop the drug!

We stress *nasolacrimal occlusion* in our practice because we firmly believe that if we are going to commit a patient to a lifetime of treatment he should use the drug in the safest and most efficacious manner. Also, nasolacrimal occlusion allows us to lengthen the interval between drug applications and significantly decrease the cost of medical therapy[2,3]. We think this is a very important concept.

When a drop is placed on the eye, it can quickly leave the tear film. After one or two blinks, over 95% of the drug is in the nasolacrimal system and is no longer against the surface of the eye or being transported to targeted receptors. Once the drop enters the nasolacrimal system, it goes to the nasopharynx with its high surface area covered by the most vascularized mucous membranes in our body. On exposure to this area, there is irritation which causes one to sniff, putting the drug in a mist and distributing it throughout the entire nasopharyngeal area.

This has been likened to an i.v. injection with extremely fast egress into the systemic vasculature. Approximately 60% of a lipid-soluble drug and 25% of hydro-soluble drug is absorbed for systemic circulation. Because of the point of entry, these drugs absorbed for systemic circulation miss hepatic first-pass metabolism. We deliver a significant amount of topically applied ocular drugs to the systemic circulation. That is why we see slowing of the pulse and decrease of the blood pressure with certain ocular hypotensive drugs.

Returning to our therapeutic index ratio, the first thing we wish to do is to decrease the amount of applied drug that gets absorbed systemically. We cannot think of any situation where a systemic load from an eye-drop is desirable. In a series of studies, we have been able to show that, with good nasolacrimal occlusion in place before and for two minutes after a drop is applied to the eye, approximately two-thirds of the drug that would normally enter the systemic circulation can be prevented from doing so[1]. If we can decrease by two-thirds the amount of drug available for systemic circulation, we can decrease significantly the severity and frequency of systemic side-effects due to topical ocular drug application.

Early in the testing of nasolacrimal occlusion, we discovered another unexpected benefit of this procedure. Returning to our ratio concerning the therapeutic index, we noticed that with good nasolacrimal occlusion the numerator (efficacy) could be significantly enhanced. In studies, we were able to show that pilocarpine 2% with good nasolacrimal occlusion would give the same ocular hypotensive effect as pilocarpine 4%[2]. By doing nasolacrimal occlusion, we keep the medication in the tear film longer and increase drug corneal contact time. Therefore, more drug is driven into the eye and more drug is available to interact with the targeted receptors. This allowed us to decrease the frequency of drug application. Instead of having to use pilocarpine 4% every six hours, we were able to achieve the same diurnal IOP control using pilocarpine 2% every 12 hours. It is much easier for the patient to use a drug twice a day instead of four times a day and possibly compliance would improve.

When you consider the therapeutic index again, you can see that nasolacrimal occlusion has changed the therapeutic index by a factor of 8 for pilocarpine. We reduced the number of doses for 24 hours by half; we reduced the concentration by half; and of the applied medication, nasolacrimal occlusion prevents over half of it from reaching the systemic circulation. We believe that this simple maneuver, that can double or quadruple the therapeutic index of the agent you have chosen to use, is well worth your time and effort to help patients achieve good nasolacrimal occlusion when they instill their medication.

Note that nasolacrimal occlusion needs to be in place before the drop is applied and needs to remain in place for at least two minutes. For most patients this means applying their drug to one eye with nasolacrimal occlusion for two minutes, and then applying that same drug to their other eye with a similar procedure.

If, after the patient has learned to do good nasolacrimal occlusion, you commit him to twice daily pilocarpine or once daily beta blocker, it is best to check the patient in the morning office hours before he has used the medication that morning. This will measure IOP at pharmacological trough in that you will have less active drug than at any other time during the 24-hour period. Furthermore, the IOP in most patients tends to be highest in the morning hours. If under those conditions the IOP is at a level you deem safe, then you can be fairly assured that you have that patient controlled at that level or better for the full 24 hours of treatment.

We think that involving family members in the treatment of this problem also improves compliance greatly and gives the patient much needed home support. In this situation, a person could put nasolacrimal in place OU and then have a family member apply the medication in the inferior cul-de-sac in both eyes. This would shorten total drop application time to two minutes from four minutes.

Also, a nasolacrimal occlusion device is being developed which is put in place so that the hands are free to treat both eyes. At the end of two minutes, the lid margins and lashes can be wiped with a tissue and the nasolacrimal device removed. In closing, we think that this is our responsibility to treat and reinforce NLO if we are going to commit a patient to life-long therapy.

Before we move to the drugs, let us add another little section that we call 'office pharmacology'. Taking care of glaucoma patients is difficult and we should try to enlist all the help we can get. A ready source of help is your office personnel. They can certainly do a lot of things to make the care of your glaucoma patients go more smoothly. For instance, you should have in-service meetings and talk about compliance in glaucoma patients. We all know that non-compliance can be as high as 60-70% and very often has to be considered a reason for treatment failure. Your office staff should be aware of this and readily reinforce the proper use of medications to each patient. You and your office personnel must always remember to stress the 'big picture'. Merely to say to the patient that the test came out fine and that the treatment is working, is possibly a reinforcement of poor compliance that the patient has been practicing! During the in-service with your staff, you can enlist them to help educate and reinforce. They should be able to readily supply information concerning testing, procedures, and medication use as the patient requests this information. Your office staff can help you tremendously in the educational and reinforcement part of improving compliance.

Your front office should be aware of the special procedures that need to be done yearly on all glaucoma patients. They could readily be taught to remind you when it is time to do these procedures. For instance, if you are seeing a patient every few months, on one visit you would do your routine plus gonioscopy. On the second visit, you might do your routine plus visual field testing. On the third visit, your routine plus dilation, examination of the optic nerve and photographs. This could be done with a reminder on the chart for that particular glaucoma patient or even by providing you with the gonioprism. Along this same line, one of the desired pieces of information from your chart would be a good diurnal curve. We know that if we bring a patient into the office and keep him there all day or put him in the hospital, the diurnal curve does not always reflect what is going on in the patient's 'normal' life. One way your office staff can help you is to make sure that they bring the patient back at different times of the day on subsequent visits. If you record the time of day that you took the pressure on each visit and record the times that the patient took their ocular hypotensive drugs, then at the end of six, seven, or eight visits, you have a very nice in-office diurnal curve related to when the patient uses this medication. Not only do you get duration of action information, but you can also do a dose-response curve over that same period of time by decreasing the concentration of the medication. This is much more information than knowing exactly what this patient's IOP is at 3:00 p.m. every visit.

You and your office personnel should stress that the patient wait five to ten minutes between different drop applications to the same eye. In drugs that are used in combination, you should also use an epinephrine or a beta blocker first followed by the other drugs. These adrenergic agents 'roughen' the corneal epithelium somewhat and possibly allow better penetration of drugs that follow. All drugs should be used b.i.d. tailored to the patient's lifestyle. All drugs (except Timoptic XE and Pilopine H.S.) should be used with nasolacrimal occlusion and you and your staff should reinforce this on every visit.

Furthermore, good communication should be established between you and the patient's primary care physician. This is not only excellent care for the patient, but it may preserve your practice base in the future. We cannot stress enough that if you are going to commit a patient to lifetime treatment, it is your responsibility to do it correctly.

Finally, we will look at the agents, go over our old friends, and look at some of the recently introduced agents and agents to be introduced in the near future.

The beta blockers

This section will not be all inclusive, but will focus on new information and/or differences between the agents in this class. The topical beta blockers were first introduced in September 1978. The five drugs available are timolol in its old familiar and its two new forms, levobunolol, metipranolol, carteolol and betaxolol.

In general, the drugs timolol, levobunolol, and metipranolol are very similar when one considers efficacy and systemic and ocular side-effect profiles. The other two drugs, carteolol and betaxolol, have distinguished themselves because of different pharmacological characteristics. When developing drugs or trying to improve a class of drugs used for a particular problem, one again considers therapeutic index. With the therapeutic index in mind, the individual drugs in a class are examined to see if there is a difference which might hypothetically improve the use of this class of drugs.

With beta blockers, the first pharmacological difference is selectivity. Selectivity is the characteristic which identifies betaxolol among the group of beta blockers that we have available. It was hoped that by studying a β_1-selective drug, such as betaxolol, we might maintain the same efficacy while decreasing the systemic side-effects. Also, it might be possible to affect the blood supply to the back of the eye differently than does a non-selective beta blocker.

Experience with betaxolol has shown it to be slightly less efficacious, but it definitely has an advantage in patients prone to bronchiospastic disease. There may be other advantages in its effect on quality of life in the elderly.

The next group of beta blockers to show a different characteristic were those that had intrinsic sympathomimetic activity (ISA). It was hypothesized that the ISA might create a 'softer beta blocker' as far as systemic side-effects were concerned. Studies in Japan and the United States have shown less heart rate change with ISA beta blockers. Furthermore, the ISA beta blockers seem to have a real advantage when blood lipids are considered. Beta blockers in general deleteriously affect blood lipids. Beta blockers with ISA affect these blood lipids less than beta blockers without ISA. When one considers ten or 20 years of treatment with these agents, this less deleterious effect on the blood lipids by ISA beta blockers might have some meaningful advantage for the total health of the patient.

Another advantage of carteolol (which is the only ocular ISA beta blocker in the United States) is its hydro-lipid solubility profile. Carteolol is more hydro-soluble than most of the other beta blockers and therefore does not cross some membranes as well as do the more lipid-soluble beta blockers. Certainly, studies have shown that with the concentrations of carteolol used, very similar ocular hypotensive efficacy can be achieved. Of interest though, once the drug enters the nasopharyngeal area, is that only approximately 25% of this hydro-soluble drug is absorbed for systemic distribution, whereas 60% of a more lipid-soluble drug like the other beta blockers is absorbed for systemic distribution. This might be a real advantage once again in the amount of drug delivered systemically over a ten- or 20-year period.

It is conceivable that the ISA characteristic may have a different effect on the blood flow to the back of the eye compared to the cardioselective and/or the nonselective beta blockers. At this point, let us consider the blood flow studies and the state of the art of this fascinating new area of research.

Blood flow studies may well represent the next great frontier. We believe this area of research will provide useful information concerning the pathophysiology of this disease and the treatment of glaucoma. Most agree that any extrapolation from the currently available studies to the actual treatment of a glaucoma patient is premature. Let us look at some of the information and see if we can quickly bring ourselves up to speed concerning this important area of research.

Basically, blood flow studies have been carried out for years in rabbits and other laboratory animals. Most recently, monkeys and humans have also been studied. If one, for instance, takes timolol alone and examines its effect on blood flow, you can find conflicting data depending on the method used and the species used. For instance, concerning autoregulation, timolol spares it in the bovine eye and overrides it in the human eye.

There are currently many methods that are being used to measure blood flow: bidirectional laser Doppler velocimetry (BLVD), monochromatic fundus photography (MFP), microsphere (radioactive) and video fluorescein angiography. There are also many things that are being measured: blood velocity, volumetric flow rates, center-line red cell velocities, ophthalmic artery blood pressure (OABP), choroidal blood flow, venous diameter, a-v passage time, retinal circulation time, and arm to retina circulation time. There are a number of different places where the measurements are taking place: optic nerve (prelaminar, laminar and retrolaminar), retina (A&V), choroid, ciliary arteries. Let us return to basics and ask the question: Is glaucoma really an ischemic process? Most of us believe that ischemia has a lot to do with it, but we do not have any direct proof. If glaucoma is an ischemic process, where is that critical area? Should that area become ischemic, do we see the clinical findings of glaucoma? Most of us would probably answer that it is somewhere in the optic nerve, but are we talking about prelaminar, laminar or retrolaminar optic nerve? Do these three zones of the optic nerve have different blood supplies? If they do, are they closely interrelated? The point of all this is that we do not know what to measure, where to measure, what method to use, and whether or not any of this is really correlated with what we call glaucoma.

Other questions are brought forward by microvascular researchers who talk about autoregulation in this area and the tremendous amount of compensatory reserve. We must bear in mind that this is neural tissue and autoregulation and compensatory reserve always play large roles. In drawing conclusions from studies that have been done to date, one might easily say that if a certain drug improves the circulation in a particular zone by 100%, it is possibly stealing blood from the critical zone and worsening the disease. That hypothesis makes as much sense as concluding that, since we have increased retinal blood flow, we must be benefiting the glaucoma.

We believe this research area is going to bring us tremendous information concerning both the cause, the pathophysiology, and the treatment of glaucoma. Our point is that it is simply too early to be drawing conclusions concerning a clinical condition. (For an up-to-date summary of this area, please see the *Survey of Ophthalmology* December 1994 and the *Journal of Glaucoma*, Vol. 4, No. 6, December 1995.)

At this point in time, it is our opinion that vasoactivity does not mean vasopathology or vasoactivity does not mean vasobenefit. It will take long carefully controlled studies looking at the clinical findings of optic nerve head change and visual field change eventually to prove that one beta blocker is superior to another beta blocker as far as neuroprotection or vascular protection in the disease glaucoma.

Timoptic XE is our old friend Timoptic in a new vehicle. This vehicle has the advantage of greatly increasing the ocular residence time of timolol. Basically, the vehicle is a gel-forming solution. The key ingredient is Gelrite™ which is derived from gellan gum and was first used as a food additive. It is a heteropolysaccharide in solution form which in the presence of cations changes to a gel. The patient has to be reminded to shake the bottle before application in order to ensure its liquid form and ease of application. The drop comes out of the bottle as a liquid, but upon meeting the sodium and other cations in the tears, turns into a gel and layers out in the inferior cul-de-sac. This gel-forming solution can significantly increase the ocular residency in humans. For instance, in comparison studies a saline solution has an ocular residence half-life of approximately 22 seconds in the tear film. An hydroxyethel cellose (HEC) has a half-life in man of approximately 80-90 seconds. The half-life of Gelrite solution is greater than 1000 seconds or approximately 20 minutes compared to 1.5 minutes with the HEC. It was hoped that this increased ocular residence would drive more drug into the eye and greatly extend the duration of action of the active ingredient, Timoptic.

Timoptic XE

In direct comparison studies, 0.5% Timoptic XE was compared with 0.5% Timoptic solution. The Timoptic XE was used only once in the 24-hour period, whereas the Timoptic solution was used in the usual manner which was every 12 hours or twice in the 24-hour period. These comparison studies convincingly showed that both drug forms had very similar efficacy throughout the 24-hour diurnal curve. These same results were found at the lower concentrations (*i.e.*, 0.25% Timoptic XE *versus* 0.25% Timoptic). These studies were done in the United States and internationally. There were also switch-over studies done from Timoptic to TXE without loss of efficacy. Of course, the beauty here is that the same 24-hour diurnal efficacy was achieved by exposing the patient to half the amount of active ingredient. This, as we have discussed, should double the therapeutic index. Hopefully, that would make this drug twice as safe systemically as any of the currently used twice a day beta blockers[4].

As far as tolerability goes, approximately one out of three patients will complain of short-lasting, blurred vision. This is most likely due to the gel. Certainly the same adverse effects are possible with this form of Timoptic and all the contraindications should be observed. Only time and careful follow-up will prove or disprove the hypothesis of doubling the therapeutic index by this new form of Timoptic.

Betimol

Betimol is timolol hemihydrate. This is very similar to timolol maleate except for the absence of maleate in Betimol. Betimol performs very similarly to timolol maleate in comparison studies. It is entering the market with a lower wholesale price than Timoptic. As Timoptic is about to go off patent protection, we will no doubt see a number of generic timolol maleates. Betimol is an attempt to enter this arena with a different structure that can also give cost savings to the patients. Although the drug may have a significantly lower wholesale price to the pharmacist, this does not always get reflected in savings to the patients. The pharmacy often views this as an opportunity to gain additional profit. We advise all our patients whenever we start them on any drug to sit down with the yellow pages and call pharmacies in their area. They should ask the cost of the medication that has been prescribed and after considering issues such as delivery, location, and hours, decide which drugstore offers them the best value.

All studies to date have shown no difference in efficacy between Betimol and Timoptic with a very similar side-effect profile both ocularly and systemically. Certainly, until more information is available, the contraindications and precautions for Betimol should be the same as the other beta blockers. Cost might be a significant factor in the care of your patients.

Dorzolamide (Trusopt™)

Acetazolamide was discovered by Thomas Maren, MD, in 1954 and later in that year was shown by Bernard Becker, MD, to lower IOP. This essentially started a 40-year search for a topical carbonic anhydrase inhibition. Certainly, many researchers have realized for years that this class of drugs would be much better tolerated in a topical form than it is in the oral form. As useful as this class of drugs was for the treatment of glaucoma, our enthusiasm was certainly dampened by the serious side-effects. Our old friend, the therapeutic index, would be greatly served if we could deliver this to the eye in adequate concentrations and in much smaller amounts to the body. Early investigations trying to develop a topical ocular form were met with negative results and a dogma surfaced that it was impossible to develop topical carbonic anhydrase inhibitors as that form of delivery would never reach concentrations high enough to inhibit all the carbonic anhydrase in the ciliary epithelium. Other reasons were given, such as to the insolubility of all sulfonamides and the inability of these agents to work from the aqueous side. Low inhibitory activity compared to the high rate of activity of the carbonic anhydrase system was a problem, as well as the rapid turnover of agents such as these in the highly vascularized ciliary epithelium. Based on the above 'insurmountable' problems, most researchers turned away from expending further effort in developing a topical carbonic anhydrase inhibitor. Dr. Maren stuck to the task and eventually made the breakthroughs that ultimately made a topical carbonic anhydrase inhibitor possible.

Several candidates were looked at in the early 1980s and dropped because of one problem or another. It was not until 1986 that MK927 was developed. A series of other drugs was studied and eventually MK507 was the one chosen for marketing. This drug is currently marketed in the United States and most of Europe as dorzolamide, trade named, Trusopt.

Three key studies were done which were to compare monotherapy against placebo, monotherapy against beta blockers, and adjunctive therapy with beta blockers. During all these studies, clinical tolerability was also monitored. Dorzolamide was shown significantly to lower the IOP at peak and trough compared with baseline. When compared with the beta blockers, timolol was slightly more effective at trough than either betaxolol or Trusopt, but there was no significant difference at peak between these three drugs. In this huge, long-term study, Trusopt held its ocular hypotensive effect for a full 12 months. In the adjunctive study with beta blockers, Trusopt showed a very nice additivity with timolol.

Clinical tolerability was followed closely in all phases of study and showed a high rate of patient acceptance, with only five patients in the combined studies withdrawing due to side-effects. Furthermore, these clinical studies showed no changes in the electrolytes, no changes in acid base balance, and minimal to no changes in heart rate and blood pressure. Approximately one-quarter to one-third of the patients described a bitter taste in the mouth after application and this was thought to be minimized by nasolacrimal occlusion. Also, approximately one-third of the participants in the studies complained of stinging and burning on application. This is short-lived and was seldom a reason for withdrawal, but needs to be kept in mind when introducing this agent to a patient. A simple statement, such as, "this is going to sting and burn when you put it in, but this does not mean that it's hurting your eye" will often save a phone call to your office. Even though this drug appears to be safe and well tolerated, it still has to carry all the warnings and precautions of the carbonic anhydrase inhibitors. Only time and close scrutiny will tell us exactly what the side-effect profile of this agent is. The cornea and the lens will have to be monitored in Phase IV studies to ensure that the inhibition of the carbonic anhydrase enzyme system is not deleterious to these two structures. Furthermore, systemic side-effects such as blood dyscrasias or the Stevens-Johnson syndrome will have to be monitored also in Phase IV studies. Germane to this is the recent study that suggests that contralateral ocular hypotensive effect is possible with Trusopt unless nasolacrimal occlusion is used[5]. This means that there is enough circulating in the red blood cells possibly to affect other systemic organs. If this drug is used as monotherapy, it is recommended at three times daily although there is a good effect when used twice daily, especially with nasolacrimal occlusion. Furthermore, a recent study has shown that, in combination with the beta blocker, this drug has maximal effect when used in a b.i.d. or q 12-hour format[6]. We hypothesize that the decrease in the rate of aqueous production and, therefore, turnover in the anterior chamber allows a longer intraocular residence time which increases the duration of action of this agent. Of greatest importance is a recent study that shows that, in a clinically diverse population of glaucoma patients taking varying doses of oral carbonic anhydrase inhibitors, IOP control was maintained when topical dorzolamide 2% was substituted for an oral carbonic anhydrase inhibitor[7]. In 78% of the patients, IOP after four weeks of topical therapy was controlled as well or better. IOP was 10% above baseline in only 8% of these patients. So the reason for developing this agent, which was to replace the oral carbonic anhydrase inhibitors, seems to have been realized.

We know of no major systemic or ocular side-effects, and we are hearing results from other groups and individuals similar to those outlined above. This looks to be a most promising new agent and marketing surveillance indicates that it has become the 'first choice' adjunctive drug to the beta blockers in the U.S. Whether this drug will achieve primary or initiation of treatment status remains to be seen. Certainly those patients for whom a beta blocker is contraindicated might be started on this agent initially.

α_2-Adrenergic agonists

Apraclonidine is currently the only approved drug in this class. It was originally approved for adjunctive use with laser procedures in order to prevent the IOP spike. Apraclonidine works very well in this respect and later was approved for chronic use for up to a 90-day period.

Brimonidine is another drug in this class and is in the late stages of development. Preliminary work with this agent has shown promise that this might be a better α_2-adrenergic agonist. This class, the α_2-adrenergic agonists, is a very interesting addition to our glaucoma armamentarium. As often happens, the first drug from a new class may not be the best one. As we see more drugs emerge, we believe that an excellent drug will be developed.

The α_2-adrenergic agonist, in general, decreases IOP by decreasing the production of aqueous humor. A recent study by Toris *et al.* suggests that brimonidine may have an effect on the uveal scleral outflow system[8]. This study suggested that, although Brimonidine decreases aqueous humor production, it may also increase uveal scleral outflow. Brimonidine is a very potent agent for lowering IOP and has been shown to be additive with maximal medical therapy.

Apraclonidine, the first drug in this class to be used for the treatment of glaucoma, has several significant limitations. In some studies, an unacceptably high incidence of immunologically based allergic reaction occurred. This clears after the drug is stopped, but limits its use in general. Another problem with apraclonidine is the fact that there is a high percentage of tolerance. Tolerance is defined as the loss of effect of a drug over time. In some studies it is suggested that up to 40% may have a significant decrease in the effectiveness of the drug at about 90 days. This also is a significant limitation, but this drug can be an excellent adjunctive to maximal medical therapy if the tolerance and the allergic reaction do not occur. Brimonidine seems to have reduced these two critical limitations. Studies with brimonidine have shown no significant change in heart rate or blood pressure, but some patients in the study complained of dry mouth, fatigue, and drowsiness. Brimonidine has shown an IOP lowering effect comparable to timolol and somewhat better than betaxolol. There does not seem to be an alteration in the cardiovascular response to exercise or alteration of the FEV_1 with this agent. Brimonidine is somewhat more selective for the α_2-adrenergic receptors than apraclonidine.

Prostaglandins

We have long awaited a drug from this class. It is well known clinically that uveitis, through the prostaglandins, can either increase the IOP, not change the IOP, or decrease the IOP. Subsequently, it was discovered that PGF_2 in fact, nicely lowered the IOP by increasing uveoscleral outflow. This agent has a profound effect on uveoscleral outflow and can even decrease normal IOP to single digits, below episcleral venous pressure. This is one of the most potent agents ever developed for the treatment of glaucoma. The leading candidate in this class currently is a prostaglandin analog from Sweden. A number of people deserve credit for the development of this agent, but notably the lion's share should go to Drs. Lazlo Bito, Carl Camras, and Albert Alm. It is called PHXA34 and will be marketed under the name Latanoprost.

In two recent large, multicenter studies, the IOP reduction by Latanoprost was at least as great as the IOP reduction produced by timolol[9,10]. Latanoprost does not seem to affect the pulse, blood pressure, or any of the laboratory values that were part of the study. There was slightly more conjunctival hyperemia with Latanoprost compared to the timolol group. Of concern was that the iris of some patients got darker during Latanoprost treatment. This appeared to be concentric iris heterochromia (darker centrally). Further study indicates that this does not represent an increase in the number of melanocytes, but rather represents an increase in the amount of melanin in the melanocytes. There are also several hypotheses that this might be related to a deficiency of adrenergic input not dissimilar from Horner's syndrome. This increase in pigmentation appeared only in the heterochromic hazel, green, or light brown irises.

Latanoprost shows great promise and is touted as a type of local hormone. It is hypothesized and hoped that this drug might decrease the IOP and have very few adverse ocular effects and no systemic effects. To date, the drug has been shown to be the most potent ocular hypotensive drug that we currently have, and it has an excellent ocular and systemic side-effect profile. This drug is currently in the final phases of testing and is expected to be released shortly.

Neuroprotection

For years, all we have been able to do for glaucoma is lower the IOP. We do that with drugs, we do it with lasers, we do it with surgery, and that basically has been the only intervention we have available when a patient is losing vision from glaucoma. We have looked for years at other ways of approaching this disease, such as increasing blood flow or protecting the neural elements in the back of the eye from glaucoma damage. Certain advances in the neurosciences have made these attempts even more attractive. Neuroscience research has discovered the following:

Hypoxia PAF → ↑ Glutamic acid   →   Neuronal
Ischemia   ↗   damage

PAF = Platelet activating factor
          Secondary messenger works at presynaptic site
Glutamic acid
          – an excitotoxic neurotransmitter

Translating the above, we see that injury either from hypoxia or ischemia, causes a release of glutamic acid known to be one of the excitotoxic neurotransmitters. Release and extracellular build-up of glutamic acid causes damage to the neighboring neurons. This turns into a cascade so that injury causes additional injury. Once you have a scheme like this, you can develop possible strategies. For instance, you could pharmacologically block the release of glutamic acid, increase catabolization, or interrupt the cascade at some other link. This has been done in the neurosciences with the development of an N-methyl-D-aspartate receptor antagonist which has been shown to be neuroprotective in a stroke model and a nerve crush model. Bringing this entire concept back to glaucoma, let us see why this is such an exciting and timely avenue of research. We know that extracellular build-up of glutamate is toxic. We also know that in glaucoma the first ganglion cells damaged are the larger retinal ganglion cells. Moreover, we know that these larger retinal ganglion cells are more susceptible to excitotoxins and hypoxia. Furthermore, Dreyer *et al.* found an increased level of glutamate in the vitreous of patients with chronic open-angle glaucoma compared to the glutamate level in patients that did not have chronic open-angle glaucoma[11]. This completes the circle in that there is increased glutamate in patients with chronic open-angle glaucoma, large retinal ganglion cells are susceptible to this build-up, and the large retinal ganglion cells are the first ones to go in the glaucomatous process. The neuroscience literature is growing rapidly and we should follow it with great interest. Drugs that will be developed from this research may well be applicable to glaucoma.

Along the same line is the idea of increasing blood flow to the back of the eye in order to slow or stop the glaucomatous process. The candidates that have been getting the most attention along this line have been the calcium channel blockers. The idea of using a calcium channel blocker to break up part of this cascade is one that is being tested now not only in glaucoma, but also in the neurosciences. Calcium channel blockers basically:
- block membrane-bound calcium channels
- inhibit calcium influx
- relax smooth muscle in vascular wall
- decrease vascular tone
- increase blood flow

There are several studies in Japan by Sawada and here in the United States by Netland, who have shown that there is some promise for the use of calcium channel blockers in the treatment of low-tension glaucoma[12,13]. These studies have shown that although there is no detectable effect in chronic open-angle glaucoma, there seems to be a beneficial effect in low-tension glaucoma. There will be a considerable number of additional studies done with the calcium channel blockers. Currently, if we have a patient with low-tension glaucoma who is still progressing despite a very low IOP, we call the primary-care physician and ask him to consider starting calcium channel blockers in this patient. We explain that we believe the process in the eye is like Raynaud's phenomena or migraine and would he kindly start a dose that would be appropriate to prevent vasospasms such as these. We then follow the patient very carefully and the primary-care physician follows the patient with regard to the use of their oral calcium channel blockers. Certainly, a study randomizing these patients to standard treatment plus calcium channel blockers *versus* just standard treatment is needed.

References

1. Zimmerman TJ, Kooner KS, Kandarakis AS, Ziegler LP: Improving the therapeutic index of topically applied ocular drugs. Arch Ophthalmol 102(4):551-553, 1984
2. Sharir M, Zimmerman TJ: Prostaglandin analogs as ocular hypotensive agents. Ocular Ther Management 1(2):14-18, 1992
3. Sharir M, Zimmerman TJ: Effect of nasolacrimal occlusion on dose and duration of action of topical ocular hypotensive agents. Adv Ther 10:74-85, 1993
4. Dickstein K, Torbjorn A: Comparison of the effects of aqueous and gellan ophthalmic timolol on peak exercise performance in middle-aged men. Am J Ophthalmol 121:367-371, 1996
5. Robison MY, Gamero GE, Hammon H, Goldsmith LJ, Fechtner RD, Zimmerman TJ: The effect of

nasolacrimal occlusion on the duration of action of Dorzolamide 2%. Invest Ophthalmol Vis Sci 37(3), 1996

6. Gamero GE, Robison MY, Harmon H, Goldsmith LJ, Fechtner RD, Zimmerman TJ: The duration of action of Dorzolamide 2% with concomitant use of a topical beta adrenergic antagonist. Invest Ophthalmol Vis Sci 37(3), 1996

7. Fechtner RD, Robison MY, Gamero GE, Goldsmith LJ, Zimmerman TJ: A comparison of the efficacy of Dorzolamide 2% and oral carbonic anhydrase inhibitors in clinical practice. Invest Ophthalmol Vis Sci 37(3), 1996

8. Toris CB, Gleason ML, Camras CB, Yablonski ME: Effects of brimonidine on aqueous humor dynamics in human eyes. Arch Ophthalmol 113(12):1514-1517, 1995

9. Camras CB, US Latanaprost Study Group: Comparison of latanoprost and timolol in patients with ocular hypertension and glaucoma. Ophthalmology 103:138-147, 1996

10. Watson P, Stjernschantz J, Latanoprost Study Group: A six-month, randomized, double-masked study comparing latanoprost with timolol in open-angle glaucoma and ocular hypertension. Ophthalmology 103:126-137, 1996

11. Dreyer EB, Zurakowski D, Schumer RA, Podos SM, Lipton SA: Elevated glutamate levels in the vitreous body of humans and monkeys with glaucoma. Arch Ophthalmol 114:299-305, 1996

12. Sawada A, Kitazawa Y, Yamamoto T, Okabe I, Ichien K: Prevention of visual field defect progression with brovincamine in eyes with normal-tension glaucoma. Ophthalmology 103(2):283-288, 1996

13. Netland PA, Chaturvedi N, Dreyer EB: Calcium channel blockers in the management of low-tension and open-angle glaucoma. Am J Ophthalmol 115(5):608-613, 1993

Clinical controversies: target pressures – what are they?

Moderator: Paul Palmberg

Paul Palmberg, MD: What we were reflecting on when we were talking earlier is that, when I was a fellow, I thought that probably the worst thing that could happen to a patient would be to have glaucoma and fall into the hands of an assistant professor. Consequently, I thought I had better try to get some feeling for the long-term outcome of this disease. So I would read the charts of Dr. Becker's patients, some of whom had been followed for 20 years. I noticed that the people whose pressures were down around 10, 12, or so, had full thickness filters. Even if they had terrible damage, it seemed to be stable. Some people were on medical therapy or had undergone surgery, and pressures were running in the upper normal range or occasionally low 20s. In these people, the chart often indicated that things were basically going all right. However, if you looked back ten or 20 years, they were losing significant ground. I thought perhaps our approach to glaucoma, that of just trying to get people down into the upper normal range and considering that controlled, might not be right. I was a little too timid to say anything about it and so it ended up being many years later that other people proposed that perhaps we needed to be lower.

This session is about target pressures. Where did this term come from? I invented the term in about 1989. Al Summer had put together a committee for the preferred practice pattern of the American Academy of Ophthalmology and we were told that there were three phases of Medicare. Phase one was to make care available to all the senior people. Phase two was to cut costs. I have not noticed that they have stopped that yet. And the hypothetical phase three, according to Dr. Roper, was that they were going to start looking at quality. Clerks were going to come and look at your charts and decide if you were doing a good job or see how your cataract patients turned out, or your filter patients. And we really could not think of very much that you could look at regarding what a doctor was doing for glaucoma to find out whether good quality was being provided or not. What I came up with was that doctors should have some considered opinion about what pressure they think they would like to take the patient to, and should feel strongly enough about that that they would be willing to keep doing things until they got to that pressure, or they would notice if they were not meeting that goal. They would write it in the chart and therefore the clerk could come and look and it would say target pressure 18. If the patient came in with a pressure of 26 and the doctor says come back three months, that would not be good quality care! But if it says 18 and the pressure is 17 and they said "meets target, come back three months", you would have some feeling that the person was awake at the switch for their patients. That is where the idea of target pressure comes from. Besides its hokey purpose for dealing with the government, there was actually a positive purpose of making it a summary of your considered opinion about the patient. You had con-

Peril to the Nerve – Glaucoma and Clinical Neuro-Ophthalmology, pp. 87–95
Proceedings of the 45th Annual Symposium of the New Orleans Academy of
Ophthalmology, New Orleans, LA, USA, April 25-28, 1996
edited by Barry J. Leader and Jonathan C. Calkwood
© *1998 Kugler Publications, The Hague/The Netherlands*

sidered the literature available about the relationship between pressure and damage. You had looked at the amount of damage present in the patient, how rapidly the damage had developed between maybe a normal visit in the past and this time, had considered the family history of blindness and the life expectancy of the patient. Taking all that into account you are going to make a guess, and that is all it is going to be, a guess about target IOP.

The idea from this preferred practice pattern was that after documenting the baseline status, you would choose a target pressure. You would have to reassess that from time to time. You would treat to try to control the pressure to that range. You would have to decide the next step you might consider if you are not quite at the target pressure. You might be willing to watch the patient, but it would be a considered opinion. Or you would keep going until you controlled the pressure. You would monitor them for stability to see if you had to change your assessment. Maybe they were going to need a lower pressure than you thought would be adequate. You would try to minimize the side-effects of therapy and get the patient engaged in it.

It has been mentioned that Hart and Becker showed that 73% of people at Washington University had gotten worse on their visual field during a ten-year follow-up. Often not a whole lot worse, but 25% of the patients had gotten at least 50% worse in one eye during that time. This was with a mean pressure of 20. And I was happy to hear Harry say that maybe only 18% of their patients had gotten worse, although in a shorter period of time, at maybe somewhat lower pressures and with more aggressive treatment. And Mickelberg and Drance had shown the same thing. Thor Odberg in 1987 had given us a very nice study from a private practice. He followed patients for five to 18 years and found out that when the pressures were in the low normal range, there was a benefit. Those people did not get worse as quickly as people who had sometimes been or were all the time over 20. And that getting into the upper normal range may not be enough for the patients in his study who had fairly severe glaucoma to start with. I collected data, particularly George Spaeth's very important study where he had randomized patients to getting topical steroids or not at the time of filtering surgery. As a result, five years later the mean pressures had come down to 19 after filters done without steroids and 14 after topical or topical and systemic. Only 6% of the people had progressed versus 58 in other studies. Al Kolker at Washington University, Werner and Drance and Rollins and Drance in Vancouver, Kidd and O'Connor in London, Grave and Dake in The Netherlands, within their studies seemed to show some sort of a dose-response relationship, suggesting that the nerve was more likely to be stable in the lower normal range than the upper normal. So the idea was that we were not just trying to get to the normal range, but somehow well down into it for people with a lot of damage.

Let us take a patient and see how the panel feels about this and how they approach it. Let us start off with the most straightforward kind of case. Here is a typical one. The patient comes in. The pressure is 27 in the right eye, 24 in the left. The cupping is 6 and 4. What kind of a pressure reduction would you want to achieve in this patient? First of all, is there anybody who would just follow this patient? I should say that the visual field shows about a 3-dB decrease in the eye with the larger cup and the higher pressure than the other eye. Would anybody here just watch them for a while to see if they got worse?

George L. Spaeth, MD: There are all kinds of other factors, how old the patient is and whether they are allergic to every kind of medication, etc., etc.

Dr. Palmberg: This patient is 65 years old. We have no history of allergies or systemic drug problems. A pretty straightforward case without complicating factors. In general, what would you want to try to accomplish with a patient like this? George, let me start with you. If you have not got any contraindications to therapy, you are convinced that there is a little nerve damage and there is some visual field loss that correlates, and it is in the eye with a higher pressure.

Dr. Spaeth: It is interesting that the title of this is target pressures, but really what we ought to be talking about of course is target goals. And the goal is to keep the patient visually functioning and not damage him along the way, and the likelihood is that if this patient were never treated at all, 15 years later he or she would still be doing fine. So I think the thinking is, well, maybe the patient is going to get hit in the left eye, it makes sense to try to preserve the right eye. Why do we not treat the patient gently, try something like a beta blocker 1/4% twice daily, one eye therapeutic trial, and see if that lowers the pressure in comparison to the pressure in the other eye. I do not think I would set a really strict target pressure, but something like 21.

Dr. Palmberg: So that would be about a 25 to 30% reduction?

Dr. Spaeth: Yes.

Don Minckler, MD: I was just going to comment that I think the concept of a target pressure is a real good one in terms of helping us to organize our thinking or maybe to be sure we are thinking. But I think it can also be a bit of a trap. The problem is if you take it too seriously, that the complications of some therapies, particularly surgical, can be far worse than what you might have experienced in terms of the natural progression of the disease. That is just a comment related to the rigid adherence to what you have predetermined to be a reasonable pressure.

Dr. Spaeth: Paul, to add to that, Ken Richardson has a great distinction between what he calls the target pressure or the index pressure, I think it is, and the acceptable goal pressure. In other words, you set in your own mind what you think you really want the pressure to be, but then you set another pressure that is realistic.

Dr. Minckler: There are some patients, I think, in whom you have a sort of clinical experience or track record because of asymmetrical problems in the two eyes. I guess pseudoexfoliation might be one example, or maybe chronic open-angle glaucoma, which just happens to be very different in the two eyes. You have a track record during which, at whatever pressures were maintained, you clearly lost ground in one eye and the other eye at a significantly lower pressure was stable. So I think, in that situation, that one eye has taught us maybe what that particular person's vulnerability level is.

Dr. Palmberg: It is one reason that I presented a patient who did not have any damage in the other eye.

Harry A. Quigley, MD: If I thought the patient was an ocular hypertensive who was not yet damaged in either field or nerve fiber layer, I have a conversation in which I briefly tell him that you have a circumstance where you might not get worse for quite some time. But there are two kinds of people in the world. There is the kind who would do anything to stay off medicines because they hate medicines and they probably will not take them; and there is the kind who would go to bed tonight worried because they had lost four more nerve fibers, and who would take medicine and buy twice as much liability insurance as they normally would need. Which kind are you? And then there is a pregnant pause, and I sort of look over at them. And if they say, well, I would rather be treated, then they go the therapeutic trial route, and if not, none.

Dr. Palmberg: Thom, you were quoted recently as saying somebody who goes from a 6/10 to 8/10 cupping during their life will probably be happy and die seeing well. Is this the kind of patient you might watch for awhile, or would you treat this patient as long as the therapy was not causing any side-effects?

Thom J. Zimmerman, MD, PhD: I think all the comments that have been made are quite germane. One of the problems, and Dr. Spaeth alluded to it, is that we do not know the natural history of this disease. We cannot look at that patient and tell you where they are going to be in ten or 15 years. We can back up and look at some studies. I think the OHTS that Mike Kass is running is going to give us some good information. I think that some of the other studies will give us good information. We could do a retrospective and discover who are the blind people from glaucoma, as Harry mentioned today, who are the people that are visually handicapped? Can we identify them? Should black Americans be treated more aggressively and earlier? We can get some guidelines like that, but all the statements are really saying that what you have to do is to individualize it for that particular patient. Until we back off and do a study where we treat half the people and do not treat the other half, and we find out what happens over a 25-year period, and I do not know if that study will ever get done, we will not know what we are doing. As Mike Kass points out, prediction is a difficult art.

Dr. Quigley: One more quick comment. That would be, if I chose to treat this patient, I would not start the therapy on that day. Typically you have very little information on which to base the baseline pressure. I have seen hundreds and hundreds of charts where there was one pressure measured before therapy started and then 15 years of treated pressures, when I do not really know what they would have been without it. So I say to the patient, we are going to start treatment, but first, would you call at the office on two more days, whatever day you can show up, whatever time of the day you can show up. A technical person will help me by measuring your pressure and you are out of here. On the third day, you will be starting the unilateral drop trial, after I have three measurements.

Dr. Zimmerman: Once you commit to meds, you do not have to do that for the rest of their lives. You can back off after three, four or five months and look around town a little bit and have a further discussion with them. Having them involved in taking care of themselves not only improves compliance, but also sets up a dialogue for education. They can understand what you are trying to get done, and what you two as a team are trying to accomplish. That dialogue is extremely important and I think should be started long before therapy.

Dr. Palmberg: I think in this patient that I would treat them. I would be reassured that the other eye was not damaged by 24. I would figure if I got him down 30%, that would probably be good enough, just judging by how the other putt rolled on that green. I would not push it with any medications that caused them problems until I saw some kind of progression, or least got back up in this neighborhood.

Dr. Minckler: I am still surprised at how many patients I see for the first time who are already on multiple medications, who have no idea, at least admit to no clue, as to whether or not even the first medicine actually affected their pressure. So I have assumed that it is still common, at least in my area, for physicians to add medicine without ever really judging whether or not there has been a response. I do not think there is much pharmacological logic, if you will, to do that.

Dr. Palmberg: So you would do a one-eyed trial to see?

Dr. Minckler: If you are going to try something, I would try it, make a decision that this did or did not work. If it did not work or did not work adequately, get it out of there and try something else.

Dr. Palmberg: Yes, stop something that does not work.

Michael A. Kass, MD: The only thing I think is maybe a little excessive is 30%. I do not think you need to lower this person's pressure 30%, because I do not think you will get there most of the time with simple therapy. I would think if you got this down even 20%, if you could get this person's pressure down to 22 or 21, I think that is plenty. It is not easy to get somebody's pressure down 30% from here, and I think it will either push you to rather intolerable medicines or to more aggressive treatment. I think if you got even 20% here, if you took this person's pressures down let us say to 22 in the right eye, that would be a good response as far as I am concerned. I would sit awhile and wait and see how they did with this. That is really a pretty reasonable response for somebody with this degree of damage.

Dr. Palmberg: Now that we could add Trusopt and probably even Latanaprost, after a while it may be that we will be able to get that kind of reduction with medications that do not cause much that the patient notices.

Dr. Kass: Maybe. We do not know about latanaprost yet. I certainly would not commit this patient to three medications. I would try to do something with one and see how they do.

Dr. Zimmerman: I agree, but Paul's point is exactly what the marketing survey of Trusopt is showing now, that Trusopt does not cut into the pilocarpine market yet. It has nailed the oral CAI market, but it is basically being added onto beta blocker people who have pressures of 18 in order to drop them to 16 or 15, and that is how the marketing surveillance goes. So Paul, your point is well taken, that as we get more different and better accepted meds on the market, people are going to be going for 14 when they would have lived at 19 or 18.

Dr. Palmberg: Obviously, we do not know long term whether this patient would do better at 15 than they would at 19, or whether they would do better than 22. Probably most patients would do all right at 20 or 22, as Mike points out. The other eye did at 24. Let us say latanaprost ends up knocking people down nine points and can be taken once a day, and turns out to be safe. Would we have more aggressive treatment of glaucoma with medical therapy if we did not have side-effects? I think it is sensible to add a second drug with Trusopt. I do with these kinds of patients, as long as it does not hurt the patient in any way.

Dr. Kass: I just want to make one last general point. I think we have gotten trapped in glaucoma treatment into this business of putting patients into two classes. There were those who were stable and those who were worse. And I think this has been a great trap and has served us and our patients poorly. In most patients there is nothing terrible if 15 years later, you are slightly worse. As long as they can function well. And I think we need to get away from this dichotomous outcome of either you are stable or something terrible has happened to you. If somebody leads out their natural life and they are slightly worse in one eye, that should be called a good result, not a bad result.

Dr. Palmberg: Maybe not an optimal result, but a good result. Here is a patient with somewhat more damage.

Dr. Spaeth: Paul, that is probably an optimal result. Because you have saved the patient a lot along the way. Everything you do in the way of treatment costs. It costs in terms of expense, it costs in terms of decreased end expiratory volume that you do not know about until you stop, fatigue, until you are off the medication. I think that is a great result. That is an optimal result.

Dr. Palmberg: Well, okay. I always thought optimum was when you prevented all the damage.

I want to go on to another patient. This patient has something that more of the panel would be willing to agree, is starting to get towards impacting on the patient. They have a visual field defect, they complain of a little fogginess of vision, they have got a little more focal damage, the pressures are 23 and 19. Now how do people feel about this? Do you take an approach that, in this kind of situation, you want a 30% reduction, do you want a 50%, do you want to be down to 15, or what goes into your thinking process on this patient with 23 in this eye and the other eye has a little suspicion of a thin cup, and the pressure is 19? It does not look as if either eye is tolerating the pressure they have completely. And this one is really not. Still not terrible damage.

Dr. Minckler: Well it looks to me like you have got a convincing field defect, at least on this one study, and I think some correlating changes in the disc. I presume you have just encountered this patient, and the question is what to do and do we know what medications they are on, or what the pressure is...

Dr. Palmberg: This patient is on no medication. It is a fresh case of glaucoma, 23 in this eye and 19 in the other.

Dr. Minckler: In this situation I would ideally want to collect a lot of pressure measurements, a mini-diurnal, or whatever. It is a great opportunity to get a good baseline and then to start some therapy.

Dr. Quigley: I have a rule that if the first field is abnormal, repeat it, but if the first field is normal believe it. So we would want to do the field test another time. I would want to see a little further into the retina to be sure there is no histo spot sitting over there that is responsible for the field defect. But this is someone who by and large I would treat, yes.

Dr. Palmberg: What would your goal be? Would you have a target pressure of 23?

Dr. Quigley: Yes, 25% is a nice number. What I would treat them with is another story. There is another talk as to what am I going to give you for lowering this 25%? Is it medicine, laser, or surgery?

Dr. Zimmerman: I would look at this hard. I do not like the fact that the high pressure that you are recording is 23 basically on no meds. The defect is closer to fixation than I like to see it. I would be all over this patient for follow-up and diagnostic stuff; wondering if I knew what was going on here. I would be pretty aggressive and maybe be aiming at a lower target pressure. I might decide I want to be under 16, 15 area or so.

Dr. Palmberg: That is what I want to try to bring out. Is there some point when you stop wanting a percentage reduction from what they had before and you are looking at this field business and you want to try to get to the low normal range? Any other comments on this patient?

Dr. Quigley: Did you tell us how old this patient was?

Dr. Palmberg: 65.

Dr. Kass: What if this patient is 94 and has terrible coronary artery disease? Does that change this discussion? Of course it does.

Dr. Palmberg: Yes, see him in two years.

Dr. Kass: Wish him a good life. Give him refraction, give him bifocals, that is probably all he needs.

Dr. Palmberg: We are running down to the end of the time. Let me throw a couple of other things at you. This patient with normal-tension glaucoma, if you will, shows up and his initial pressures were 19 and 17. He has corresponding fixation splitting disease. He has lost his inferior nerve. He is an 80-year-old rabbi, but he is going to live to be 100 because God told him he was going to be able to finish his commentary on the Jerusalem talmud and he produces one book a year. As a matter of fact, he is now 93. What are you going to do for this patient with normal-tension glaucoma, about 8.5 cup in one eye, 8 in the other, fixation split and he shows up with 19 and 18? Mike, you already gave the talk, but what would you want to do?

Dr. Kass: Do you know at what period of time this occurred? Again, you need a little more information. How much do his pressures vary? Is this the highest he has ever had, the average, the lowest. Who has followed him up to now, and over what period of time has this occurred, and so on?

Dr. Palmberg: It has been ten years since his last examination. He was normal then. We have got several more pressures. They were never over 19 or 20. A couple of years later they were 25 and 22. And that was on therapy.

Dr. Kass: You did not catch him at the highest point. I think that is always a trap. If you go through the history, the examination, and you have no other explanation, the only thing you can offer him is a reduction in pressure. He is 80, but apparently healthy in other regards, so I would then probably treat because of his split fixation and all. I would aim for a 25 or 30% fall in pressure, and I would probably go through medical means first. If I could do it with simple medical means, fine, or laser, or even up through a filtering operation in one eye at least, depending on how I could get there for him.

Dr. Palmberg: As it turns out, he did not respond to medicine. We did laser. It got him down to 10 or 12 for about eight years and then he went back up and he had a cataract by then, and we did combined procedures. Now pressures are 8 and he is stable.

Dr. Kass: He'll probably dedicate the volume to you.

Dr. Palmberg: He's on volume 17. One last consideration. If the patient has cataract or has corneal opacity, or if the patient has macular degeneration, it is going to make it hard to do fields. If the patient has drusen that are already perhaps also influencing the field, what do you do in this kind of a situation in trying to choose a target pressure? You believe they have glaucoma, because let us say they have an afferent defect in this eye, or they have visual field defect as well. But you know it is going to be hard to follow. Any special wisdom?

Dr. Spaeth: I have no special wisdom. These people are among the most difficult that we have to take care of, because we just do not really know what to say. That brings us back to Harry's point which was so very well made in the very first patient. In this sort of situation, I think you have to tell the patient to some extent of your uncertainty and involve them hugely in the decision making. Depending upon whether they are people who really believe in glaucoma treatment and want it, in that case I think you are obligated to give it to them full force. Especially the patients you have just described, the patients with drusen who have field defects. They look like glaucoma, they get worse, and you do not have any idea whether it is the glaucoma getting worse or the drusen getting worse. I think you just have to go on the old fashioned population-based information of lowering the pressure a certain amount and involving the patient in the decision.

Dr. Palmberg: Finally, I wanted to get your thinking about something that perhaps is controversial. We have talked about target pressures. To some extent we use them, although it is obvious that we use them in somewhat different ways. There is certainly nothing solid in the literature, so that you can look at those two tables and the preferred practice and know that everybody should be 15, which is sometimes attributed to me and it is not what it says. It does say that people with very advanced disease may do better when they are in the low normal range than in the upper normal range. We are now going to have enough modalities: 5-fluorouracil or mitomycin on a primary filter, and if you should choose to, add Trusopt to Timoptic, and latanaprost to these other medications. Now we may be wanting to think of not just a target pressure, but a different idea, which is the maximum benefit target pressure. If there was something you could do that would get the pressure down and did not have any adverse effects, would you really want everybody to be down around 10 or 12, especially people who have moderate to severe damage to start with rather than a 30% reduction? Are we going to use these other modalities that are becoming available to us, either at the time of filtering surgery with antimetabolites, the first filter, or are we going to perhaps add the second or third drug? What is your feeling on that? How do you plan to use these things?

Dr. Minckler: Everybody should be at 8.

Dr. Quigley: I would love to answer your question, Paul, but I cannot imagine a real world circumstance where that applies. Timolol was not known to do anything bad to anybody in 1978 when it came out. Superficial punctate keratopathy and asthma and cardiac effects and cholesterol effects were all there. There has not ever been a surgical procedure invented that did not have a side-effect. And the only reason I think laser trabeculoplasty has almost no side-effects is because it is relatively mild in terms of its beneficial effect. I do not know that I can actually answer your question.

Dr. Zimmerman: I do not know.

Dr. Spaeth: Your question brings up consideration of medical ethics: non-maleficence and beneficence. You do not want to harm, and I could not agree more with Harry. Every treatment harms to some extent, and you want to help, so you have just got to balance. You push it down as low as you think you can in a way which is going to benefit maximally and harm minimally.

Dr. Kass: I would add that in this current day one must consider money. You have to have some reasonable use of medical resources. You cannot put everybody on three drugs, even if they were harmless. You have now tripled the cost. If you are going to operate on everybody and whatever is going to happen from that, there has to be some consideration of the societal costs for all these things as well. We can no longer operate as free agents. I think there has to be some thought on your part about reasonable expectation of benefit rather than some kind of theoretical goal of strawberry fields forever. Would it not be nice if we could get everybody to some level?

Dr. Palmberg: Just briefly, I would say I think the answer is that long-term therapy has to be guided by long-term results and that a number of very good long-term clinical trials are going on. In our case, we are trying to follow a very large number of patients who have had filtering surgery with antimetabolites, and those who have not. We hope to find out who is doing better in ten years, and what kind of side-effects they have had, what kind of benefits they have had. The answer is we do not have the answer, but we are getting there.

Glaucoma: where have we been, where are we now, and where should we be going?

George L. Spaeth

Wills Eye Hospital/Jefferson Medical College, Philadelphia, PA, USA

It is not fair to attribute it all to Galen, that ancient classifier of disease. Nor can we point the finger solely to the great pathologists such as Virchov, or classifiers such as Linnaeus. Some credit (or blame) should go to Locke, the 18th century Enlightenment philosophers, and Comte and the logical positivists. What they all did was to classify and objectify.

Medical art was transformed into medical science. Patients have benefited hugely. But patients also suffered hugely.

This presentation will sketch the evolution of some of these changes, especially as they relate to 'glaucoma'.

Until the time of the rise of science, knowledge was largely experiential. The subjective (what I think and feel) was not separated from the objective (what actually is, unrelated to me). For example, a person knew he was sick because he felt sick, not because the doctor did some objective test and pronounced him ill. The patient did not answer in response to the question, "How are you?" "My doctor says I'm fine". A whole new sense of reality developed when we learned, starting around the 1800s that what we thought we knew was really just a mish-mash of biases and prejudices. The only valid way to establish knowledge was by using so-called 'objective' methodologies (such as mathematics) to eliminate subjective considerations.

What do these thoughts have to do with our subject, "Glaucoma: Where have we been, where are we now, and where should we be going?"?

Two thousand years ago, glaucoma was essentially what a person describing it thought it to be. It was not until the 1800s, with Bannister and Von Graefe, Muller, and Von Jaeger, that glaucoma became codified and classified, a direction that has continued up to the present time[1-4]. These changes are, of course, not limited to glaucoma.

Where we were a long time ago, up until the rise of science, was in a world where disease literally meant 'disease', where knowledge was anecdotal and empirical, where what really existed was primarily subjective. Where we are now is in a world that distrusts the subjective and attempts as much as possible to be ob-

Address for correspondence: George L. Spaeth, MD, Wills Eye Hospital/Jefferson Medical College, 900 Walnut Street, Philadelphia, PA 19107-5598, USA

Peril to the Nerve – Glaucoma and Clinical Neuro-Ophthalmology, pp. 97–108
Proceedings of the 45th Annual Symposium of the New Orleans Academy of
Ophthalmology, New Orleans, LA, USA, April 25-28, 1996
edited by Barry J. Leader and Jonathan C. Calkwood
© *1998 Kugler Publications, The Hague/The Netherlands*

jective. The Ocular Hypertension Treatment Study (OHTS) is a quintessential example of where we are now. Thousands of persons are considered homogeneous, because they have an intraocular pressure (IOP) above a particular level, but do not have visual functional damage as demonstrated by a computerized examination of the visual field. These thousands of supposedly similar objects are then randomly divided into those who will be treated in an objective way which will limit any possible variations within the population, and those who will be untreated. Then, they will be measured objectively with a totally standardized definition of what qualifies as a 'change' of significance. [For example, a decrease in the visual fields of three points that are separated from each other is not a change, whereas it *is* a change if the points are contiguous. This criterion is based on the belief that when glaucoma defects develop in the visual field, they develop at a particular location rather than simultaneously in several different locations. Is this correct? Do some patients develop defects in one area and others in several areas? The answer is almost certainly that some patients develop visual fields one way, and others in another way. But to admit to that would mean that: *1.* a loss of definition, and *2.* an increase in variability and a decrease in the ability to discriminate. Consequently, even though the validity of the definition of visual field change has not been established, it is utilized because it is 'more right than wrong', or 'the best estimate'.] When the data are in, and the results of the OHTS are analyzed, the conclusion will be that, if a person has an IOP above x, he is less (or more) likely to develop visual field loss if he is treated (or untreated). This conclusion will be generalized to all other similar objects (people with elevated IOP or 'glaucoma'). An objective study will have provided objective data that can be generalized.

But, back to the evolution of the concept of 'glaucoma'. With increasing objective study, the definition of glaucoma became much clearer. Specifically, since glaucoma was related to the IOP, glaucoma became a condition in which IOP was above a specific, statistically significant number[5-8]. But as it became apparent that more people with IOP above that level never got damaged by the IOP, and many people who showed the type of damage that was thought to be characteristic of high IOP, never had elevated IOP,

it became clear that defining glaucoma on the basis of a specific level of IOP did not work[9-15].

Since glaucoma could not be validly defined by IOP, a better way was to define the disease on the basis of a standard type of damage. The same basic methodology, that is, defining an objective, universally appropriate standard was then applied to a different criterion, specifically, visual field loss. The disease was present if and only if a statistically significant, machine-measurable quantity of visual field was lost. But it became apparent that visual field loss was not the initial sign of damage, but only a response to other types of damage, presumably damage to the optic nerve[16,17]. Therefore, the same methodology was applied to the appearance of the optic nerve, specifically, the determination of objective changes differed by a certain amount from the average. The appearance of the optic nerve is a quantifiable characteristic that can be machine-measured and mathematically analyzed. But the correlation between quantifiable disc characteristics and functional damage is so poor that it has become clear that the use of disc parameters such as cup volume and rim area do not discriminate well between those with functional damage and those without. This led to measurement of a more specific parameter, specifically the retinal nerve fiber layer (RNFL) thickness. But this also does not work;

RNFL thickness varies with age and cup size. So now the same methodology is being applied at a more molecular level – to neurons, chromosomes, and to genes. The next step will be application of the same methodology to the components of genes, the nucleic acids, etc.

Where we are now, then, is in a world that attempts to define glaucoma on objective, generalizable data. This, of course, applies to all medical practice. Furthermore, and more importantly, this reflects the evolution of our sense of knowledge and our organization of reality, *i.e.*, our epistemology and our metaphysics. We believe that objective science is the only source of valid knowledge and that objects (including persons) can be known objectively and objectively classified into categories such as normal, abnormal, obese, glaucomatous, febrile, hypertensive, liberal, conservative, Afro-American, Catholic, WASP, pro-choice, and pro-life.

The underlying assumption behind all of this evolution, as it relates to glaucoma and disease and health, is that there are attributes able to be understood in the same way scientists thought they could understand reality, specifically, by an objective dissection of the whole into its parts. There are, however, fundamental flaws in that assumption, especially for conditions as complex as glaucoma in human beings.

One major problem is that totally objective scientific measurement is extremely difficult. Many scientists believe now that objective measurement is, in fact, impossible. The very act of measuring itself involves a subjective component that affects the final measurement. Uncertainty principles are now the rule, not the exception. Heisenberg's Uncertainty Principle, stating that it is not possible to determine at any precise moment where an electron is, is now old hat; so are theories that describe the limitations of mathematics. Throughout history, some have commented on the limitations of human knowledge. Job[18] recognized that "such knowledge is too great for me" when asked, "Where were you when I laid the foundations of the earth?" Two thousand years later, Russell's classic on the limitations of human knowledge came to the same conclusion. Berkeley and Croce long ago argued that reality was unknowable. Now some believe that there is *not* an immutable, quantifiable world out there. Reality is like Heisenberg's electron: it exists in motion and change; if it were frozen in time, it would cease to exist. Its very existence demands tension and change. The direction and nature of that change can never, and will never, be able to be fully apprehended.

One flaw in the current system of objectification, then, is that total objectivity is not and will not ever be actually possible.

A related flaw in current application of 'objectivity' is the attribution of hardness to data that are considered objective but in actuality are not. For example, we measure IOP and we assume that a measurement of 10 mmHg really means 10 mmHg. Frequently it does; but not always. Is the number rounded up or rounded down? If rounded up the first time and down the second time, the IOP will seem to have fallen 20% between the two measurements. Of course, such a change is spurious. When we consider variable data such as the visual field, the validity of the data is even more suspect. The 'reliable' visual field that shows a mean defect of 12 dB on the first test and 15 dB on the second test is described on the print-out as showing a definite deterioration. Of course, that is not what the test shows. It merely shows that there is a greater likelihood that the second visual field is different from the first visual field than that the two visual fields are alike. This second flaw in 'objectification' is primarily a flaw in inappropriate application of the theory, falsely considering data to be objective and then using mathematical means of manipulating them, when in fact the data are not objective. Magnificently skilled mathematical manipulation of invalid data does not result in valid conclusions. 'Statistically significant' changes in visual fields are not necessarily changes at all.

A third flaw is also a flaw in application rather than in fundamental theory. Specifically, there is a huge propensity to study only those things that can be considered 'objectively' and to ignore characteristics that are more difficult (or even apparently impossible) to measure. Consider the question: "Is the optic nerve damaged?" To answer that question, characteristics of the nerve are considered that can be manipulated mathematically: cup-to-disc ratio, rim area, etc. The question that is not considered is: "Does the optic nerve 'look damaged'?" That is, is the pattern of the nerve healthy or damaged? This question is almost impossible to answer objectively, because it is based on a subjective, almost intuitive evaluation. This analog aspect is in fact possible to handle using scientific, mathematical methods, but the challenges to this are so great that such questions simply do not get asked, much less answered.

For example, when studies are being done to determine what constitutes an appropriate reimbursement for a physician, the most appropriate question to ask, obviously, is: "What is the value of the service to the patient?" But this is specifically not even considered in the method currently being utilized, specifically the resource-based: Relative Value Scale. It is not believed that the question is inappropriate, but the question is not asked, because it is considered too difficult to quantitate. How does one get such data? If one were able to acquire such data, how would one manipulate it? This third flaw of prioritizing questions on the basis of the ease with which they can be answered is of real concern when considering patients with glaucoma. What is the only question that really needs to be answered when dealing with such patients? Specifically, the only real question of importance, is "How are you doing?" with the subordinate questions such as, "How is your visual function?" and "Are you having any troublesome side-effects from the medication you're using?" But these questions are not amenable to multiple-choice type answers. These questions are rarely even addressed. In contrast, the patient's IOP is measured and the visual field 'quantitatively determined'.

The current buzzword in medical (and elsewhere) is 'outcomes'.

But the value of outcome research depends completely on whether the outcomes being studied are in fact meaningful.

A fourth flaw in the objectification trend is also a flaw in application, not in the science itself. This is perhaps the most important issue to consider when pondering the question of: "Glaucoma: where have we been, where are we now, and where should we be going?" The problem here relates to the failure to recognize the differences between populations and individuals.

Current medical science maintains that with most characteristics there is a distribution bunched around a mean, and that the number of individuals decrease as one gets further and further away from the mean. The current concept of disease is largely based on the belief that it is possible to determine the average frequency or nature of a particular characteristic and then determine the well-being of an individual based on how similar that individual is to that average characteristic. The principle is utilized in every field. The Gaussian curve, then (Fig. 1), serves as the basis for determining the normalcy or abnormalcy of each individual within a

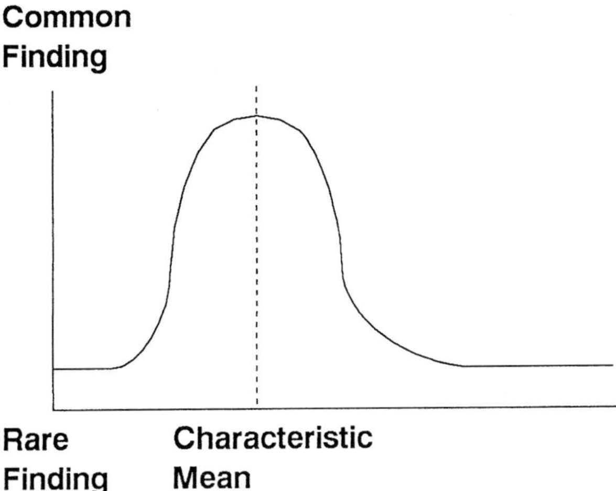

Fig. 1. The Gaussian curve serves as the basis for determining the normalcy or abnormalcy of each individual within a population.

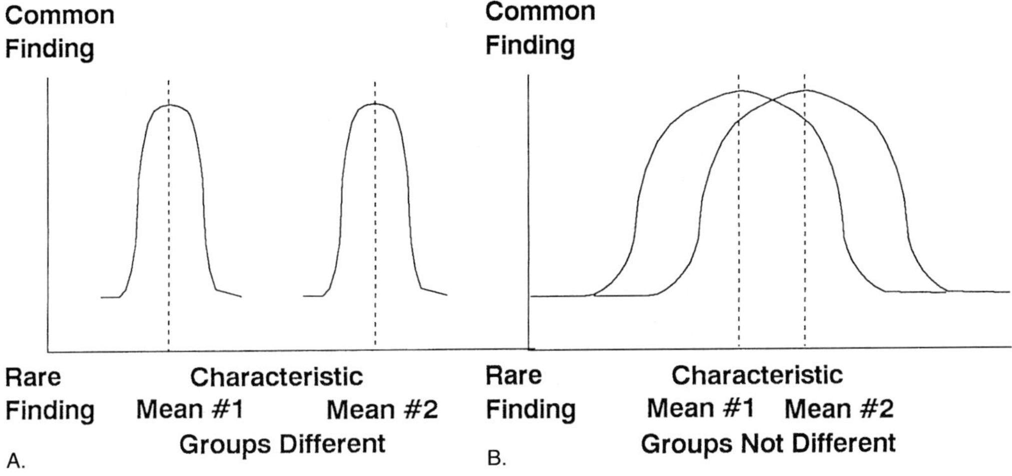

Fig. 2. Comparison of two (or more) Gaussian curves is used to differentiate between two (or more) different populations, and to determine the effects of interventions of all sorts.

population. Comparison of two (or more) curves is used to differentiate between two (or more) different populations, and to determine the effects of interventions of all sorts (Fig. 2).

For example, a normal or healthy IOP is easily determined. One thousand individuals have their IOP measured and the standard distribution curve developed (Fig. 3). If the effect of an intervention is to be determined, the same 1000 individuals have an intervention (say treatment with pilocarpine) and the characteristic undergoing consideration (here, IOP) evaluated and a standard distribution curve developed. If both curves have a sufficiently close bunching around their mean, and the means of each individual curve are sufficiently far apart (Fig. 2A), then it is be-

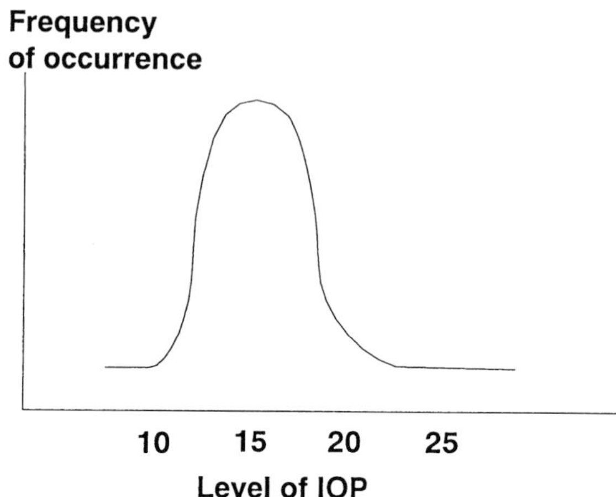

Fig. 3. The standard distribution curve of 1000 individuals with a healthy or normal intraocular pressure.

lieved that the intervention (treatment with pilocarpine) has had a causal effect on the population being studied. If they overlap considerably, then the treatment is considered ineffective (Fig. 2B).

As another example, one could develop a standard distribution curve of IOP in a population of people with glaucoma, all of whom were 50 years old, and compare that with a standard distribution curve for a population of glaucoma patients, all of whom were 25 years old. If the two curves were identical, it would be assumed that whether a person with glaucoma was 25 or 50 years old would not affect the level of IOP.

Current medical science stresses that the population-based model does not work when the population (or populations) being considered is (or are) not truly homogeneous, even when the intervention and the method of measuring the effect of the intervention is standard. In actuality there is no such thing as a homogeneous population, much less two homogeneous populations. There are no two people with exactly the same constitutional make-up – not even rare cases of 'identical twins'. When it comes to studies of populations of dissimilar individuals, the two populations are certainly not identical.

But, current population-based methodology argues, of course, that the people in population A are not identical; however, they are *sufficiently* identical that the differences between them are not 'significant'. Furthermore, if one is looking at two different populations allegedly composed of all A's, the slight differences between the two will be the same in the two populations and those differences will cancel each other out. Both comments, however, are assumptions and are unverifiable. How alike must patient A and B be or population A and population B be, so that A and B really respond to intervention Q in exactly the same way? Nobody knows. Presumably, the more similar, the more likely they will be to respond similarly, but no quantification is possible.

Theoretically, one could consider all of the ways that A is different from B and do a systems analysis so that one could quantitate the differences and the similarities. One could consider the probability curve, *e.g.*, for all those factors known to affect the development of a particular condition such as glaucoma. With regard to glaucoma this would include IOP, genetic make-up, perfusion pressure of the optic nerve, topography of the optic nerve, genetic make-up, race, body make-up, etc. One problem, however, is that none of these factors is binomial, that is, related in a yes-or-no fashion. They are all variably related: linearly, logarithmically, etc. Additionally, the exact shape of these relationships is either not known at all or at best only approximately understood. Consequently, it is not possible to combine the various ways in which A and B are different to come up with a meaningful estimate of just *how* different they are. For example, if one is trying to combine three different linear curves and the exact slope of the lines are not known, the combination would be meaningless. Where the shape as well as the slope of the curve is unknown, combining the curves becomes increasingly meaningless. Additionally, to continue the example of glaucoma, not only are the slopes and shapes of the curves not well known, but it is not known how heavily each attribute should be weighted – which is more important, IOP or family history? Further, it is not even known what attributes are missing from the equation that describes the development of glaucoma in a particular individual. It is obvious, however, that it is more than just IOP, race, abnormality of the 1-Q gene, and perfusion pressure of the optic nerve. When one considers the actual human being (or other animals) with a few fairly well characterized, well-known curves, and a vast number of unknown curves, it follows that it is impossible to quantify how similar A is to B, or how dissimilarly A and B will respond to exactly the same intervention.

The significance of this concept is vast. It invalidates for the individual the epistemology on which 'scientific' medical care is based.

It also invalidates the methodology of health economics that says, for example, "The cataract diagnostic-related group is ABC, and the cataract extraction in current procedural terminology is ABCD; hence, evaluation of a patient with ABC should be worth X dollars in reimbursement for procedure ABC; and for ABCD should be Y dollars". For, in fact, a cataract is not just ABC. In the first place, no two cataracts are identical. In the second, nobody in whom the unidentical cataracts are located is identical. And, lastly, no person (a far more complex creature than a body) in whom those unidentical characteristics reside is identical with any other.

Is there a better way to determine 'healthy' and 'not healthy'? Many models of disease have been proposed and others have suggested the concept of the person-based model[19-24]. In the person-based model, the person serves as his or her own control. Rather than consider a specific criterion as healthy or unhealthy based on comparison with a presumably similar population, the criterion is compared with a previous or subsequent criterion in the same individual, or to how the criterion is conceived by the individual. For example, the person whose visual acuity was 20/15 and is now 20/30 is presumably getting worse, in contrast to the person whose visual acuity was 20/30 and is still 20/30. The person who felt well but now feels ills is presumably getting worse in contrast to the person who for many years has always felt ill. The person who wants to see 20/20 and who presently has vision of 20/40 needs to have that wish addressed, whereas the person who is content with 20/40 vision does not need to have that wish addressed.

How can one determine the nature and responses of individuals? The character of each individual is established on the basis of as objective an evaluation as possible of all of the aspects that make that individual a unique person: age, race, sex, eye color, blood pressure, genetic structure, hopes, fears, expectations, life-style,

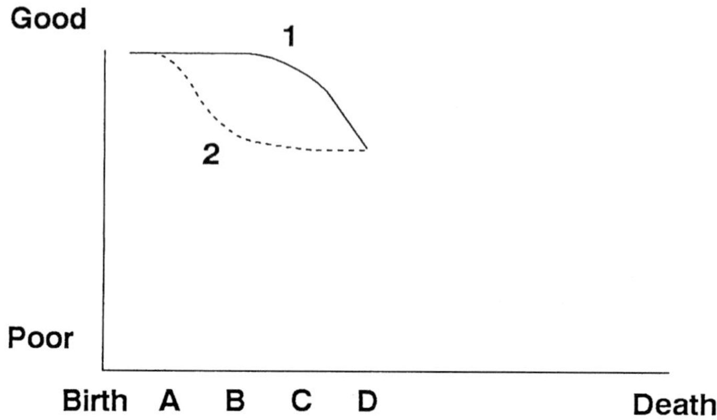

Fig. 4. Graph illustrating the clinical course of the health of two distinct individuals (#1 and #2). On the vertical axis is a measure of the extent of health, 'completely healthy' being at the top and 'completely diseased' at the bottom. On the horizontal axis is the patient's life, birth being at the left and death at the right.

etc. If the consideration with which one is most concerned is the individual patient's health, then it is self-defining that those characteristics to which the physician or other caregiver must pay most attention are those that are most closely related to the patient's health.

As such, the patient's own perception of his or her health is the primary priority.

To ascertain that perception of health is a surprisingly difficult task, which requires establishing a sense of trust between the caregiver and the patient and helping the patient draw out of himself or herself thoughts and feelings that may be frightening and which probably have never been well articulated. This is the job of 'history-taking', which continues to be the most challenging and the most important part of the evaluation of any patient. It is hard to conceive of any instrument that could ever do this adequately.

Patients do not exist in one point in time and they are not concerned with just that moment in which they are in the caregiver's office, but they are also concerned about what will happen in the future. That is, health and disease are kinetic, and it is essential that the physician develop a model that incorporates the changing nature of the patient. One way in which this can be done is by plotting a graph in which the variable being considered is on the y axis and the longevity of the patient's life on the x axis (Fig. 4). The most global attribute to consider is 'health', although this could be less general; perhaps the consideration would be visual function or, more specifically, visual acuity of one eye, or the volume of the cup of the optic nerve, or the velocity of flow of blood in the short ciliary artery.

The patient's clinical course is based on developing a series of points that de-

$\rightarrow$

Fig. 7. The graph of Figures 6 and 7 with an additional point added. This additional point has a small degree of variability. This additional information, added to the prior three points, with their variabilities, provides the strong suggestion that the attribute under consideration is decreasing over time.

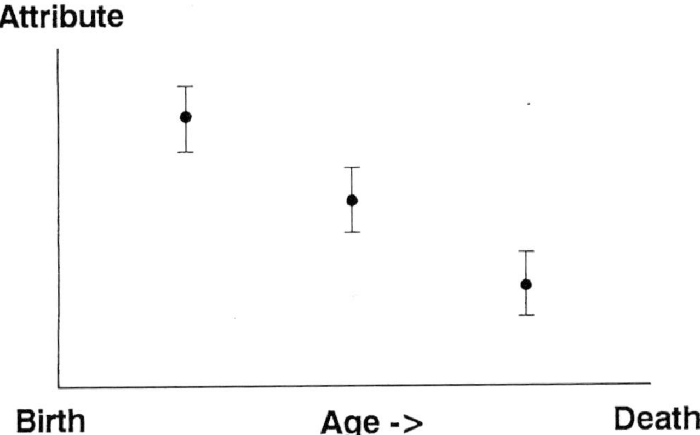

Fig. 5. Graph representing a particular characteristic decreasing over time, with a small degree of variability. It is highly likely that there is a significant decrease between the first and the third point.

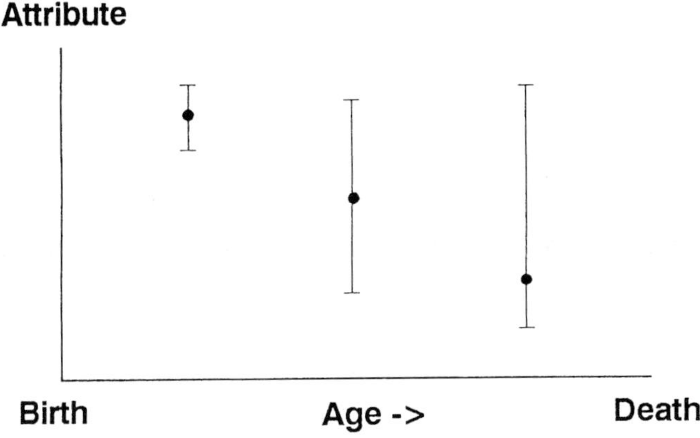

Fig. 6. Graph representing a particular characteristic decreasing over time, but with a much greater degree of variability than that illustrated in Figure 5. Even though the three *individual* points are decreasing at the same rate, it is not possible to say with certainty whether any actual change has occurred in the characteristic.

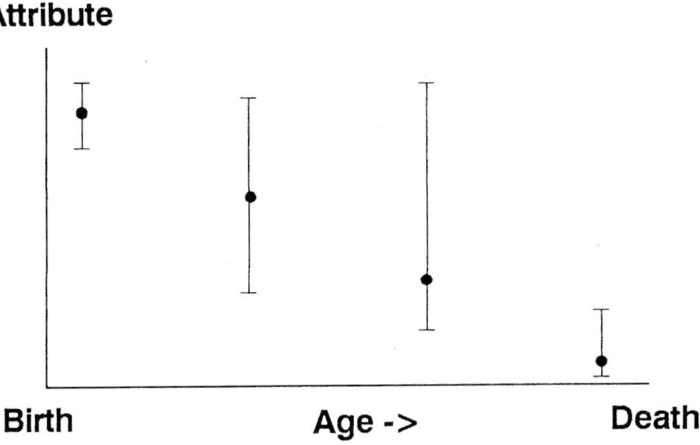

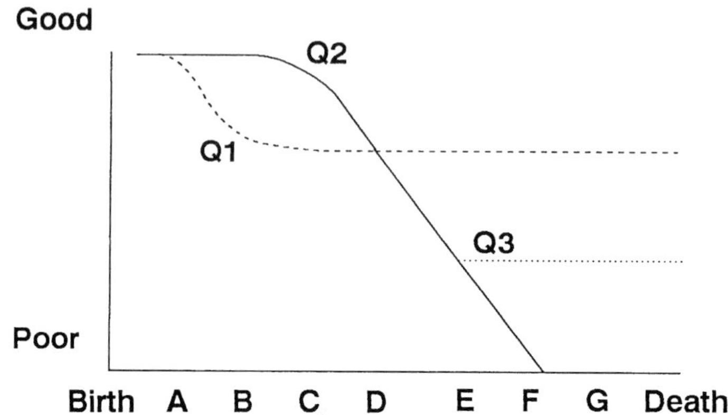

Fig. 8. In this graph the curves are extrapolated out towards the time of the patient's death. Even though both patients 1 and 2 are at about the same point at the age of 30 (D), it is likely that patient 2 will become completely diseased, probably around the age of 65 (F), prior to his death. In contrast, patient 1, who at age 10 (A) was getting worse, but at age 30 was apparently stable, may reasonably be expected to remain in his or her current state of health until the time of death at about age 80 unless some other change occurs.

scribe where on that graph the characteristic under consideration lies. For example, Figure 4 illustrates the clinical course of the health of two distinct individuals: individual number 1 and individual number 2. On the vertical axis is a measure of the extent of health, 'completely healthy' being at the top and 'completely diseased' at the bottom. On the horizontal axis is the patient's life, birth being at the left and death at the right. For example, in Figure 4, both patients start out at birth being totally healthy. Let us assume that the patient will die at the age of 80. That figure cannot be established with certainty, but a fairly good idea of the anticipated age at which the patient will die can be established. In Figure 4, then, patient #1 has gotten worse during his first 30 or so years; whereas patient #2 got rapidly worse at the age of about ten years and has not changed since.

The accuracy of the clinical curve is limited by the validity of the individual points. Thus, the more one can apply scientific methods of statistics to the data obtained, the more accurately one can draw a valid curve. Consider Figures 5, 6, and 7 in this regard. In Figure 5, a particular characteristic is decreasing over time, with a small degree of variability, and it is highly likely that there is a significant decrease between the first and the third point. In contrast, in Figure 6, there is a much greater degree of variability and even though the three individual points are decreasing at the same rate, it is not possible to say with certainty whether any actual change has occurred in the characteristic. In Figure 7, an additional point is added, and this additional point has a small degree of variability. This additional information, added to the prior three points, with their variabilities, provides the strong suggestion that the attribute under consideration is decreasing over time.

The specific diagnosis, then, is based on a compilation of multiple individual characteristics. The accuracy of the diagnosis is based upon the validity and the completeness of the characteristics.

The future course of the individual may be extrapolated from the course that has been described by the acquisition and representation of the series of points shown in Figure 4. In Figure 8, the curves are extrapolated out towards the time of the patient's death. Even though both patients 1 and 2 are at about the same point at the age of 30 (D in the Figure), it is likely that patient 2 will become completely diseased, probably around the age of 65 (F), prior to his death. In contrast, patient 1, who at age 10 (A) was getting worse, but at age 30 was apparently stable, may reasonably be expected to remain in his or her current state of health until the time of death at about age 80, unless some other change occurs. Consider that when patient 2 was 25 years old (point C) an intervention (Q2) was made; subsequent testing proved the intervention to be ineffective. It would be appropriate, then, after the ineffectiveness of Q2 was demonstrated to consider a different intervention. If this new intervention, Q3, made at about age 55 is effective (as shown in Figure 8), then patient 2 will maintain that current state of health until his demise at age 85, although his state of health for those last years of his life will be worse than it would be for patient 1.

Where have we been? In a subjective world where knowledge was experiential, measurement inaccurate, evaluations personal. Where are we now? In a world which attempts to be scientific, objective, and standard; where the mean is the healthy and the goal is to standardize as completely as possible. Where are we going?

I hope we are going to a world in which both the subjective and the objective are valued and appropriately utilized,

– in which populations are studied and compared but not used as the basis for determining what is healthy for individuals. In the new world, I hope that individuals will become their own controls, and that the goal will be to maximize the potential of each unique individual, to treat the ills of each unique individual, to treat that person's idealized conception of himself or herself as the goal for that unique person. For glaucoma, this means the physician's job is to determine what is healthy for the individual patient, not judged against the means of populations, but judged against the person's own baselines, the person's own needs and wants. The most appropriate treatment for a person who has an IOP of 30 mmHg, a visual acuity of 20/400, and far-advanced cupping of the optic nerve may be as different as: 1) no treatment; 2) medicinal therapy to lower IOP; 3) surgery to lower IOP; or 4) removal of the eye.

We must stop using the mean of a population as the basis for diagnosis and management. We must stop misusing objective methodologies to evaluate non-objective findings. Until we start using both objective and subjective methods to evaluate individuals, with the person as his or her own model, we will continue to do unnecessary damage, and we will continue to miss our noble calling of being healers.

References

1. Bannister R: A Treatise of 113 Diseases of the Eyes and Eyeliddes. London 1622
2. Von Graefe A: Vorläufige Nortiz über das Wesen des Glaucoma. Graefes Arch Clin Exp Ophthalmol 1:371, 1854
3. Von Graefe A: Amaurose mit Sehnervenexcavation. Graefes Arch Clin Exp Ophthalmol 3:484, 1857
4. Müller H: Glaukom und Excavation des Sehnerven. I. Über Glaukom. Sitz Ber Phys Med Ges Würzburg 2, 1856
5. Müller H: Beiträge zur Ophthalmologie: über Nervean-Veränderungen an der Eintrittsstelle des Sehnerven. Arch Ophthalmol 4:1, 1858

6. Von Jaeger E: Über Glaucom und seine Heilung durch Iridectomie. Z Ges Aerzte Wien 14:465, 1858
7. Elliot RH: A Treatise on Glaucoma. London: Frowde, Hollder and Stoughton 1918
8. Harrison R: Annual review: glaucoma. Arch Ophthalmol 72:865, 1964
9. Elschnig A: Der normale Sehnerveneintritt des menschlichen Auges: klinische und anatomische Untersuchungen. Denkschriften der K.K. Akademie der Wissenschaften. Mathem Nature Kl 70: 219, 1899
10. Bankes JLK, Perkins ES, Tsolokis S et al: Bedford glaucoma surgery. Br J Ophthalmol 1:791, 1968
11. Linner E, Stromberg U: Ocular hypertension: a five-year study of the total population in a Swedish town, and subsequent discussions. In: Leydhecker W (ed) Glaucoma: Tutzing Symposium, p 187. Basel: Karger 1967
12. Perkins ES: Recent advances in the treatment of glaucoma. Trans Ophthalmol Soc UK 86:199, 1966
13. Wilensky JT, Podos SM, Becker B: Prognostic parameters in primary open angle glaucoma. Arch Ophthalmol 91:200, 1974
14. Hollows FC, Graham PA: Intra-ocular pressure, glaucoma, and glaucoma suspects in a defined population. Br J Ophthalmol 50:570, 1966
15. Graham PA: The epidemiology of glaucoma. In: Heilmann, Richardson KT (eds) Glaucoma: Conceptions of a Disease, p 7. Stuttgart: Thieme 1978
16. Read R, Spaeth GL: Practical clinical appraisal of the optic disc in glaucoma: the natural history of cup progression and some specific disc field correlations. Trans Am Acad Ophthalmol Otolaryngol 78:255-274, 1974
17. Quigley HA: Better methods in glaucoma diagnosis. Arch Ophthalmol 103:186, 1985
18. The Bible. Job 38:4
19. Merskey H: Variable meanings for the definition of disease. J Med Philosophy 11:215-233, 1986
20. McCullough LB: Thought-styles, diagnosis, and concepts of disease: commentary on Ludwik Fleck. J Med Philosophy 6:257-262, 1981
21. King JB: Illness attributions and the health belief model. Health Ed Quart 103:287-312, 1984
22. Bergner M: The sickness impact profile formulation. II. Development and final revision. Med Care 19(8):787-805, 1981
23. Bergner M, Bobbitt RA, Kressel S, Pollard WE, Gilson BS, Morris JR: Conceptual formulation and methodology for the development of a health status measure. Int J Hlth Serv 6:393-415, 1976
24. Zaner RM: Medicine and dialogue. J Med Philosophy 15:303-325, 1990

Surgical treatment of glaucoma

Contents

Surgery: realities, expectations and indications

George L. Spaeth

Wills Eye Hospital/Jefferson Medical College, Philadelphia, PA, USA

Introduction

"Do you believe in early surgery for glaucoma?" "How much antimetabolite do you use when you do glaucoma surgery?" "How many patients are made worse by glaucoma surgery?" "Do you think glaucoma surgery interferes with the patient's quality of life less than the use of medications?"

All of these are important questions. But all are also senseless questions. They are all so broad and undefined that no meaningful answer can be given.

The first thing that must be done when one considers a standard question such as "What are the indications for glaucoma surgery" is to clarify the language, to define the question so as to permit a meaningful answer.

Definition of glaucoma

Glaucoma is a condition in which there is damage to ocular tissue at least partially related to intraocular pressure (IOP). Various tissues can be damaged. The extent to which they can be damaged varies widely. The mechanism by which the damage occurs varies widely, and the clinical course of the conditions associated with damage varies widely. Meaningful consideration of the realities, expectations, and indications for surgery in patients with glaucoma demands understanding that every patient with glaucoma is unique and the only universally applicable guideline is that patients must be treated as unique individuals.

Appropriate outcome measures

Before one can assess potential benefits of glaucoma surgery, one has to decide what outcome measures are appropriate. Is it IOP, visual field loss, cupping of the optic nerve head, thinning of the retinal nerve fiber layer? The traditional criterion has been the level of IOP. Indeed, much glaucoma surgery has as its primary goal lowering IOP. Certain types of surgery, however, such as peripheral iridotomy when performed for a partially closed angle in a patient with normal IOP, have

Address for correspondence: George L. Spaeth, MD, Wills Eye Hospital/Jefferson Medical College, 900 Walnut Street, Philadelphia, PA 19107-5598, USA

Peril to the Nerve – Glaucoma and Clinical Neuro-Ophthalmology, pp. 111–117
Proceedings of the 45th Annual Symposium of the New Orleans Academy of
Ophthalmology, New Orleans, LA, USA, April 25-28, 1996
edited by Barry J. Leader and Jonathan C. Calkwood
© 1998 Kugler Publications, The Hague/The Netherlands

goals unrelated to lowering IOP; in such cases, the goals include deepening the anterior chamber and preventing further angle-closure attacks. In most cases of glaucoma today, the goal *is* related to an effect on IOP, but possibly *lowering* the IOP may not be the most appropriate goal. It may be that *stabilization* of IOP with elimination of spikes and troughs is more important than actual IOP lowering itself.

Some patients following glaucoma surgery appear to have had no change in the mean IOP, nevertheless, will have an apparent change in their clinical course, with stabilization of their condition following the surgery in comparison to deterioration prior to the surgery. Additionally, it may be that some of the apparently beneficial effects related to argon laser trabeculoplasty, as demonstrated by the Glaucoma Laser Trial, is a function of stabilization of IOP caused by the trabeculoplasty rather than lowering of pressure[1]. This is, of course, all speculation. But it is *not* speculation that IOP is *not* the primary appropriate outcome criterion. It is at best an indirect precursor of the damage which is the essential component of glaucoma. And this is the point. *Damage, then, is a more appropriate outcome measure.*

With regard to glaucoma damage, two important indicators are the optic disc and the visual field.

Even a fairly short while ago it was believed that the discs or visual fields could not 'improve'.

However, one study showed improvement in around one-third of those having a 30% reduction of IOP[2], and a more recent investigation reported 85% of patients demonstrating improvement in the appearance of the optic nerve following a 40% reduction in IOP[3]. It has even been suggested that such improvement constitutes the only sure demonstration that IOP has been lowered adequately in the particular patient under consideration[4,5].

If lowering IOP can be achieved without any side-effects, then assessing damage to the optic nerve would itself be a fairly satisfactory outcome measure. Lowering IOP surgically, especially with traditional surgery such as a guarded filtration surgery (trabeculectomy), causes many different effects. Appropriate assessment of the benefit or lack of benefit of such surgery must take these other effects into account. It is disturbing that despite pleas in this regard for many years, such considerations are still largely or even totally ignored[6].

Again it should be stressed that the specific type of outcome measure chosen relates to the type of glaucoma, the person, and the type of glaucoma surgery. For example, when peripheral iridotomy is performed for an asymptomatic narrow angle, deepening of the anterior chamber angle would be an appropriate outcome measure. Change in IOP, disc, and field, are inappropriate. In contrast, where peripheral iridotomy is performed for the pigment dispersion syndrome, change in anterior chamber angle is only an indirect and relatively unimportant outcome measure. The goal of the iridotomy is lowering IOP and improving disc and field. Thus, even the same procedure may have different appropriate outcome measures in different situations. Visual function is a more global and more valid outcome indicator for most situations than is mere assessment of the optic disc and visual field. However, it is also a much more difficult measure to assess quantitatively. Nevertheless, difficult or not, it is much more important to evaluate. If the patient has had an improvement in visual field, but a decrease in visual function, the patient has not been assisted. For example, the patient whose IOP is markedly lowered but whose cataract progresses may have a diminution of visual function, as might a patient whose IOP is lowered but who develops a thin, irritating filtering bleb with associated photophobia and ptosis.

The most global and the most valid outcome measure for every type of glaucoma surgery is the effect of such surgery on the patient's sense of health. This involves quality of life, but is not limited to the patient's estimate of his or her quality of life. Health is a perception of wholeness. The only global valid indicator of the worth of glaucoma surgery to the patient is how such surgery affects his or her health, that is, how the surgery influences the patient's perception of wholeness.

Realities

What, then, are the realities associated with glaucoma surgery, especially as they relate to the patient's sense of health? The only honest answer is that we do not know the answer well because it has never been (repeat, never) been studied. Nevertheless, though never subjected to a systematic study, every ophthalmologist who does his or her job properly has always considered the effect of glaucoma surgery on the patient's health as an important outcome criterion. It does not take a prospective, controlled, randomized clinical trial to reach a valid conclusion. In fact, the conclusions of such clinical trials, despite their virtually universal acclaim, must always be qualified and must be considered in terms of their applicability to the unique individual to whom care is being given. Those in research not infrequently are highly critical of clinicians' failure to utilize the results of clinical trials[7]. That they are so critical is an indication of their failure to understand that individual patients are not subjects in homogeneous populations, but rather unique individuals whose needs and wants may be very different from those in the clinical trial.

The reality of glaucoma surgery is that in almost every instance it substitutes one problem for another problem. Even that procedure which is one of the most exemplary in medicine, the performance of a peripheral iridotomy for angle-closure glaucoma, has aspects of damage associated with its performance. Argon laser iridotomy virtually always is associated with the development of a localized cataract, and, unless specific measures are taken, is followed by posterior synechias. Both argon and YAG laser iridotomies may cause a bothersome ghost image due to refraction of light by the tear film at the edge of the upper lid, which serves as a prism deflecting light through the small iridotomy, even when it is underneath the lid. This is usually a minor symptom, but in some individuals it is very troublesome.

The point, however, is that all glaucoma surgery causes problems. It is the excessive focus of the surgeon that results in the problems associated with glaucoma surgery being overlooked, ignored, or, frankly, disqualified. While examining the patient with an IOP of 10 mmHg, an unstable refractive error, photophobia, and ptosis, that very unfortunate phrase reminiscent of medical student satire comes to mind: "The operation was a success, but the patient died".

The first reality, then, is that

glaucoma surgery is never to be undertaken lightly and never with the mistaken impression that the patient will be 'cured'.

The partial exception to that comment is the patient with the narrow or partially closed anterior chamber angle in whom a peripheral iridotomy is performed for the release of relative pupillary block. When performed properly with a neodymium

YAG laser, so that the iridotomy is tiny (*i.e.*, barely visible and located under the upper lid), the likelihood of improvement of the patient's abnormal anatomy is great, and the likelihood of troublesome postoperative symptoms is extremely small. The benefit is lasting and the likelihood of such an iridotomy closing in the uninflamed eye is close to zero.

Another essential reality regarding the surgical treatment of many types of glaucoma, is that surgery can be beneficial: the configuration of the angle can be improved, progressive visual field loss can be slowed or prevented, visual recovery can occur, improvement in optic nerve appearance can occur, and improvement in the patient's quality of life is a reality in many individuals. The challenge, then, is to determine in whom the benefit is most likely to occur and how the surgery can be fashioned to show that the reality of that benefit is most likely.

Expectations

The expectations of the patient and the surgeon may be very different. The usual cause for unhappiness in the postoperative patient is an unfulfilled expectation. Where the patient anticipates a result quite different from what the surgeon anticipates, the outcome is almost certainly going to be an unhappy patient.

Due to the physician's obsession with IOP, many patients also consider part of the measure of success or failure of the surgical failure in terms of the postoperative level of IOP. However, far more important to the patient is the effect of the surgery on how well the patient feels. The patient with a pressure of 10 mmHg, a stable visual field, and a large ischemic bleb, adjacent to which is a dellen, is an unhappy patient. The ophthalmologist may consider the surgical procedure a triumph, but the patient does not share the ophthalmologist's enthusiasm. The patient is photophobic, he cannot obtain a proper refraction, his eye tears constantly, and he may even be incapacitated. As the bleb becomes increasingly thin and the symptoms increase, the drooping lid becomes more prominent, the visual acuity becomes worse due to hypotony and changing refraction, and the patient becomes increasingly convinced that he made the wrong decision in having surgery. When the blebitis develops and in some cases the endophthalmitis, the patient looks back with deep regret on his decision to have surgery performed. The proper measures of outcome are discussed in detail in this Chapter, because these constitute the expectations and they must be clearly understood by the patient and the physician prior to the surgery.

With regard to retention of function, it is important for the physician and the patient alike to recall that a certain number of neurons are lost merely through aging. For an individual who has a million neurons coursing through his optic nerve, the loss of 5000 or so neurons a year is not noted. However, in the patient with far-advanced glaucoma, who may have only 50,000 neurons left, a loss of 5000 neurons is noticeable and may result in total loss of vision. Consequently, it is appropriate to advise a patient with far-advanced glaucomatous nerve damage that continuing visual loss may occur, even after surgery has lowered IOP to a level that the surgeon believes is ideal.

'Wipeout' is rare but real[7,8].

Recent studies indicate a frequency between 1% and 5% of guarded filtration procedures. Clearly, the incidence of 'wipeout' is closely related to the preoperative state of the eye. It is extremely rare if it occurs at all in patients with healthy visual fields. It only appears to be a problem in patients in whom the visual field extends directly up to or into fixation. In patients who have already lost fixation, wipeout is not an expected problem. It can probably be minimized by avoiding hypotony.

Loss of vision due to an IOP spike following surgery, is not properly called 'wipeout'. In such a case, there is an explanation for the loss of vision, specifically, progression of the glaucomatous nerve damage caused by elevated IOP. Furthermore, loss of vision due to macular edema in association with hypotony is not properly considered 'wipeout'.

It is reasonable to expect that continuing deterioration of visual field can be halted in around 80% of those with primary open-angle glaucoma who have a standard guarded filtration procedure without an antimetabolite[9]. This figure is lower in patients of black African origin, those below the age of 20 years, those having had previous anterior segment surgery such as cataract extraction, and those with any type of inflammatory glaucoma. In some series, the success rate in terms of preservation of visual field is even higher. In an eye having had a successful guarded filtration procedure, it is reasonable to expect continuing control of IOP for at least ten years. Life table analyses show gradual loss of control of IOP, and such loss of control is partially related to the nature of the filtering bleb. The loss of control of IOP following a guarded filtration procedure is sufficiently long in developing that it is reasonable for the ophthalmologist and patient to expect that a successful procedure will probably not require reoperation within the patient's lifetime. This is not true in secondary types of glaucoma, such as the glaucoma associated with chronic uveitis and Chandler's syndrome. In patients having had filtering procedures or tube-shunt procedures for neovascular glaucoma, the rate of failure is much higher, and most procedures will fail within five years. The duration of filtration procedures and tube-shunt procedures in children has not been well established, but it is not similar to that in adults, and it is not reasonable to expect that a procedure will work for more than ten years.

Patients who have full-thickness procedures or guarded filtration procedures performed in conjunction with an antimetabolite can expect to have difficulties with their filtering bleb, with increasing tearing, increasing hypotony, and an increasingly uncomfortable eye. Where the antimetabolite has 'done its job' and resulted in a totally avascular bleb, the long-term outlook for the patient is gloomy.

Indications

The indication for glaucoma surgery is the need to intervene surgically in order to enhance the patient's health. Since health cannot be measured in terms of IOP, anterior chamber depth, or any other similar single parameter, consideration of the entire patient is essential. With regard to chronic glaucomas, the indications require: considering the *stage* of the glaucoma, the *stability* of the glaucoma – and, if it is unstable – the rate at which the glaucoma is changing, the mechanism of the glaucoma, the *anticipated duration of the patient's life,* and *the needs and wants of the patient* as defined by the patient.

The stages of glaucoma can be divided into four categories: Stage 1: findings, Stage 2: damage, Stage 3: symptomatic damage (*i.e.,* disease); and Stage 4: deteriorating disease.

A *'finding'* is something that predisposes a patient to developing damage. *'Dam-*

age' is a change that is definite, but which has not yet produced symptoms; a significant notch associated with a unilateral paracentral scotoma represents *'damage'*, but is frequently asymptomatic. *'Disease'* is that condition in which the damage has progressed to the point that the patient is aware something is wrong, that is symptomatic. *'Deteriorating disease'* is present when the patient is aware that whatever is wrong is getting worse.

Regarding *stability*, the condition could be 'improving', 'unchanging', or 'deteriorating'. This is determined by history or by appropriate serial evaluations such as evaluations of corneal endothelium, visual field, optic nerve, the retinal nerve-fiber layer.

The *rate* at which change is occurring must also be established. In the early stages of most glaucomas the determination of rate of change is made by serial evaluations such as repeat gonioscopy or repeat quantitative analysis of the optic nerve topography. In the early stages, history is overwhelmingly the most important aspect of determining the rate of change.

An estimate must be made of how long the patient is likely to live. This entails personal history, family history, and evaluation of the patient's general health and lifestyle. Lastly, the realities of what the patient really wants and needs must be appropriately evaluated. Some patients are perfectly content to lose a small amount of visual field. Such loss is usually not associated with a significant change in the patient's ability to function until the field loss is so advanced that any deterioration is noticed. The proper goal of glaucoma therapy is not to prevent patients from losing visual field but to keep the patient feeling healthy. For some patients, it is preferable for them to avoid surgery even though they have progressive damage.

The last consideration deals with the needs and wants of the patient. These are unique to each individual.

Laser trabeculoplasty

A few words about argon laser trabeculoplasty also appear appropriate. Argon laser trabeculoplasty, performed in patients who have idiopathic open-angle glaucoma, open-angle glaucoma in association with the exfoliation syndrome, or open-angle glaucoma in association with the pigment dispersion syndrome, also is a procedure likely to cause few side-effects, at least when performed properly. If the burns are placed over the ciliary body or if the power utilized is so great that it causes a marked inflammatory response, the consequence is frequently a uveitis and peripheral anterior synechias. If the patient has a markedly decompensated trabecular meshwork, significant glaucomatous cupping, and the trabeculoplasty results in release of considerable pigment, the chance of a pressure spike causing further optic nerve damage is high enough to be a concern. In patients with a decompensated trabecular meshwork, marked pigmentation of the trabecular meshwork, and advanced cupping, it is mandatory to pre-treat and post-treat the patient with agents that are effective in minimizing pressure spikes; additionally, such patients should usually be treated with a maximum of 50 applications over 180°, a subsequent treatment of the remaining 180° being performed later if IOP lowering is not judged adequate.

The major problem with trabeculoplasty, however, is that the amount of IOP lowering produced by the procedure is not great enough to prevent further deterioration in a significant percentage of patients.

The exact percentage will vary with the type of patient and the skill with which the trabeculoplasty is performed. A very rough guideline is that approximately 50% of patients in whom an argon laser trabeculoplasty is an appropriate procedure will have a clinically significant benefit from the procedure, that is, clinically beneficially in terms of IOP decrease and planned diminution of diurnal variation of IOP. Related to this problem is the unpredictable duration of effect. A rough guideline is that approximately 10% of patients in whom trabeculoplasty is performed will escape the deleterious effects of the trabeculoplasty each year, so that at the end of five years, one half of the treated individuals will continue to have a clinically useful response, and at the end of ten years, about one-tenth of the individuals will continue to be benefited. This lack of universal effect and the lack of permanent effect has been frequently used as a critical commentary on argon laser trabeculplasty. It is easy to reverse that and to point out with considerable enthusiasm that half the patients have been spared the problems associated with conventional surgery and fully one-tenth of the patients have been spared such problems for ten years. That is a major accomplishment, and the advantage of such a benefit is inadequately appreciated.

The benefit of repeating a trabeculoplasty has been quite well studied and has been reported to occur in at least 30% and probably closer to 50% of individuals who are appropriate candidates for trabeculoplasty to start with. Repeating trabeculoplasty in the individual who initially had a satisfactory response in terms of pressure control is a sensible procedure which I believe is underutilized. Performing a third trabeculoplasty in an individual who had an initially satisfactory response to the first and the second trabeculoplasty is also appropriate. The argument that the trabecular meshwork may be damaged in such a case, necessitating filtration surgery, is, of course, specious, because the procedure to be performed in the place of trabeculoplasty is almost invariably a filtering procedure anyway.

References

1. GLT Research Group: The Glaucoma Laser Trial: 1. Acute effects of argon laser trabeculoplasty on intraocular pressure. Arch Ophthalmol 107:1135-1142, 1989
2. Spaeth GL, Katz LJ, Poryzees E et al: Is improvement of the optic disc or visual field in patients with glaucoma a sign of clinical importance? Invest Ophthalmol Vis Sci 30:421, 1989
3. Shin D: Removable-suture closure of the lamellar scleral flap in trabeculectomy. Ann Ophthalmol 19:51-53, 1987
4. Caprioli J, Spaeth GL: Looking for better ways to measure the optic disc. Ophthalmic Surg 18:866, 1987
5. Spaeth GL: A new management system for glaucoma based on improvement of the appearance of the optic disc or visual field. Fortschr Ophthalmol 85:614-619, 1988
6. Spaeth GL, Fernandes E, Hitchings RA: The pathogenesis of transient or permanent improvement in the appearance of the optic disc following glaucoma surgery. Doc Ophthalmol 22:111-125, 1980
7. Kolker AE: Visual prognosis in advanced glaucoma: a comparison of medical and surgical therapy for retention of vision in 101 eyes with advanced glaucoma. Trans Am Ophthalmol Soc 75:539-555, 1977
8. Costa VP, Smith M, Spaeth GL et al: Loss of visual acuity after trabeculectomy. Ophthalmology 100:599-612, 1993
9. Costa VP, Wilson RP, Moster MR: Hypotony maculopathy following the use of topical mitomycin C in glaucoma filtration surgery. Ophthalmic Surg 24:389-394, 1993
10. Araujo SV, Spaeth GL, Roth SM, Starita RJ: A ten-year follow-up on a prospective, randomized trial of postoperative corticosteroids after trabeculectomy. Ophthalmology 102:1753-1759, 1995

Grand Rounds II

Topics: filter location, combined procedures, one incision or two?, anti-metabolites, saving blebs, beta blockers and iritis, correct dosing in the aged, punctal occlusion

Moderator: Katherine Loftfield

Katherine Loftfield, MD: *The first question is directed toward Dr. Palmberg. It is a two part question. First, why is your incision at the limbus for your combined so large, and why do you wait until after the case is done to put the mitomycin on instead of putting it on before you enter the chamber?*

Paul Palmberg, MD: The conjunctival incision is so large because when we tried making a pita pocket entry of only a couple of clock hours and then tried to close it with a couple of 10-0 nylon mattress kind of stitches, they are in a location where the lid rubs on them because they are not quite at 12 o'clock and they are irritating to the patient. All that mechanical action over them has torn some of them and caused them to leak. So every time I have tried to make a smaller incision, it does not work for me and the one that is out six clock hours, although it seems excessive, is quite comfortable for the patients; it heals well, it does not leak. And so I finally do not know of a better way to fix it.

The other question was about mitomycin. I think that the key thing is not to get the mitomycin inside the eye. I do not like having it on if it were going to be exposed to any kind of a wound that I wanted to heal, like on an extracap. I always put it on just after fashioning a scleral flap in those extracapsular cases. In the phaco cases, there is really no other wound that I worry about affecting in an adverse way. I was a little concerned about dragging instruments back and forth through that area into the eye and taking cells with mitomycin on or in them into the eye. I knew that I had a watertight seal. I put fluid in, the pressure in the eye feels like 20 or so at that point. I put a stitch in to boot. If any fluid were going anywhere, it would be coming out. So I think it is quite safe to do it the way that I do it. It was just a fear that putting it on at the beginning, things are going in and out of the eye, that maybe I would carry some in. People who do put it on at the beginning instead do not seem to have any trouble, so it probably does not make any difference as long as there is no way for mitomycin to get in the anterior chamber. As Harry has shown very well, it is not a nice thing to have in there.

Dr. Loftfield: *Maybe a brief comment about other people's views on that.*

Don Minckler, MD: I was just going to remind the audience that there is an alternative to a single incision, and I would argue with Paul's choice of 12 o'clock. It

Peril to the Nerve – Glaucoma and Clinical Neuro-Ophthalmology, pp. 119–124
Proceedings of the 45th Annual Symposium of the New Orleans Academy of
Ophthalmology, New Orleans, LA, USA, April 25-28, 1996
edited by Barry J. Leader and Jonathan C. Calkwood

seems to me you inevitably plough up a lot more ground placing the incision there, in terms of preserving the adjacent tissue for subsequent filtering attempts.

I guess I am not as confident in the outcome as Paul is, and I would still advise placing the incision in one or the other quadrants. Whether you do a single incision combined procedure or my preference, which is a temporal phaco and completely separate trabeculectomy, usually upper nasally, in which case you can use mitomycin just as you would during a routine trabeculectomy.

Dr. Loftfield: *Any other comments?*

Dr. Palmberg: I think when we did not use mitomycin that your point of going supranasal and saving another location is well taken. I think with mitomycin blebs we have more trouble when the blebs stick out underneath the edge of the lid a little bit. So I hope you are saying to put it at 11 o'clock or something, not 10:30 or 10:00, because you really do not want a mitomycin bleb exposed. You do not want to do them down below where the risk of endophthalmitis is three times as much, and the patients we have had who seem to have problems with irritation, with leaking blebs, are much more often the ones in whom it is not right at 12. The success is so high that we do not usually need to do anything more and that is the reason I switched, and I am happy with the switch. But if you do not use mitomycin, you had certainly better put it to one side so that you will have another opportunity.

Dr. Minckler: We have had some late mitomycin failures. Some of them are going to fail and the point is that it is not going to last forever in everybody, that is for sure. In fact we might point out that there is really no significant long-term followup on the use of mitomycin in trabeculectomy. If you use the Wills' experience that George talked about as a kind of a control, the success rate was fairly good without antimetabolites. If we take that as a control, we need comparable long-term followup with mitomycin before we can be all that confident about the permanence of these procedures.

George L. Spaeth, MD: I would like to follow up on that, Don. We do have some fairly short-term studies. I think it is helpful to remember that Dong Chin's study now published quite a while ago did not show any significant difference between the antimetabolite and the non-antimetabolite treated eyes. At the last ARVO meeting, there was a presentation by Samuelson, a nice prospective, randomized, masked study, in which one group of patients was randomized to standard phacoemulsification with guarded filtration procedure without antimetabolite. The other was with mitomycin, fairly standard methodology, and at the end of over a year, that is short term, as Don pointed out, there was no difference between the two groups. This is new surgery. Whether or not mitomycin is really beneficial or necessary in that type of procedure still has not been determined.

Dr. Palmberg: I think it is quite clear in the study what Dong Chin did with a small piece of sponge, being very careful not to push on the sponge in any way, which does not get as much stuff out of the sponge, and that he found no effect. I think there are a lot of us who are getting average pressures of 10, not average pressures of 15, who have 86% of the people off medication, where it is clear that our surgery does not accomplish that without the mitomycin. So it is not the time and the concentration alone; it is how much leaves the sponge that makes a difference. You can do a randomized control trial: if you do not get the stuff out of the sponge, you will see no effect. If you get it out of the sponge, you will. So it is very clear that it works. If you have done several hundred cases without it and several hundred with it, this is very clear, and it does not take a randomized control trial to tell the difference between a pressure of 10 and a pressure of 15 average, and getting blebs in the vast majority or not. Whether it is a good idea or not long term, in terms of complications and benefits, I would agree with them. We have an obligation to look at it carefully, consistently for at least ten years before we know whether this lowering of pressure really benefits the patient and how much we are paying for it. And I could not agree more about that. But it certainly does work.

Dr. Loftfield: *One other question regarding the combined surgeries. If you have a functioning filter that is working well and they now need a cataract surgery, has anyone found that the use of adjunctive antimetabolites at the time to protect that filter is useful?*

Michael A. Kass, MD: People have tried a variety of things: 5-FU injections. Recently what we have done is just take a sponge with mitomycin and put it over the bleb, let it sit for a few minutes, irrigate it off, and then go ahead and do the operation. Other people have actually injected small doses of mitomycin into the bleb. Once again, however, I am not aware of any real good long-term trials on this. There is no question that you will lose some blebs when you take a cataract out, or that some of them will also shrink and the control will be less than you might have hoped for.

Dr. Loftfield: *The next question is – there are some people who are doing their combined surgeries – a trabeculectomy in one site and a clear corneal incision in another completely separate site. Do any of you have experience with that, and if you are doing it, why do you think it is better?*

Dr. Minckler: That is my preference. In a patient who needs cataract surgery, who may be a subsequent candidate for filtering surgery, whether you do it at the same time or not, it makes sense to protect the option of doing surgery superiorly. So a temporal cataract, whether it is clear cornea or not, makes sense to me. I believe actually that the Japanese have a huge experience with this type of approach. In fact, I have heard it referred to as the Japanese incision approach. The astigmatism one winds up with after temporal cataract surgery has been small. There are several reports about that, so it is favorable from that point of view. It simply gives you the most flexibility, I think, in terms of subsequent surgery.

Dr. Palmberg: If you just need to take a cataract out, surely the idea of doing a temporal phaco and leaving the conjunctiva alone is a good idea. If you are doing them both at the same time, there may be some cases with a very deeply set eye in which doing a phaco superiorly would be difficult, and you would be wise to do a temporal phaco and then do your filter up above, because otherwise you would be working in a pit, which would be very hard to do. But if there is no special consideration, I do not see any reason for having two wounds when you could do it all through one, and the time saving in the operating room would be considerable just to do three punches in a phaco wound and have a filter. You are not going to sacrifice any more tissue or any more approach that way than you would with the others if you are doing simultaneous. So I do not see why one would want to separate them, with the possible exception of people with a lot of astigmatism that you were hoping to reduce by doing the phaco temporally. A lot of the astigmatism depends on the tightness of the stitches in your wound. If you use a safety valve incision rather than a scleral flap based at the phaco, you have very little need for tension on those stitches. Most of the resistance comes from the valve-like incision and those stitches are not tight and they do not induce much astigmatism. If you make a scleral flap, a triangle or a square, and make a punch under it in what was a phaco incision, then of course you are going to have considerable astigmatism induced in some cases. You might want to have done the procedure separately for some consideration of astigmatism.

Dr. Minckler: Paul alluded to one of the disadvantages of the two-incision approach, which is the time it takes, and obviously that is an important issue these days. Another practical problem is if you do not have gurneys or operating room tables that are fixed so that you can comfortably sit at the patient's side, then it becomes quite an awkward business. I have heard descriptions of doing side phaco while sitting at the head of the patient. In fact, Walter Stark has described that, even using his right hand across the nose to operate on the patient's left eye by simply rotating the eye temporally. There are a lot of ways to get around these mechanical problems.

Dr. Loftfield: *Maybe one or two more questions before we have to move on. The next one is addressed to Dr. Zimmerman. Two parts: number one, with the beta blockers, do you feel that there is any use for peak flow meters, and do you recommend they be routinely used? Secondly, regarding Optipranalol, does it work as well as the other beta blockers and medically/legally, should we be using it because of this question of uveitis?*

Thom J. Zimmerman, MD, PhD: On the first one, the flow meter, certainly Alcon has been around with their flow meter. We have had little clinical experience with it. We did hand it over to our pulmonologist who, surprisingly, after he tested it in a number of patients, came back and told us not to waste our time, just to send the patients to him and, for a small fee, he would do the appropriate testing for us. Actually, he said that there is tremendous variability and that, unless you have a dedicated technician cheerleader who can practice with the patients and work hard, the results were not very good for a good part of the time.

I think there are a lot of other things you ought to be doing, such as maybe blood pressure and pulse and stuff like that. Before I turn it over to other panel members like George, who has just moved forward to talk about the flow meter, let me answer the Optipranalol question. There is no doubt that there is a small number of patients who will have a frank uveitis on Optipranalol. The largest series I know of is through the Kaiser group where they found four or five out of thousands and thousands of patients per year on Optipranalol. Optipranalol is attractive to a lot of large volume buyers because of its pricing, which is why it is used in the Kaiser Foundation and other groups like that. The VA system has embraced it also. I think this is peculiar to this beta blocker. Although other beta blockers have shown a uveitis like this, Optipranalol does it more frequently. You should be alert; you should have it in the back of your computer that, should a patient on a beta blocker complain of uveitic symptoms, you ought to think about Optipranalol and move them to a different beta blocker. I do not think it is a contraindication for it is general use. I do not think that you are exposed medical/legally. It is definitely as potent.

Dr. Spaeth: We have had some experience with the flow meter and I want to second and reinforce Thom's comments. It is variable. You learn how to use it; if you expire into it very suddenly you can be a superman with a huge flow. If you blow rather slowly, you wonder if you are going to make it through the day. I do not think it has any role in clinical practice until it is either refined or handled in a different way from that suggested so far.

Dr. Minckler: I would like to ask Thom a question related to aging and the potential for systemic toxicity. At least two of these agents, betagan and timolol, come in two different concentrations. Is it important, do you think, to get the elderly patient on as low a dose as possible? My impression is that if you ask questions related to potential toxicity, particularly cardiovascular functioning, and a variety of other things, people in their 80s particularly are getting toxic from these things. So it makes sense to me to reduce the dose whenever possible.

Dr. Zimmerman: That is right in my wheelhouse. I have been preaching it for years. My feeling, although there is new evidence that I may be wrong, is that all the lower dose beta blocker solutions are of the same potency as the higher dose ones. Let us just consider timolol for instance in that 0.25 is going to give you the maximal effect for just as long as 0.5. There is no difference in the dose response curve, and I would love to catch up with the idiot who did the initial dose response curve that showed that there might be a difference. There is some evidence now on betamol comparison with timolol that both the betamol and the timolol lower dose is different as far as dose response and duration of action than the higher doses are concerned. I am looking at those data hard and I want them to repeat that, because I do not believe it is true. The point is nicely taken. You ought to start with the low concentration and if it gives you what you want, leave it there. Unfortunately, in the United States for marketing surveillance, the prescription rate is 80 to 20, 0.5 to 0.25%. There is also a 'big stick' psychology: if a little bit is good, then a lot is better, and that is not necessarily true. It is the denominator or the side-effects we are worried about. Don's point on aging is right on target. Everything slows down. I have noticed a few examples myself. But certainly the catabolic process in the liver and the way we handle drugs pharmakinetically, their distribution, all changes with age. Marvin Sears first pointed out that he had a number of patients controlled on timolol 0.25% in their 80s once every three or four days. And so the duration of action can be huge in the elderly. If they are at 0.5, drop them down to 0.25 for a bottle or two, and see whether that really does make a difference in the pressure. Nasolacrimal occlusion in the elderly I think becomes extremely important. One of the things we are doing now is involving family members. We think that promotes compliance and support at home for their treatment.

Dr. Spaeth: One clue about punctal occlusion. Thom and others have been talking about this. It really makes a difference. But it is hard to incorporate it in your practice until you get an easy way to do it. If you ask your technicians or you yourself, when you are getting the history, on every patient simply to put down 'POP' or 'PNOP', then you know it has been asked about. Patient occluding puncta or patient not occluding puncta. So then when you see the patient you know whether they have been asked about it because it is like any other educational thing, it has got to be reinforced time and time again.

Harry A. Quigley, MD: You watch out as well, George, for what medicines the patient is taking and which ones are for shortness of breath or wheezing or asthma. There is a good study by Jerry Avorn that shows that patients in the New Jersey health care system, who were prescribed a topical beta blocker for glaucoma, wind up having an increase in the number of medicines they use to control their shortness of breath and lung disease. Why they were receiving beta blockers when they already had lung disease is, of course, an interesting question, but if you are asking each time you see the patient what other medicines are you taking for your general health, and you see medicines for shortness of breath popping up, it may be as good as the flow meter or better.

Dr. Kass: One other thing you can sometimes do, I guess it never snows down here, but some day when you have some natural disaster going on, and only three patients show up in your office, and you are bored, is have the patients put the drops in as you watch them. It is a horrifying experience. If you have never done this, you will wonder why every postoperative cataract patient does not have endophthalmitis. They jab themselves in the eye and they contaminate every time, and I think there is an enormous amount of teaching: it is amazing to me how often I see patients and I say to them, here is how you put it in, and they say, God, I have been going to eye doctors for 15 years and nobody has ever told me how to put in the drops. So, it is a useful and somewhat horrifying experience.

How to suspect, detect, and treat a person with angle-closure glaucoma

George L. Spaeth

Wills Eye Hospital/Jefferson Medical College, Philadelphia, PA, USA

Introduction

The proper diagnosis and management of the angle-closure glaucomas involves the same three components seen in all medical decision-making: history, examination, and specialized testing. The most critically important part of the evaluation of every patient is the history. This is also true for patients with narrow-angle or angle-closure glaucoma. In addition to taking a history competently, the physician caring for patients with narrow angles or angle-closure glaucoma must be competent in an aspect of the physical evaluation of the patient which is frequently ignored, improperly performed, or misinterpreted, specifically gonioscopy, the appearance of the anterior chamber angle. Gonioscopy is the key when it comes to diagnosing and treating angle closure.

The initial, scientific, approach to understanding glaucoma was centered on the anterior segment, on the inflow and outflow of aqueous humor. Tonography, for example, at one time was considered by some to be the most important part of the evaluation of a glaucoma patient[1-3]. Nevertheless, the scientific, critical evaluation of the appearance of the anterior chamber angle itself has received short shrift. Even glaucoma specialists vary considerably in their approach to examining and interpreting the anterior chamber angle. For example, not all glaucoma specialists use indentation gonioscopy.

The angle-closure glaucomas continue to cause visual loss. In some parts of the world, such as the Arctic and most of the Far East, they are among the leading causes of blindness. How can this be when the conditions are so easily diagnosed and can be so effectively treated? The angle-closure glaucomas continue to cause blindness, because 1. they are not suspected; 2. they are not appropriately detected; and 3. they are not appropriately treated. These three issues will be discussed now: First, who is at risk for developing angle-closure glaucoma; second, how the angle-closure glaucomas are properly diagnosed; and third, what constitutes appropriate treatment for the angle-closure glaucomas.

Address for correspondence: George L. Spaeth, MD, Wills Eye Hospital/Jefferson Medical College, 900 Walnut Street, Philadelphia, PA 19107-5598, USA

Peril to the Nerve – Glaucoma and Clinical Neuro-Ophthalmology, pp. 125–140
Proceedings of the 45th Annual Symposium of the New Orleans Academy of
Ophthalmology, New Orleans, LA, USA, April 25-28, 1996
edited by Barry J. Leader and Jonathan C. Calkwood
© 1998 Kugler Publications, The Hague/The Netherlands

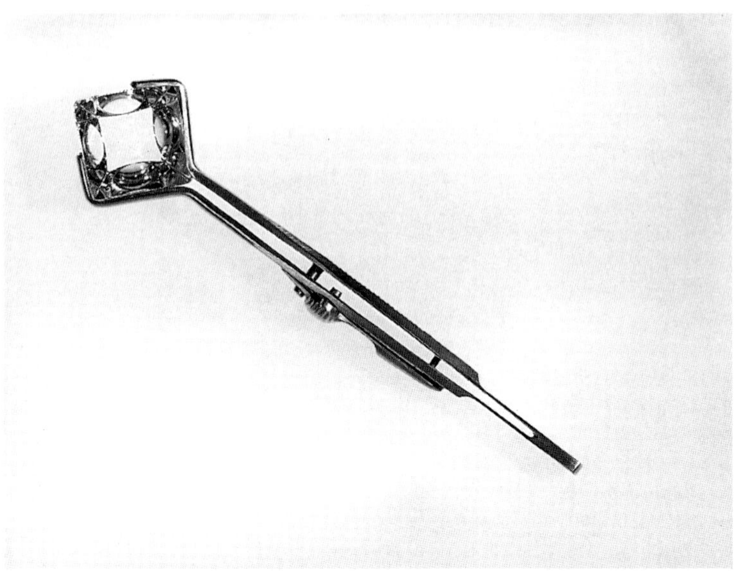

Fig. 1. Zeiss 4-mirror gonioscopic lens on an Unger handle. This type of lens is essential for performing gonioscopy quickly and conveniently, without the need to use a viscous solution to bind the lens optically to the cornea.

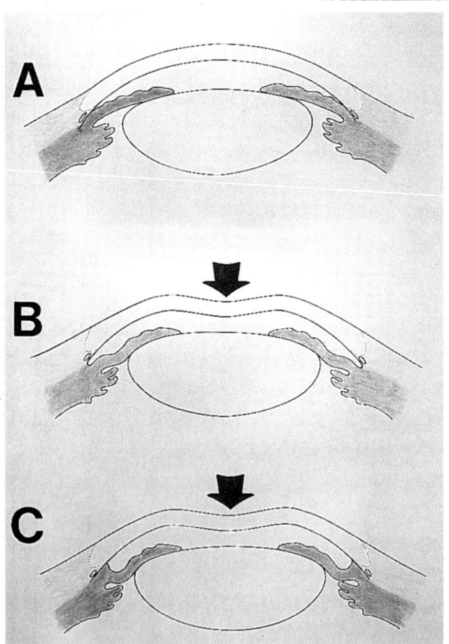

Fig. 2. Indentation gonioscopy: A. The Zeiss 4-mirror goniolens is pushed posteriorly against the cornea, displacing aqueous to the periphery of the anterior chamber. B. The iris moves posteriorly where it is not supported by the lens, revealing that the contact between the iris and the endothelial surface shown in 'a' is merely appositional and not synechial, as the angle recess opens, allowing visualization of the ciliary body. C. Here, as the iris is put on stretch, the presence of synechias can be noted. (Modified from Spaeth GL: *Ophthalmic Surgery: Principles and Practice.* Saunders, 1981).

Problems with current methodology

The answers to these three concerns – who to suspect, how to detect, and how to treat – revolve almost exclusively around two separate issues, gonioscopy and the proper performance of a neodymium YAG laser peripheral iridotomy. Both will be described in detail.

Gonioscopy is rarely performed with sufficient frequency, is often performed incorrectly, and the findings from it are frequently misinterpreted. At the root of the problem with gonioscopy are improper gonioscopic technique and the continuing use of a conceptual framework based on an obsolete and inadequate method of describing the anterior chamber angle. Consequently, at the central core of understanding how to detect and treat the angle-closure glaucomas is an improved system of gonioscopy, technically and conceptually[4,5].

Technically, the matter of how to perform gonioscopy is easily answered: employ a Zeiss 4-mirror gonioscopic lens (Fig. 1). This type of lens allows *1.* accurate gonioscopy without the need to use a gonioscopic solution that causes the patient's vision to be blurred following gonioscopy and makes examination of the eye by the physician difficult following gonioscopy; *2.* accurate gonioscopy to be performed quickly (within about one minute); *3.* easy comparison of the anterior chamber angles between the two eyes; and *4.* indentation gonioscopy. The only instrument that fulfils all these criteria is a lens such as the Zeiss 4-mirror gonioscopic lens. Of the 4-mirror lenses, the Zeiss lens, on the Unger handle, is the longest-lasting, best designed, and easiest to use. It is glass, so it can easily be sterilized and wiped without being scratched. The angle of the handle permits the hand to hold the lens properly in the eye without awkwardness of indenting.

Comments made by some ophthalmologists disqualifying Zeiss gonioscopy on the basis that it is too difficult or too prone to cause errors, are similar to comments made by those who disqualify phacoemulsification; they are comments on the commentator's incompetence.

It should no longer be necessary to comment on the need to perform indentation gonioscopy. Without indentation gonioscopy, it is impossible to distinguish mere apposition between the iris and the cornea from actual adhesion between the iris and the cornea[4] (Fig. 2). With indentation, this determination usually is easily made. If the angle is apposed (*no* synechias), the treatment is peripheral iridotomy. If the iris is adherent to the cornea anterior to Schwalbe's line, then a peripheral iridotomy usually will not be of benefit. Distinguishing between the two is important.

Conceptually, the matter of improved gonioscopy is, paradoxically, much more difficult. Old thought patterns are difficult to change. A new method of considering the anterior chamber angle involves changing the way ophthalmologists have – for the last 30 years – thought about the appearance of the anterior chamber angle, which has basically been determined by the system of gonioscopy. I will describe the appearance of the anterior chamber angle in detail, and also discuss how to examine it, and how to record the results of that examination.

Who to suspect (or who is at risk for developing angle closure?)

All angle-closure glaucomas are secondary[6]. A classification of angle-closure glaucomas is shown in Table 1. It is obvious from this Table who is at risk for developing a primary angle-closure glaucoma. A helpful contribution in this regard

Table 1. The angle-closure glaucomas

A. Anatomical features (inherited or congenital)
    1.   Small anterior segment
         a.   hyperopia
         b.   nanophthalmos
         c.   microcornea
         d.   microphthalmos
         e.   retinopathy of prematurity
         f.   hereditary narrow angle
    2.   Anterior iris insertion
         a.   Eskimos
         b.   Asians
         c.   Black Africans
    3.   Shallow anterior chamber
         a.   women (as opposed to men)
         b.   the elderly
         c.   plateau iris syndrome
         d.   loose or dislocated lens
         e.   large lens
B. Obstruction of the aqueous humor at the pupil
    1.   Normal iris-lens contact
    2.   Contact between iris and pseudophakos, vitreous, or other material such as silicone
    3.   Adhesion between iris and other material (lens, pseudophakos, vitreous)
    4.   Obstruction of aqueous humor posterior to pupil or traumatic angle damage and
         adhesions secondary to surgery
C. Ciliary block (malignant glaucoma, aqueous misdirection)
D. Anterior rotation of ciliary body
    1.   Retinal vein occlusion
    2.   Other obstruction to venous outflow
    3.   Cyclitis (as follows cyclophotocoagulation)
    4.   Choroidal effusion
    5.   Scleral buckling
E. Anterior displacement of the lens-iris diaphragm
    1.   Parasympathomimetic agents (miotics)
    2.   Aqueous misdirection
    3.   Pressure from the posterior segment
         a.   tumor
         b.   expanding gas
         c.   angioma, etc.
    4.   Loose or dislocated lens
F. The exfoliation syndrome[29,30]
G. Adherence of iris to trabecular meshwork unrelated to pupillary block
    1.   Chandler's syndrome
    2.   Essential iris atrophy
    3.   Cogan-Reese syndrome
    4.   Neovascularization of anterior segment
    5.   Inflammatory adhesions secondary to uveitis or inflammation
    6.   Adhesion secondary to angle recession or hyphema
    7.   Adhesion secondary to surgery

was made recently by an evaluation of results of the Baltimore Eye Study[7]. Clearly, the nature of the anterior chamber angle is a factor in the development of angle closure[8-15].

Table 1 indicates the features that predispose to angle closure. For example, any 90-year-old person is at risk for developing an angle-closure glaucoma related to relative pupillary block; that risk increases if the person is a woman, increases more if the woman is a hyperope, and increases still more if the elderly hyperopic woman is Korean. The diagnosis of an anterior displacement of the lens-iris diaphragm and an angle-closure glaucoma should immediately come to mind for an individual who has a unilateral elevation of intraocular pressure in association with a shallower anterior chamber following the use of pilocarpine. It should be obvious that the sudden elevation of intraocular pressure associated with inflammation and pain and a deep anterior chamber in a person with diabetic kidney disease is most likely caused by neovascularization of the anterior chamber angle and a neovascular glaucoma.

The suspicion of the presence of an angle-closure glaucoma is a direct function of knowing who is predisposed. By and large, one only sees what one looks for and one only looks for what one knows!

Signs and symptoms of angle closure and damage caused by angle closure

A variety of signs and symptoms all lead one to suspect that angle-closure glaucoma may be present. A positive family history of 'sudden glaucoma' should alert the physician, as the propensity to primary angle-closure glaucoma is inherited as an autosomal dominant[5]. Recurrent headaches, especially in association with reading or in the evening but never in the morning on awakening, episodes of misty or smoky vision, especially in association with eye pain or headaches, and recurrent spectral halos, are all flags that suggest recurrent angle closure. The signs of angle closure have also been well described, including asymmetric or irregular pupils, local iris atrophy, the presence of fine new vessels in the pupillary margin, a shallow anterior chamber angle, and anterior subcapsular lens changes (the so-called 'Glaukomflecken'). Obviously, it is also important to note the level of intraocular pressure, whether there is inflammatory disease, and the state of health of the optic nerve. While these may not help determine the mechanism of pressure elevation, they all influence the treatment markedly. For example, if the intraocular pressure is around 80 mmHg, *i.e.*, above the level of blood pressure in the ophthalmic artery, treatment is urgent, perhaps even requiring a paracentesis immediately. If the optic nerve is damaged, so that glaucomatous cupping is present, either the patient has had recurrent elevations of pressure or has two conditions: a normal anterior chamber angle *and* a separate cause for optic disc cupping; the state of the disc, then, is essential to be understood so that treatment can be directed appropriately. But, actual detection of angle closure itself is based almost exclusively on the appearance of the anterior chamber angle, *i.e.*, on gonioscopic evaluation.

Gonioscopy and gonioscopic classification

As T.S. Eliot once said, "I gotta use words when I talk with you." Those words or symbols define and limit the way we think and communicate. Our present concept of the anterior chamber angle is not just simple, it is simplistic. Saying that an angle is 'open' or 'closed' is like limiting description of the retina to 'flat or 'detached' or the visual field to 'normal' or 'abnormal'. Consideration of the pigmentary aspects of the anterior chamber gives us an idea of how we fail to examine carefully, because we do not look for what is already known. There is a vast amount still to learn, not just in the way of correlations, but also in the way of observations. For example, a light dusting of black pigment lying on the surface of Schwalbe's line is probably the first detectable sign of the exfoliation syndrome, long preceding the classic exfoliative changes on the iris or lens. Recognition that

Table 2. Aspects of the anterior chamber angle that need evaluation at the time of gonioscopy

Site of adhesions of the iris to the cornea, angle recess, ciliary body
Site of contact between the iris and the cornea, angle recess, or ciliary body
Angular approach to the recess
Configuration of the peripheral iris
Nature and amount of pigmentation in the posterior trabecular meshwork
Pathological changes:
   angle recession
   hyphema
   cyclodialysis
   foreign body
   abnormal Schwalbe's line
   exfoliated material
   Sampaolesi line
   neovascularization

the patient has the syndrome is important, because it changes management; it encourages early trabeculoplasty, and alerts the ophthalmologist that the patient has a glaucoma in which marked deterioration occurs far more rapidly than in most of the other types of glaucomas. In contrast, a dense brown deposit of pigment superiorly indicates the presence of the pigment dispersion syndrome, especially in connection with a posteriorly concave iris. The distinction between the two conditions, the exfoliation syndrome and the pigment dispersion syndrome, is important, because treatment of the two is different.

Aspects of the anterior chamber angle that deserve being looked for are listed in Table 2.

Grading the anterior chamber angle is important, because how we describe the angle defines and limits our understanding of the anterior chamber angle. The grading system must be easy to use, reproducible, reliable, and allow easy recording. It should also be quick and convenient. Various systems have been used, such as those of Becker and Shaffer[15] and Scheie[31]. Excellent descriptions of gonioscopy have been published[16-23]. These were advances, but they considered only two aspects of configuration. Here I describe a more comprehensive and reproducible system[24-26].

The Spaeth gonioscopic grading system uses three different descriptors to indicate the configuration of the angle (Fig. 3), and one to describe the amount of pigmentation of the posterior trabecular meshwork. Other characteristics are, of course, also important, and should be appended where appropriate. However, in all cases, the configuration and the pigmentation are necessary.

The first descriptor indicates the site of iris insertion, *i.e.,* where the iris is adherent to the inner wall of the eye (Fig. 4). Because this cannot always be determined without indentation, this descriptor comes in two 'forms'. The level of actual adherence between the iris and the inner wall of the eye is indicated by a capital letter, either A, B (Fig. 5), C (Fig. 6), D (Fig. 7), or E, A being the most anterior, and E the most posterior. But in some cases it is not possible to visualize this level because of a narrow angular approach to the angle recess or anterior bowing of the iris. In such cases, the actual site of insertion can be determined only by using Forbes indentation gonioscopy. Where the actual site of insertion cannot be determined without indentation gonioscopy, then the examiner uses an additional descriptor, specifically, a capital letter placed in parentheses (Fig. 8). This indicates the most posterior portion of the angle that can be visualized without indentation. Thus, in a patient with a marked anterior bowing of the iris, so that without inden-

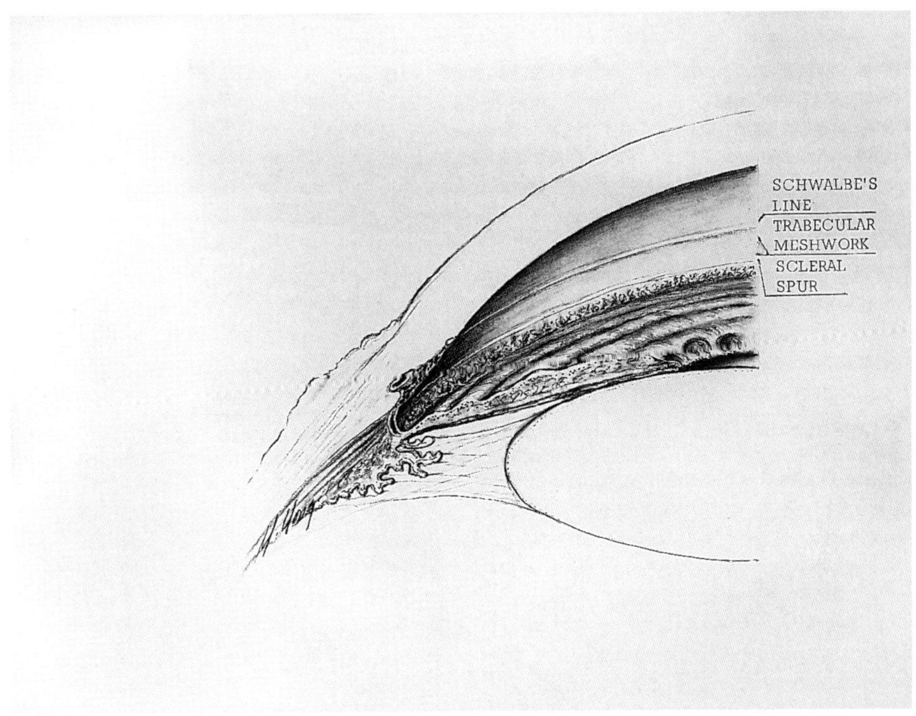

Fig. 3. Gonioscopic appearance of normal anterior chamber angle. *Note*: pupil border; peripheral iris, a. insertion, b. curvature, c. angular approach, ciliary body band; scleral spur; trabecular meshwork, a. posterior, b. mid, c. anterior, Schwalbe's line. (See also Fig. 4) (Reproduced from Spaeth *et al.*[25], by courtesy of Slack Inc.).

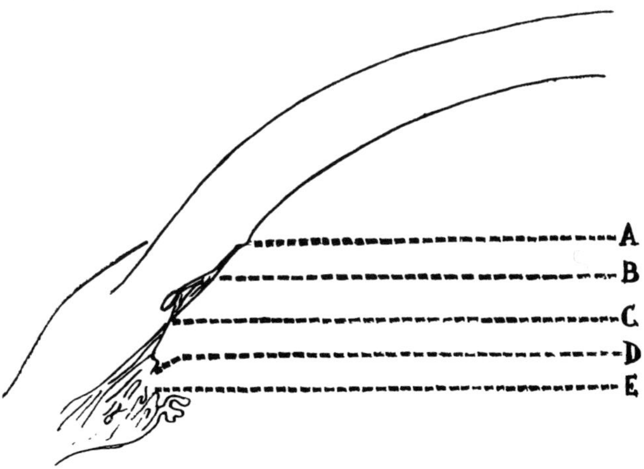

Fig. 4. Schematic drawing of five possible locations where the iris 'inserts' onto the inner wall of the globe. 'A' signifies contact between the iris and corneal endothelium in the area of Schwalbe's line. Where the iris adheres to the trabecular meshwork behind Schwalbe's line, it is expressed as 'B.' 'C' describes the situation where iris attaches to the anterior portion of the ciliary body so that scleral spur is just visible. 'D' signifies the normal deep, open angle. 'E' indicates an even deeper angle recess. (A helpful way to recall the code letters is: A - anterior, B = behind Schwable's line, C = can't see ciliary body, D = deep, and E = extremely deep).

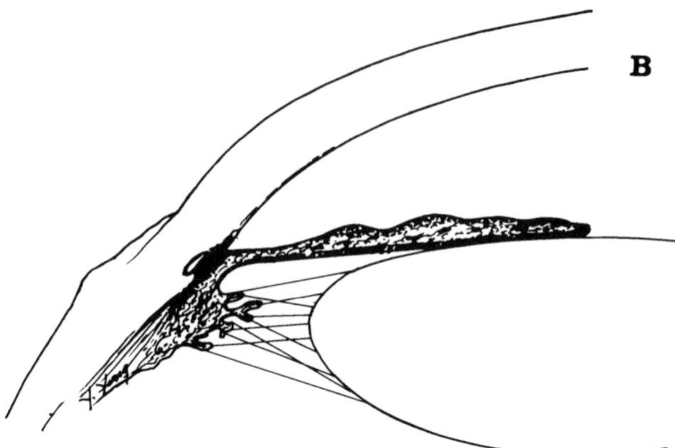

Fig. 5. Note that the depth of the anterior chamber is similar to that seen in Figure 7. Yet Figure 7 is normal and the angle in this figure is definitely pathologic, with adherence of the iris just posterior to Schlemm's canal. This angle would be graded as a B-30-r.

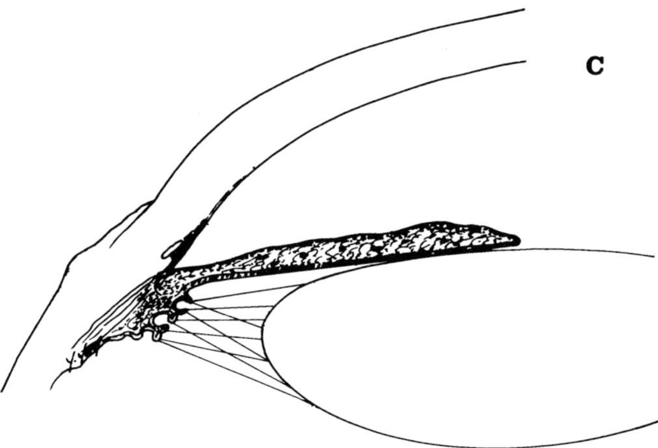

Fig. 6. The iris adheres just at the level of the scleral spur. This is an infrequent appearance, but may occur normally, most often in the brown-eye individual younger than 20 years of age.

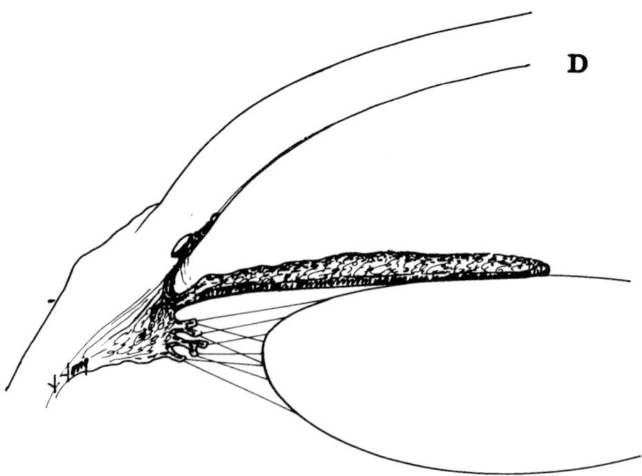

Fig. 7. A normal anterior chamber angle; this would be graded D-40-r.

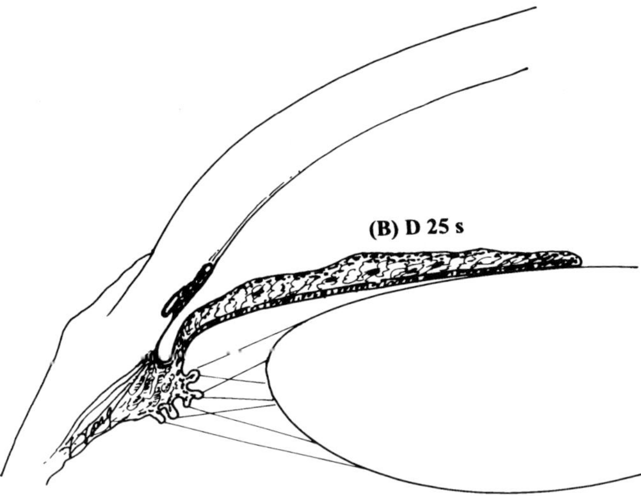

Fig. 8. This angle would be graded (B) D-20-s. The anterior chamber angle is of average depth. However, there is a sudden, steep, sharp rise of the peripheral iris(s). This produces narrowing of the angle and decreased visualization of the recess. The observer could not see past the scleral spur without indentation gonioscopy. However, the iris insertion is normal (D). Placing parentheses around 'B' indicates that the iris appears to be inserting at the scleral spur, but in actuality inserts in the ciliary body in a normal fashion.

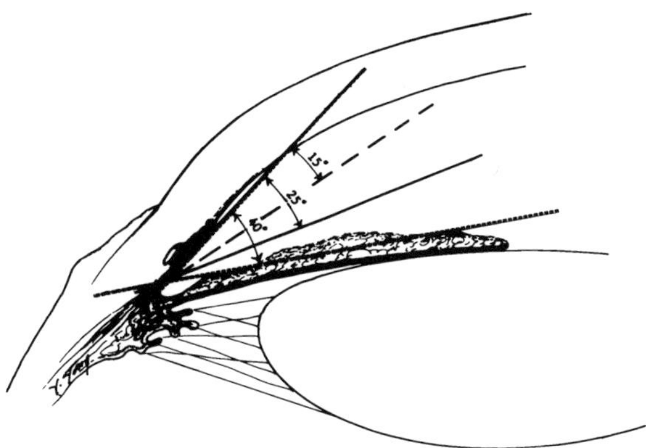

Fig. 9. Angular width of anterior chamber recess. The depth of the anterior chamber is estimated by constructing a tangent to the anterior iris surface about one-third of the distance from the most peripheral portion of the iris and joining it to a tangent to the cornea at the area of Descemet's membrane. The anterior chamber recess illustrated here would be graded as approximately a 40° angle. Two narrower approaches are also indicated.

tation gonioscopy the most posterior portion of the angle that can be visualized is Schwalbe's line, the examiner would indicate that by recording '(B)'. In that same eye, when the examiner employs indentation gonioscopy and determines that the site of actual insertion of the iris to the inner wall of the eye is actually posterior to the scleral spur, so that the ciliary body is visible, that aspect of the angle would be designated with a capital D. Thus, the initial portion of the description of the angle would be (B)D.

The next characteristic is the angular approach, measured just anterior to

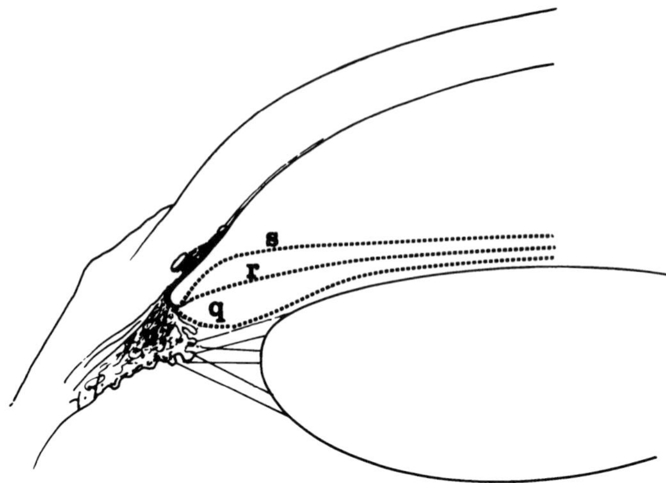

Fig. 10. Characterization of the curvature of the peripheral iris. One of the three configurational aspects of the angle recess. The peripheral iris may have an anterior convexity, as indicated schematically by s. In most individuals there is little curvature (r). A posterior concavity is signified q. s = steep, r = regular, and q = 'queer.'

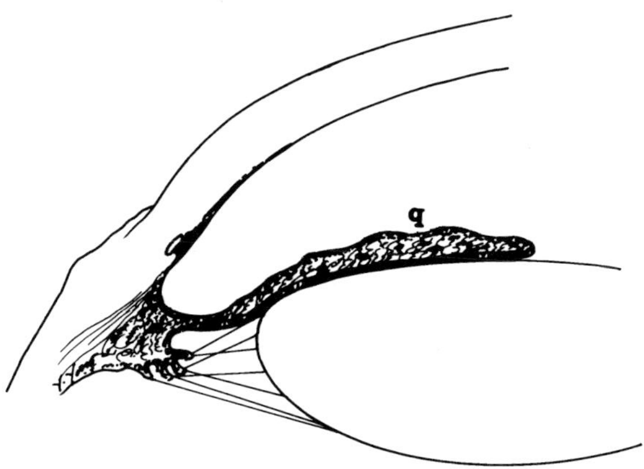

Fig. 11. A posteriorly concave bowing of the peripheral iris is designated 'q'. This can be artifactually produced by indentation.

Schwalbe's line (Fig. 9). This is recorded as a simple number indicating the degrees of the angle that separates the tangents from the corneal endothelial surface and the anterior surface of the iris. In the example just given (Fig. 8), in which there was a marked anterior iris bowing, the angle is slightly narrower than usual, perhaps 25°. Thus, the examiner would record the number 25, and the grading would be (B)D25.

The last descriptor of the iris configuration refers to the configuration of the peripheral portion of the iris (Fig. 10). Again, in the example given, if the iris bowed anteriorly very steeply and then flattened out into a plateau, so that there was a steep, sudden anterior convexity of the iris, that would be designated by the examiner as an 's' configuration (Fig. 8). In contrast, a posterior bowing is called 'q' (Fig. 11).

Putting these all together, the angle just described (Fig. 8) would then be recorded as (B)D25s. This would completely describe the configuration.

It helps to draw a circle, and then indicate the angle configuration at one point. If the angle configuration is the same over 360°, one can simply draw an arrow around the circle indicating that. If, on the other hand, the angle is different in different areas, one places the appropriate descriptors in the appropriate positions on the circle. Consider the angle just described, which has a sudden anterior convexity and a slightly narrow approach. Consider that this occurs just superiorly. Inferiorly, without indentation, it is possible to see the ciliary body, the angular approach is deeper, around 30°, but there is an anterior convexity, similar to that seen superiorly. In this eye, then, the examiner would draw a circle, and at the top of the circle would write (B)D25s, and at the bottom of the circle would write D30s.

The last descriptor routinely used in all cases relates to the amount of pigmentation of the posterior trabecular meshwork from 0, meaning no pigmentation, to 4+ meaning the most intense pigmentation imaginable. If the amount of pigmentation of the posterior trabecular meshwork in the eye just examined were considered to be just detectable, that is, 1+ in all four quadrants, then, the standard description of the angle would be (B)D25s1+pTm to describe the superior angle, and D30s1+pTm to describe the inferior angle.

Treatment

Proper treatment depends upon proper diagnosis. Using proper gonioscopic techniques, including indentation gonioscopy and considering the factors mentioned in Table 1 should permit a proper diagnosis.

In years past, whether or not to perform a surgical peripheral iridectomy required a well-considered evaluation of many factors. Today, there are only four really significant considerations: *1*. Is the angle probably occludable? *2*. Is the mechanism of angle closure related to pupillary block? *3*. Does the person planning to perform the iridotomy have the equipment and the appropriate skills to perform the iridotomy properly? *4*. Does the patient wish to have an iridotomy performed after learning what is involved?

Is the angle occludable?

The answer to whether the angle is occludable cannot be given with definite certainty until spontaneous angle closure has developed. When spontaneous angle closure has developed, some damage has already occurred, and clearly the goal is to prevent such damage. Factors that increase the likelihood of the angle closing are an anterior insertion of the iris, a narrow angularity, a peripheral anterior bowing, and a flaccid iris. The more of these factors are present, the more likely angle closure is to occur. For example, a 'C' angle, in which the iris inserts just posterior to the scleral spur, is not likely to occlude in a brown eye with a 30° approach. However, a 'C' angle in association with a 10° approach and a thin blue iris is at high risk for closing. Angles in which the angular approach is narrower than 15° are at risk. Angles with an 's' configuration are at risk. A 'C10s' angle is at great risk for occlusion. There have been no prospective, longitudinal studies to determine which characteristics of the anterior chamber angle are certain to lead to an-

Table 3. Guidelines suggesting an anterior chamber angle is occludable

Angle characteristic	Level of risk of angle closure			
	low	moderate	high	'certain'
Iris insertion	E or D	C	B	A
Angular approach	>20	15	10	0
Peripheral iris configuration	q or r	--	s	--
Examples	E40q	E20r	E10s	E0s
	D30r	D10r	D5r	D0r
	D30s	D15s	D0s	
	C30r	C15r	C10r	C0r
			(B)C10r	(B)C0r
			(A)D10r	(A)D0r

gle closure. However, consideration of the nature of the anterior chamber angle of the fellow eyes of patients who have had spontaneous angle closure provides good clues[5,9]. Some guidelines are indicated in Table 3.

Is the mechanism of the narrow angle related to pupillary block?

It is important to determine whether the mechanism of angle closure is related to pupillary block. If it is not, clearly a peripheral iridotomy will not be of help. The type of configuration in which there is a marked sudden anterior bowing of the iris which then flattens out as the iris moves towards the pupil appears to be anatomically determined. This so-called 'plateau iris', best described by Tornquist[26], may be related to an abnormality of the ciliary processes pushing the peripheral iris forward[27]. Diagnostic ultrasound may possibly be of some help in discriminating the plateau iris and the anterior chamber that is narrow, but in which the narrowness is not caused by pupillary block. The other mechanisms for a narrow anterior chamber angle, as mentioned in Table 1, should in most cases be fairly easily diagnosed on the basis of other findings. For example, it should be clear that the eye in which the anterior chamber angle becomes narrower after the instillation of pilocarpine may have an anterior displacement of the ciliary body as the inciting cause for the narrowing anterior chamber angle.

Can the iridotomy be properly performed?

The third issue relates to the technique of performance of a laser iridotomy[28]. These include obtaining an appropriate informed consent, making sure that the indications are appropriate and that the iridotomy is needed, performing the iridotomy under the upper lid, keeping the iridotomy tiny, making sure that the iridotomy is patent, ensuring that posterior synechias do not develop postoperatively, and ascertaining that the iridotomy works to prevent angle-closure glaucoma.

An iridotomy is appropriate if *1.* the angle is considered occludable, *2.* the patient wishes to have the iridotomy performed, and *3.* the iridotomy can be competently performed.

Does the patient wish to have the iridotomy performed?

Appropriate informed consent includes warning the patient of the development of a ghost image, of the extent to which it is likely that the intraocular pressure will rise following the iridotomy, and the likelihood of success. If the iridotomy cannot be placed underneath the lid, the likelihood of a ghost image is considerable. Even when the iridotomy is under the lid, such an image may be bothersome. This image is caused by the entry of light into the eye through the iridotomy, and the tear film can serve as a prism to refract the light into the eye even when the iridotomy is under the lid. The functional ability of the trabecular meshwork is a factor in determining the likelihood of pressure rise following the iridotomy. Patients with the exfoliation syndrome, with the pigmentary dispersion syndrome, and especially patients with either of those conditions in whom the pressure is elevated preoperatively, are at greater risk for developing significant pressure spikes following the iridotomy. Patients in whom the optic disc is already cupped are at greater risk for developing further disc damage if a pressure spike develops. It is fair to tell patients with narrow angles caused by non-inflammatory relative pupillary block that it is virtually certain that their iridotomy will remain open.

Except in patients with pupillary block glaucomas such as those that occur in association with posterior synechias or pupillary block with anterior chamber intraocular lenses, there is no reason to perform an iridotomy in any position except the superior pole of the eye. The goal should be to try to place the iridotomy under the upper lid. This is not possible in all cases, since some individuals have upper lids that do not cover the cornea at the 12 o'clock position. However, in most individuals it is possible to position the iridotomy under the upper lid.

The iridotomy need not be large. As long as the opening is full thickness, virtually any visible hole will be adequate to allow enough aqueous to flow from the posterior to the anterior chamber that pupillary block will not develop.

The iridotomy must be patent. It is not adequate to guess at this. A transillumination defect in the iris is not proof of a fully patent iridotomy.

Posterior synechias tend to develop after iridotomies performed with argon lasers. Such synechias are rare in patients in whom the iridotomy is performed with an Nd:YAG laser. However, in patients who have been receiving miotics for many years and in whom the pupil is small and non-reactive, posterior synechias may develop even after a Nd:YAG laser. Therefore, it is essential to dilate the pupils of such patients and to use appropriate anti-inflammatory agents.

It is important to determine whether or not the iridotomy has accomplished its goals, specifically, deepening of the anterior chamber and prevention of closure of the anterior chamber angle.

Unfortunately, there is no artificial way to test for this, because the so-called provocative tests are not accurate imitators of what happens spontaneously. Following the iridotomy, the eye should be examined gonioscopically and compared with the preoperative appearance. If there has been no change in the angle appearance, then either the iridotomy is not patent or the cause of the narrow angle is not relative pupillary block. In either case, the patient will not have benefited from the treatment. If it is clear that the iridotomy is in fact patent and the angle is not changed in appearance, then it is highly unlikely that relative pupillary block is the cause of the narrow angle, and, consequently, the iridotomy cannot be expected to prevent angle closure from developing. It is helpful to dilate the patient with phenylephrine 2.5%, one drop, to determine if pupillary dilatation will induce angle closure and elevation of intraocular pressure. Cycloplegics such as tropicamide paralyze the sphincters of the iris and the ciliary body, allowing the dilators to work. Consequently, the cycloplegic agents have a minimal effect on increasing pupillary block. Furthermore, because of the paralysis of the ciliary body sphincter, they tend to deepen the anterior chamber angle in phakic patients. Therefore, a cycloplegic agent is not an appropriate agent to use in trying to induce angle closure. In contrast, a cycloplegic agent is the appropriate drug to use to dilate a pupil in a patient in whom one wishes to avoid inducing an angle closure. The cycloplegic does cause angle jamming and can include angle closure in patients in whom there is a plateau iris mechanism. There is usually a small rise in intraocular pressure caused by the cycloplegics, even when the angle remains open. Therefore, a small rise in pressure following dilatation with a cycloplegic is not a sign of angle closure. In contrast, mydriatic agents such as phenylephrine stimulate the dilator, but do not paralyze the sphincters. Consequently, the dilator pulls against the sphincter, increasing the degree of relative pupillary block and predisposing to a relative-pupillary-block-induced angle closure. Additionally, the mydriatics do not cause the anterior chamber to deepen. Consequently, mydriatic agents are more likely to induce angle closure in patients in whom there is a relatively pupillary block mechanism of angle closure. As such, they are not appropriate to use for dilatation purposes when trying to avoid angle closure, but they are appropriate to use following peripheral iridotomy in order to test the effect of the iridotomy. As with the cycloplegic agents, mydriatics such as phenylephrine can cause angle jamming and therefore can cause an elevation of intraocular pressure in patients with a plateau iris. Unlike cycloplegics, however, they tend to cause the intraocular pressure to fall slightly. Following an iridotomy, then, in order to dilate the pupil, prevent posterior synechias, and to test for the effectiveness of the iridotomy, it is appropriate to utilize a mydriatic agent such as phenylephrine.

The third factor relates to the technical performance of the peripheral iridotomy. An Nd:YAG laser is preferable, as it is less likely to produce posterior synechias, iritis, retinal burns, and localized cataract. The instrument should be used in the Q-switched mode, and, if an option is possible, in the 'multimode'. Appropriate power varies from instrument to instrument, but 7 mJ with a run of three bursts is an appropriate setting for most eyes.

Prior to performing the actual iridotomy patients should be told that they will feel the iridotomy and that they may jump, but that will not affect the procedure. The pupil of the eye being treated should be made miotic with pilocarpine. If there is a likelihood of pressure or of a pressure spike causing damage, the eye should be pretreated with an intraocular-pressure-lowering agent such as apraclonidine. Pilocarpine itself may be adequate. The surgeon should be sure that the patient's general health is adequate to withstand the minimal trauma of an iridotomy, and the intraocular pressure preoperatively should be known and documented.

The oculars on the laser should be adjusted to the surgeon's refractive error. A magnifying contact lens is placed on the eye and the patient requested to look down. The aiming beam is then focused meticulously on the iris surface, in the depths of a crypt if that is possible. This is done at the 12:00 o'clock position. Once the focus is entirely satisfactory, the joy stick is advanced so that the focus is approximately one-third of the way into the depth of the iris stroma. The laser is activated, and in most cases an iridotomy should be accomplished with one burst of power. In thick irides, two bursts may be necessary. Very rarely is it necessary to use three bursts. Patency is demonstrated by a sudden flow of pigment from the posterior into the anterior chamber associated with immediate deepening of the iris periphery.

Following the iridotomy, the intraocular pressure is checked and a topical steroid utilized for four to seven days.

The major technical mistakes are not having the ocular adjusted, not having the pupil miotic, not placing the iridotomy under the lid, allowing posterior synechias to develop, and not gonioscoping the patient following iridotomy to make sure that the iridotomy has done its job.

The timing of the iridotomy is important. Another major mistake is trying to perform a laser iridotomy when the cornea is insufficiently clear. This only results in traumatizing the cornea, frustrating the ophthalmologist, and frightening the patient. In a patient who has an acute angle-closure glaucoma, it is typical for the cornea to become thicker and hazier as the intraocular pressure falls. Where this is the case, it is best to wait a day or more, and perform the iridotomy after the cornea has cleared. Once the attack has been fully broken, it is not usually difficult to maintain a low intraocular pressure with aqueous suppressants. A fairly sure sign that the attack has been broken fully is that the intraocular pressure in the eye with the angle closure is lower than it is in the other eye. In such cases, it is usually appropriate to perform the peripheral iridotomy on the fellow eye, which has not had the attack of angle-closure glaucoma, and to defer the iridotomy on the affected eye until the cornea has cleared.

It is certainly possible to perform a laser iridotomy with an argon laser, but the complications are more serious, and the technique is acceptable only when an Nd:YAG laser is not available. However, in a patient who is on anticoagulants or who has a bleeding problem, it is frequently helpful to pretreat with an argon laser that area in which the iridotomy is planned to be made with the Nd:YAG laser.

The peripheral iridotomy must be fully penetrating, *i.e.*, all layers of the iris must be penetrated. It is not adequate to hope that one has achieved this. The surgeon must see the characteristic gush of aqueous coming from the posterior into the anterior chamber, carrying with it pigment. As long as the iridotomy is fully patent, it will almost never close in an eye in which there is not an inflammatory component. It is not necessary and, indeed, it is not appropriate, to enlarge a patent iridotomy.

Inflammatory pupillary block in association with an iris bombe requires a different approach. In such a case, multiple iridotomies should be performed. There is often one area in which the iris bombe is especially prominent, but it is usually not adequate to perform the iridotomy merely in that area. There are often isolated, loculated areas of pupillary block, and the iris will not flatten completely unless each one of the individual areas is treated with peripheral iridotomy. Additionally, such iridotomies need to be larger, since they tend to close off.

References

1. Becker B, Christensen RE: Water-drinking and tonography in the diagnosis of glaucoma. Arch Ophthalmol 56:321-326, 1956
2. Grant WM: Tonography: past, present and future. Ophthalmology 85:252-258, 1978
3. The answer to the question "What is the single most important aspect of evaluation of the glaucoma patient", asked at the Wills Eye Hospital Annual Conference in 1963, was 'tonography'
4. Forbes M: Gonioscopy with corneal indentation: a method for distinguishing between appositional closure and synechial closure. Arch Ophthalmol 76:488, 1966
5. Spaeth GL: Gonioscopy: uses old and new: the inheritance of occludable angles. Ophthalmology 85:222, 1978
6. Ritch R, Krupin T, Shields MB: Angle-closure glaucoma. In: The Glaucomas, 2nd Edn. St Louis, MO: Mosby 1996
7. Tielsch JM, Sommer A, Katz J, Royall RM, Quigley HA, Javitt J: Racial variations in the prevalence

of primary open-angle glaucoma: the Baltimore Eye Survey. JAMA 266:369-473, 1991

8. Mapstone R: Closed-angle glaucoma in eyes with non-shallow anterior chambers. Trans Ophthalmol Soc UK 101:218-220, 1981
9. Benedikt O: Prophylastische Iridektomie nach Winkelblockglaukom am Partnerauge. Klin Mbl Augenheilk 156:80-83, 1970
10. Swan KC: Iridectomy for closed (narrow)-angle glaucoma: anatomic considerations. The XXVI DeSchweinitz Lecture. Am J Ophthalmol 61:601-619, 1966
11. Spaeth GL: Classification and management of patients with narrow or closed angles. Ophthalmic Surg 9:39-44, 1978
12. Lowe RF: Aetiology of the anatomical basis for primary angle-closure glaucoma. Br J Ophthalmol 54:161-169, 1970
13. Clemmesen V, Alsbirk PH: Primary angle-closure glaucoma (a.c.g.) in Greenland. Acta Ophthalmol (Kbh) 49:47-58, 1971
14. Oh Y, Minelli S, Spaeth GL et al: The anterior chamber angle is different in different racial groups: a gonioscopic study. Eye 8:104-108, 1994
15. Becker B, Shaffer RN: Diagnosis and Therapy of the Glaucomas, pp 29-55. St Louis, MO: CV Mosby 1961
16. Barkan O, Boyle SF, Maisler S: On the genesis of glaucoma: an improved method based on slit-lamp microscopy of the angle of the anterior chamber. Am J Ophthalmol 19:209, 1936
17. Francois J: Gonioscopy in primary glaucoma. In: Duke-Elder S (ed) Glaucoma: A Symposium. Springfield, IL: Charles C Thomas 1955
18. Gorin G, Posner A: Slit-lamp Gonioscopy. Baltimore, MD: Williams & Wilkins 1957
19. Kronfeld PC, McGarry HI: Present limits of gonioscopy. Am J Ophthalmol 27:147, 1944
20. Shaffer RN, Schwartz A: Gonioscopy. Surv Ophthalmol 2:389, 1957
21. Sugar HS: The Glaucomas, 2nd Edn. New York, NY: Paul B Hoeber Inc 1957
22. Troncoso MU: A Treatise on Gonioscopy. Philadelphia, PA: FA Davis Co 1947
23. Chandler PA, Grant WM: Lectures on Glaucoma, pp 54-107. Philadelphia, PA: Lea & Febiger 1965
24. Spaeth GL: The normal development of the human anterior chamber angle: a new system of descriptive grading. Trans Ophthalmol Soc UK 91:709-739, 1971
25. Spaeth GL, Schwartz LW, Brown GC: Laser Therapy of the Anterior Segment: A Practical Approach. Thorofare, NJ: Slack Inc 1984
26. Tornquist R: Angle-closure glaucoma in an eye with a plateau type of iris. Acta Ophthalmol (Kbh) 36:413, 1958
27. Pavlin CJ, Ritch R, Foster FS: Ultrasound biomicroscopy in plateau iris syndrome. Am J Ophthalmol 113:381-395, 1992
28. Liebmann JM, Ritch R: Laser iridotomy. Ophthalmic Surg Lasers 27:209-227, 1996
29. Wishart PK, Spaeth GL, Poryzees EM: Anterior chamber angle in the exfoliation syndrome. Br J Ophthalmol 69:103-107, 1985
30. Ritch R: Exfoliation syndrome and occludable angles. Trans Am Ophthalmol Soc 92:845-944, 1994
31. Scheie HG: Width and pigmentation of the angle of the anterior chamber in systems of grading by gonioscopy. Arch Ophthalmol 58:510, 1957

Argon laser trabeculoplasty

Michael A. Kass

Department of Ophthalmology & Visual Sciences, Washington University School of Medicine, St. Louis, MO, USA

Introduction

In 1974 Worthen and Wickham[1] reported substantial intraocular pressure (IOP) reductions when argon laser energy was applied to the outflow structures of glaucomatous eyes. Some of their patients had IOP decreases for as long as a year after laser treatment and some were able to avoid filtering surgery. In 1979, Wise and Witter[2] reported mean IOP reductions of more than 10 mmHg following argon laser trabeculoplasty in patients with open-angle glaucoma. Over the next few years this report was confirmed by a number of investigators[3-6]. Shortly thereafter, argon laser trabeculoplasty started to be widely used in the treatment of open-angle glaucoma.

Technique

The technique that I use for argon laser trabeculoplasty includes a spot size of 50 µm, a duration of 0.1 seconds and a power of 400 to 1000 mW, adjusted to a visible tissue reaction. Forty to 50 treatments are given to one-half of the circumference of the angle, aiming the beam at the anterior border of the pigmented meshwork. While I espouse a specific technique, it is clear from reviewing the literature that argon laser trabeculoplasty is remarkably technique-insensitive. Good results have been obtained with a variety of parameters including the following:

Spot size

Most clinicians utilize a 50 µm spot size, as recommended in the paper by Wise and Witter[2]. However, there is relatively little research to suggest that this is the ideal spot size. It is important, however, to keep in mind that changing this spot size would have a major impact on the power density.

Address for correspondence: Michael A. Kass, MD, Department of Ophthalmology & Visual Sciences, Washington University School of Medicine, St. Louis, MO 314-362-5713, USA

Peril to the Nerve – Glaucoma and Clinical Neuro-Ophthalmology, pp. 141–152
Proceedings of the 45th Annual Symposium of the New Orleans Academy of
Ophthalmology, New Orleans, LA, USA, April 25-28, 1996
edited by Barry J. Leader and Jonathan C. Calkwood
© 1998 Kugler Publications, The Hague/The Netherlands

Duration

Most surgeons utilize a laser duration of 0.1 seconds, as mentioned above. However, other surgeons have utilized 0.2 seconds with good results[7,8].

Visible endpoint

Many investigators alter the energy level to achieve a visible treatment result, usually either blanching of the pigmented meshwork or small bubble formation at the site of impact. However, other investigators report satisfactory results utilizing the same energy level for all patients[9-11].

Number of burns

Most clinicians employ 50 or 100 burns per session. However, one group reported substantial IOP reductions with as few as ten burns per session[12].

Portion of the angle treatment

Most studies comparing argon laser treatment to one-half of the angle *versus* treating the entire circumference of the angle have noted similar pressure responses[5,13-19]. Some clinicians have noted good IOP responses to treating as little as one-quarter of the angle, although the effect appears to be somewhat less than would be obtained from treating one-half of the angle[20-22]. Some clinicians believe that IOP reductions are more long lived after 360° laser treatment. The results seem similar whether laser trabeculoplasty is delivered in two sessions of 180° each or in one session of 360°[23].

Location of the burn

Most surgeons aim the laser beam at the anterior border of the pigmented meshwork. However, other clinicians treat the center of the meshwork or even the posterior meshwork along the scleral spur. While all these approaches produce similar IOP reductions[12,24-26], posterior treatments are associated with more frequent and more severe post-laser pressure rises[12,27] and more extensive peripheral anterior synechiae formation[28,29].

Wavelength

Most clinicians use the blue-green laser for trabeculoplasty. However, others have reported good results using other wavelengths, including green[30,31], krypton red[32], neodymium YAG in the thermal mode[33-35], and the diode laser[36-41].

Mechanism of action

Argon laser trabeculoplasty diminishes the resistance to aqueous egress. Numerous studies have documented increased tonographic facility of outflow following laser treatment[3,5,6,18,42-45]. In addition, fluorophotometry reveals that aqueous humor formation is unchanged following this procedure[46,47].

Histological examination of human or animal eyes after laser argon trabeculoplasty demonstrates necrosis of cells and disruption of the trabecular beams[48,49].

However, argon laser trabeculoplasty does not produce full thickness direct passages from the anterior chamber to Schlemm's canal[50]. Studies demonstrate widened intratrabecular spaces with juxtacanicular tissue herniated into Schlemm's canal and increased passage of tracers through the meshwork into Schlemm's canal[51].

The theories to explain the therapeutic effect of argon laser trabeculoplasty can be grouped into two categories: *1.* a mechanical effect on the outflow channels and *2.* an effect on cellular proliferation and metabolism in the meshwork.

Mechanical effect

Wise and Witter first proposed that argon laser energy mechanically tightens the trabecular meshwork, thereby increasing outflow facility[2]. They proposed that the laser burns contract localized areas of the meshwork, thereby pulling open the surrounding areas that were not directly affected by the energy. Wise has compared this type of treatment to a 'face-lift' for the meshwork.

Cell synthesis and metabolism

Using human and animal eyes, a number of authors have noted increased cell division in the trabecular meshwork following trabeculoplasty[52-57]. Most of the cell division is found in the anterior, non-filtering portion of the meshwork. Over several days, the new trabecular cells migrate throughout the tissue[54]. The cells increase the turnover of the extracellular matrix[58,59] and are actively phagocytic[60].

At this time, there is insufficient evidence to support either or both of these theories. Additional work will be necessary to determine the mechanism of action of argon laser trabeculoplasty.

Complications

A variety of complications have been reported after argon laser trabeculoplasty (Table 1).

Table 1. Complications of argon laser trabeculoplasty

Elevated intraocular pressure
Loss of vision
Formation of peripheral anterior synechiae
Iridocyclitis
Trabecular precipitates
Hyphema/hemorrhage into the trabecular meshwork
Corneal burns
Syncope
Encapsulated blebs after subsequent filtering surgery
Higher failure rate after subsequent filtering surgery
Cataract formation or progression
Acute angle closure glaucoma
Sector palsy of the iris sphincter muscle
Herpes simplex keratitis

Most studies report that 20-25% of patients undergoing argon laser trabeculoplasty develop substantial elevations of IOP within the first six hours[42,61-63]. The frequency with which this complication occurs depends on the definition of the pressure rise and the frequency of IOP measurements. In the Glaucoma Laser Trial, 34% of the patients had a 5 mmHg or greater rise in IOP on either the first or second treatment session, and 12% of the patients had a 10 mmHg rise[64]. Typically, the elevated pressure lasts a few hours, but it can last as long as weeks following the procedure. The early pressure rise is more common in patients who have poor outflow and heavy pigmentation of the trabecular meshwork[65]. The pressure rise is also more common when the surgeon places the treatment burns posteriorly[12,27], uses higher energy levels[66,67], and treats the entire circumference of the meshwork. Some of the concern about acute elevations of IOP has been reduced by the use of α_2 agonists such as apraclonidine[68]. It is clear that treatment of patients with these agents markedly reduces the frequency and severity of the postoperative pressure rises. Apraclonidine is far more effective than other drugs such as topical beta blockers, pilocarpine[69], carbonic anhydrase inhibitors[70], and non-steroidal anti-inflammatory agents[71]. The frequency and severity of post-laser pressure rises is similar in a 360° trabeculoplasty using apraclonidine as in a 180° treatment without apraclonidine[72]. Holmwood and co-workers[73] have reported that apraclonidine instilled immediately after laser treatment is as effective as apraclonidine instilled immediately before and after laser treatment. In a similar fashion, brimonidine (another α_2 agonist) is effective in reducing IOP spikes after laser trabeculoplasty, when administered immediately before or after treatment[74,75].

When IOP is markedly elevated after argon laser trabeculoplasty, the usual treatment includes a topical beta blocker, a topical α_2 agonist, a carbonic anhydrase inhibitor, and often an oral hyperosmotic agent such as glycerine. There is anecdotal information that a strong cocktail is as effective as oral glycerine in treating post-laser spikes (personal communication: H. Dunbar Hoskins).

Peripheral anterior synechiae have been reported in 12% to 47% of patients following argon laser trabeculoplasty[5,6,28,64]. Synechiae formation is related to the use of higher power and posterior placement of the burns[28,29]. Some investigators have noted poorer success rates when synechiae form[28,76], but most others noted no association[42,64,77].

Iridocyclitis is common after argon laser trabeculoplasty[5,6]. Generally, this inflammation is mild and self limited[5]. Occasionally uveitis can be quite severe and lead to extensive synechiae formation[6]. Post-laser inflammation is treated by topical corticosteroids and non-steroidal anti-inflammatory agents. Using a laser flare-call meter, Mermoud and co-workers[78] noted that inflammation peaked two days after laser treatment. Inflammation was more common in eyes with exfoliation syndrome or pigmentary glaucoma than with primary open-angle glaucoma.

A number of investigators have questioned whether performing argon laser trabeculoplasty prejudices the results of future filtering surgery. There are a few reports that encapsulated blebs are more common when filtering surgery is performed in eyes that previously had received argon laser trabeculoplasty[79,80]. Readers should be cautious in accepting this conclusion because it is based upon historical rather than concurrent controls and has not been confirmed by other studies[81,82]. In addition, some investigators have questioned whether the rate of success of filtering surgery might be diminished by argon laser trabeculoplasty[83,84]. However, other studies have not confirmed this impression[85,86].

Results

Most studies have assessed the impact of argon laser trabeculoplasty by calculating IOP reductions. In many studies, argon laser trabeculoplasty reduces IOP by 20% to 30%, as measured six months after treatment[17,42]. Patients with higher preoperative IOPs seem to obtain larger percentages and absolute reductions in pressure[10,42,87-92]. In this way, laser trabeculoplasty seems to act more like a drug than a filtering operation. Laser treatment also flattens diurnal pressure curves[93]. Greenidge and co-workers reported a 25% decrease in mean peak IOP eight weeks following laser trabeculoplasty[93].

Following argon laser trabeculoplasty, the number of anti-glaucoma medications can often be reduced without sacrificing IOP control[17,94,95]. Patients may be able to stop taking systemic carbonic anhydrase inhibitors or miotics that are causing annoying symptoms. However, it is rare to stop all medication after laser treatment, assuming that the treatment was performed in patients receiving maximum tolerated medical therapy.

Almost all studies show a decreasing effect of argon laser trabeculoplasty over time, whether measured by mean IOP reduction or by the percentage of patients reaching a predetermined pressure goal (Table 2). As an example, Spaeth and Baez reported that laser treatment was successful in controlling glaucoma in 81% of patients at one year but only in 5% of patients at ten years[99].

Table 2. Success of argon laser trabeculoplasty over time

Author	1 year	3 years	5-6 years	7-8 years	10 years
Moulin and Haut[96]	81%		48%	17%	11%
Shingleton *et al.*[97]	77%		49%		32%
Spiegel *et al.*[98]			22%		
Spaeth and Baez[99]	81%		35%		5%
Detry-Morel and Kallay[100]	87%		33%		
Adachi *et al.*[101]			40%		27%
Ticho and Nesher[102]		70%	55%		
Lund and Zink[103]	90%	60%			
Wise[104]			56%		70%
Lotti *et al.*[105]	78%	71%	61%		40%

There is little long-term data on the effect of laser trabeculoplasty on visual function. Most short-term studies show no effect of laser treatment on visual function, or report a small decline in visual function over time without concurrent untreated controls. Spaeth noted a correlation between the IOP reduction following laser trabeculoplasty and visual field improvement[106]. In the Glaucoma Laser Trial it was reported that eyes treated with laser first had lower IOPs and better visual field status than the eyes treated initially with medication[107].

As is typical in glaucoma management, the most important factor influencing the success of argon laser trabeculoplasty is the underlying diagnosis. Some forms of glaucoma, such as primary open-angle glaucoma, are quite responsive to laser treatment. In contrast, other forms of glaucoma, such as juvenile onset glaucoma, are much less responsive (Table 3).

Table 3. Glaucoma diagnosis and intraocular pressure reduction after argon laser trabeculoplasty

Diagnosis	*Comments*
Good to excellent response to laser treatment	
Primary open-angle glaucoma	
Pigmentary glaucoma	
Exfoliation syndrome	Effect may be lost rapidly
Moderate response to laser treatment	
Low-tension glaucoma	
Glaucoma in pseudophakic eyes	
Angle-closure glaucoma	If more than 50% of angle is open
Combined mechanism glaucoma	
Fair to poor response to laser treatment	
Glaucoma with active uveitis	
Angle recession and glaucoma	
Corticosteroid glaucoma	
Glaucoma in aphakic eyes	
Congenital/juvenile glaucoma	High rate of post-treatment complications

A number of putative risk factors for failure of argon laser trabeculoplasty have been evaluated including the following:

1. *Age*: younger patients appear to respond less to laser treatment.

2. *Race*: most evidence suggests that Caucasians, Orientals and African-Americans have similar responses to argon laser trabeculoplasty.

3. *Pigmentation*: there appears to be no major difference in the response to laser treatment according to angle pigmentation.

4. *Preoperative level of IOP*: the higher the preoperative IOP generally the greater the reduction in pressure with laser treatment. In most patients, the response of one eye to laser treatment is correlated with the results in the fellow eye[108,109].

5. *Stage of glaucoma*: the stage of glaucoma is not thought to play a major role in the response to laser treatment[104,110].

6. *Previous surgery*: if a substantial portion of the angle is open, the results of laser trabeculoplasty are generally good[62,89,94,111]. Aphakic eyes are less responsive to laser treatment than phakic eyes, as are eyes that have undergone multiple previous surgeries.

7. *Previous penetrating keratoplasty*: the response is good provided that a sufficient portion of the angle is open[112].

A number of clinicians have attempted to retreat the angle following previous 360° argon laser trabeculoplasty. If a patient had a poor response to the initial laser treatment, additional laser treatments are of limited or no value. If patients had a good response to the initial laser treatment but have lost this effect over time, repeating the treatment has been reported to be effective by some investigators[113-116]. However, other investigators have noted that repeat treatment is less effective than the initial treatment[117-119]. Some observers have also noted an increased rate of complications following repeat treatment.

When to do an argon laser trabeculoplasty

When first introduced, argon laser trabeculoplasty was used as an intermediate step between maximum tolerated medical therapy and filtering surgery. As clinicians gained experience and confidence with the procedure, the indications were liberalized. Now many clinicians utilize argon laser trabeculoplasty before introducing medications (*i.e.*, miotics or systemic carbonic anhydrase inhibitors) that are associated with bothersome side-effects. Argon laser trabeculoplasty can also be utilized in patients who do not tolerate medication well or who admit to poor compliance.

The proper use of argon laser trabeculoplasty takes into consideration the patient's age, the type of glaucoma, the level of IOP desired, and patient preference. In general, older patients respond well to argon laser trabeculoplasty. Furthermore, a reduction of IOP for three to five years may preserve vision for the lifetime of an older individual. In contrast, younger patients are generally less responsive to argon laser trabeculoplasty, and reduction of pressure for a few years is not an adequate solution. As indicated earlier in this chapter, some forms of glaucoma are very responsive to argon laser trabeculoplasty whereas others respond poorly. The choice to do laser treatment in a patient with a less responsive form of glaucoma depends upon whether there is a good therapeutic alternative. If a patient has a form of glaucoma that is generally less responsive to laser treatment, it may be more effective and cost effective to proceed directly to filtering surgery, assuming a good prognosis for the procedure. Argon laser trabeculoplasty generally does not produce low levels of IOP, unless the pressure was low prior to treatment. If low pressures are deemed desirable because of advanced damage or progression at modest levels of pressure, then filtering surgery is likely to be a better choice.

There have been a number of reports of argon laser trabeculoplasty as primary therapy in open-angle glaucoma[120-125]. All these studies show a good initial response to laser treatment which, in fact, may be superior to that noted in patients who have already received extensive pre-laser medical treatment[126]. However, most of these studies are short-term and indicate that, by two to five years, at least 50% of the patients can no longer be controlled and require medical therapy[107,123,125]. At present, I rarely employ laser trabeculoplasty as primary treatment, except in patients who are unwilling or unable to utilize medication.

A number of studies have attempted to compare laser treatment to either medical treatment and/or filtering surgery[127-130]. Typically, filtering surgery produces lower IOP than the other approaches. However, the various treatments seem to have similar effects on visual function. In the Glaucoma Laser Trial, as mentioned previously, eyes treated with laser first had slightly lower IOPs and slightly better preservation of visual field than did eyes treated with medication first[107]. The Advanced Glaucoma Intervention Study (AGIS) compares the results of argon laser trabeculoplasty *versus* filtering surgery[131]. The results of this trial should have a substantial impact on the use of argon laser trabeculoplasty in the future. Migdal and co-workers have reported that patients who underwent filtering surgery had lower IOPs and less deterioration of the visual fields than patients in the laser-treated group. In this study, the patients in the medically treated group fared the poorest[132].

Summary

Argon laser trabeculoplasty is a relatively effective and safe method for reducing intraocular pressure (IOP). Typically, this treatment produces a 20%-30% decrease in IOP in favorable forms of glaucoma. However, the effect does decrease over subsequent years. Despite studies indicating the efficacy of argon laser trabeculoplasty as primary therapy, it is still my policy to use this treatment when well-tolerated medication fails to reduce IOP to desired levels. Until the results of clinical trials such as AGIS are available, the choice between argon laser trabeculoplasty and filtering surgery depends upon the patient's age, the type of glaucoma, the IOP level desired and patient preference.

Acknowledgment

Supported in part by an unrestricted grant from Prevent Blindness America, NY.

References

1. Worthen DM, Wickham MG: Argon laser trabeculotomy. Trans Am Acad Ophthalmol Otolaryngol 78:371-375, 1974
2. Wise JB, Witter SL: Argon laser therapy for open-angle glaucoma: a pilot study. Arch Ophthalmol 97:319-322, 1979
3. Pohjanpelto P: Argon laser treatment of the anterior chamber angle for increased intraocular pressure. Acta Ophthalmol (Kbh) 59:211-220, 1981
4. Sutton GE, Christensen GR, Records RE: Trabeculotomy with continuous argon laser. Trans Ophthalmol Soc UK 101:118-120, 1981
5. Schwartz AL, Whitten ME, Bleiman B, Martin D: Argon laser trabeculoplasty in uncontrolled phakic open-angle glaucoma. Ophthalmology 88:203-212, 1981
6. Wilensky JT, Jampol LM: Laser therapy for open angle glaucoma. Ophthalmology 88:213-217, 1981
7. Blondeau P, Roberge JF, Asselin Y: Long-term results of low power, long duration laser trabeculoplasty. Am J Ophthalmol 104:339-342, 1987
8. Hugkulstone CE: The effects of different energy levels in argon laser trabeculoplasty. Acta Ophthalmol (Kbh) 67:271-274, 1989
9. Rouhiainen H, Terasvirta M: The laser power needed for optimum results in argon laser trabeculoplasty. Acta Ophthalmol (Kbh) 64:254-257, 1986
10. Thomas JV: Laser trabeculoplasty. In: Belcher CD, Thomas JV, Simmons RJ (eds) Photocoagulation in Glaucoma and Anterior Segment Disease, pp 61-86. Baltimore, MD: Williams & Wilkins 1984
11. Wilensky JT: Laser trabeculoplasty: technique. In: Wilensky JT (ed) Laser therapy in Glaucoma, pp 18-19. East Norwalk, CT: Appleton-Century-Crofts 1985
12. Douglas GR, Wijsman K: Effect of laser trabeculoplasty on intraocular pressure in the medically untreated eye. Can J Ophthalmol 22:157-160, 1987
13. Weinreb RN, Ruderman J, Juster R, Wilensky JT: Influence of the number of laser burns administered on the early results of argon laser trabeculoplasty. Am J Ophthalmol 95:287-292, 1983
14. Horns DJ, Bellows AR, Hutchinson BT, Allen RC: Argon laser trabeculoplasty for open angle glaucoma: a retrospective study of 380 eyes. Trans Ophthalmol Soc UK 103:288-295, 1983
15. Heijl A: One- and two-session laser trabeculoplasty: a randomized, prospective study. Acta Ophthalmol (Kbh) 62:715-724, 1984
16. Lustgarden J, Podos SM, Ritch R et al: Laser trabeculoplasty: a prospective study of treatment variables. Arch Ophthalmol 102:517-519, 1984
17. Fazio P, Werner EB, Krupin T: A randomized prospective study comparing 180° vs 360° argon laser trabeculoplasty in open angle glaucoma. Invest Ophthalmol Vis Sci (Suppl) 29:235, 1988
18. Eguchi S, Yamachita H, Yamomoto T et al: Methods of argon laser trabeculoplasty, complications and long-term follow-up of results. Jpn J Ophthalmol 29:198-211, 1985
19. Juhas T: Argon laser trabeculoplasty methods, results and complications. Česk Oftalmol 46:106-115, 1990
20. Schwartz LW, Spaeth GL, Traverso C, Greenidge KC: Variation of techniques on the results of argon laser trabeculoplasty. Ophthalmology 90:781-784, 1983
21. Wilensky JT, Weinreb RN: Low dose trabeculoplasty. Am J Ophthalmol 95:423-426, 1983

22. Takenaka Y, Yamamoto T, Shirato S: One-quadrant argon laser trabeculoplasty and its indication. Jpn J Ophthalmol 31:483-488, 1987
23. Elsas T, Johnsen H, Brevik TA: The immediate pressure response to primary laser trabeculoplasty: a comparison of one-and two- stage treatment. Acta Ophthalmol (Kbh) 67: 664, 1989
24. Dake CL, Bos PJM: Treatment of glaucoma simplex with argon laser coagulation of the scleral spur (L.SS.C.). Doc Ophthalmol 55:41-46, 1983
25. Higgins RA: Two years experience with laser trabeculoplasty. Aust NZ J Ophthalmol 13:237-241, 1985
26. Rouhiainen HJ, Terasvirta ME, Tuovinen EJ: The effect of some treatment variables on the results of trabeculoplasty. Arch Ophthalmol 106:611-614, 1988
27. Thomas JV, Simmons RJ, Belcher CD: Complications of argon laser trabeculoplasty. Glaucoma 4:50-52, 1982
28. Rouhiainen HT, Terasvirta ME, Tuovinen EJ: Peripheral anterior synechiae formation after trabeculoplasty. Arch Ophthalmol 106:189-191, 1988
29. Traverso CE, Greenidge KC, Spaeth GL: Formation of peripheral anterior synechiae following argon laser trabeculoplasty. Arch Ophthalmol 102:861-863, 1984
30. Smith J: Argon laser trabeculoplasty: comparison of bichromatic and monochromatic wavelengths. Ophthalmology 91:355-360, 1984
31. Makabe R: Comparison of krypton and argon laser trabeculoplasty. Klin Mbl Augenheilk 189:118-120, 1986
32. Spurny RC, Lederer CM Jr: Krypton laser trabeculoplasty: a clinical report. Arch Ophthalmol 102: 1626-1628, 1984
33. Schrems W, Glaab-Schrems E, Krieglstein GK, Leydacker W: Zur Wirkung der Neodym-YAG-Laserbehandlung beim Offenwinkelglaukom. Fortschr Ophthalmol 82:382-384, 1985
34. Schrems W, Hofmann G, Krieglstein GK: Therapie des Offenwinkelglaukoms mit dem Argon- und-Neodym-YAG-Laser. Fortschr Ophthalmol 85:119-123, 1988
35. Kwasniewska S, Fankhauser F, Larsen SE, Cruz-Orive LM: The efficacy of cw Nd:YAG laser trabeculoplasty. Ophthalmic Surg 24: 304-308, 1993
36. McHugh D, Marshall J, Ffytche TJ, Hamilton PA, Raven A: Diode laser trabeculoplasty (DLT) for primary open-angle glaucoma and ocular hypertension. Br J Ophthalmol 74:743-747, 1990
37. Brancato R, Carassa R, Trabucchi G: Diode laser compared with argon laser for trabeculoplasty. Am J Ophthalmol 112:50-55, 1991
38. Vicary DL: Diode laser trabeculoplasty. Aust NZ J Ophthalmol 19:305-307, 1991
39. Moriarty AP, McHugh JP, Spalton DJ, Ffytche TJ, Shah SM, Marshall J: Comparison of the anterior chamber inflammatory response to diode and argon laser trabeculoplasty using a laser flare meter. Ophthalmology 100:1263-1267, 1993
40. Brooks AM, Gillies WE: Laser trabeculoplasty argon or diode? Aust NZ J Ophthalmol 21:161-164, 1993
41. Juhas T, Corbova M: Nd:YAG laser trabeculoplasty Česk Oftalmol 50:41-44, 1994
42. Thomas JV, Simmons RJ, Belcher CD: Argon laser trabeculoplasty in the pre-surgical glaucoma patient. Ophthalmology 89:187-197, 1982
43. Amon M, Menapace R, Papapanos P, Radax U: Effect of argon laser trabeculoplasty on unrestricted outflow of aqueous humor in eyes with simple glaucoma. Klin Mbl Augenheilk 200:25-29, 1992
44. Giers U, Stodtmeister R: Okulopressionstonometrie nach Argonlasertrabekuloplastik. Klin Mbl Augenheilk 200:21-24, 1992
45. Krawczykowa Z, Gos R, Trzcinski J, Gontarz W, Felicka W: Our results of laser trabeculoplasty in simple glaucoma. Klin Oczna 91:167-168, 1989
46. Brubaker RF, Liesegang TJ: Effect of trabecular photocoagulation on the aqueous humor dynamics of the human eye. Am J Ophthalmol 96:139-147, 1983
47. Aliseda Perez P, Fernandez Vila PC, Beneyto Martin P: Study on the aqueous humor flow measured by fluorophotometry after argon laser trabeculoplasty. Int Ophthalmol 16:315-319, 1992
48. Alexander RA, Grierson I, Church WH: The effect of argon laser trabeculoplasty upon the normal human trabecular meshwork. Graefes Arch Clin Exp Ophthalmol 227:72-77, 1989
49. Alexander RA, Grierson I: Morphological effects of argon laser trabeculoplasty upon the glaucomatous human meshwork. Eye 3:719-726, 1989
50. Rodrigues MM, Spaeth GL, Donohoo P: Electron microscopy of argon laser therapy in phakic open-angle glaucoma. Ophthalmology 89:198-210, 1982
51. Melamed S, Pei J, Epstein DL: Delayed response to argon laser trabeculoplasty in monkeys. Arch Ophthalmol 104:1078-1083, 1986
52. Bylsma SB, Samples JR, Acott TS, Van Buskirk EM: Repopulation of the trabecular meshwork after argon laser trabeculoplasty (abstract). Invest Ophthalmol Vis Sci (Suppl) 29:129, 1988

large indication range for us doing combineds. Let us pare it down just a little bit. Mike Kass, let us say that they are well controlled on two topical medications. They are tolerating the topical medications very nicely. They have moderate damage. They have got a 25-year life expectancy and you know new meds are being developed, what are you going to do?

Michael A. Kass, MD: In terms of their tolerating the medication, you present a good scenario there. They are well controlled and they are tolerating them. I think it would depend on the level of damage they have. If they have a long life expectancy and they already have a significant amount of field loss, or if it is near fixation, I would do it. If they have a nasal step someplace and that is it, I probably would not do a combined procedure. Although, I do think the downside risks of the combined procedures are now less than they used to be.

Dr. Zimmerman: That is an excellent point and that is kind of where we are going to head with this, and ultimately kind of answer the risk-benefit of doing a combined procedure. It was not so long ago, probably ten or 15 years, that this panel discussion would have been entirely different, and there would have been people separating these two operations, recounting the horror stories that happened if you tried to combine them. Things have changed significantly now. How many on the panel would, if a patient is on two meds and well controlled...we do have to consider the economics and 25 years of meds, tolerance, and other meds and other diseases...how many would think of doing a combined, knowing that there is 25 years' life expectancy?

Dr. Palmberg: How much damage?

Dr. Zimmerman: They have a Bjerrum in one eye and glaucoma field loss in the other eye, not as bad as the Bjerrum.

Dr. Spaeth: But the disc looks pretty bad or pretty good?

Dr. Zimmerman: The disc in the Bjerrum eye reflects that and in the other eye you have an 0.5, 0.6, without terrible damage.

Don Minckler, MD: You have not told us much about the cataract.

Dr. Zimmerman: You have decided that you are taking it out. They are in California so their vision is 20/25.

Dr. Minckler: This is the true ocular emergency, an out-of-town cataract patient with cash.

Dr. Zimmerman: That is right. He has no health insurance but is from Saudi Arabia. Harry, please save me.

Harry A. Quigley, MD: I want to explain my vote. What I do depends on what the patient wants me to do. I have a conversation with patients who have glaucoma with damage. I am not going to differentiate between the level of damage. They have a visual field defect on Humphrey perimeter, which means they are outside normal limits on a hemifield test. They are under therapy. I say to them, you know, we are going to do a cataract operation on you, and your eyes are going to be anesthetized, and in an additional ten or 15 minutes, I could give you a 50% chance or better that you will not have to use drops again for a very long time. The potential risk of doing this is that there is a very small chance, well under 1% per year, that you might get an infection that you would never have gotten otherwise. This can happen, and it is a risk you will have to consider. So weighing those two, which would you prefer that I do? I wait to hear from them. About 85 or 90% of them would like to have a combined procedure under these conditions. I do not know whether my colleagues agree with this, but that is what I have been doing.

Dr. Zimmerman: Harry, I do not know doctor, what would you advise me to do?

Dr. Kass: That is exactly what I was going to say. About 90% of my patients would say, gee doctor, that is pretty confusing, what do you think I ought to do?

Dr. Quigley: Then I would tell them that we actually have not had one of those infections happen in a combined procedure. We think probably that is because the pressure does not go very low and the blebs are not very good. You might still be on eye drops. On balance, I am going to recommend that you have the combined procedure. And that is what they do.

Dr. Zimmerman: Excellent. We have heard of some of the risks. Cataract surgery is extremely successful. How much do we increase the risk by adding a combined procedure? You mention that they might get an endophthalmitis, and what are the other risks that we should tack on? Oh sure, Don, after that case you presented yesterday, you know most of them.

Dr. Minckler: Yes, I am very familiar with some of the risks. Actually, I have been surprised at how well most eyes do with combined procedures in terms of not having shallow chambers and problems. I am more or less convinced that an IOL with either sulcus or in the bag placement sort of functions like a strut, and it seems to hold the eye up. Shallow chambers, flat chambers after PCIOLs I think are pretty unusual, in the context of recent filtering surgery. So that problem seems relatively minimal. You can certainly have wound leaks from the filtering bleb and problems related to that aspect of the surgery, and late infection, I think, is a potential problem. Fortunately, I have not had that problem. I think if you have reason to do a glaucoma procedure as part of the surgery, the risks are relatively reasonable. I would like to propose another type of patient for you when you get through this question.

Dr. Palmberg: Before people who have not done combined procedures rush out and start doing them with mitomycin, it is true that if you do a lot of these and you understand how to check things at the end of the case, you are not going to get flat chambers. In 300 or 400 cases you might get one. Somebody listened to a lecture I gave in Miami and then sent me his next four cases.
Two patients had been done bilaterally, both had a pressure of 30 in one eye with a failed filter, and had a pressure of 0 with a flat chamber in the other. So, make sure that you have learned the technique from somebody who is not getting into a lot of trouble. It is not necessarily that you just slap the stuff on your usual operation. It can be bad.

Dr. Minckler: I also had a horror study relayed to me by a colleague. I do not think they had heard me talk, but somebody had done a combined procedure. However, they had done the trabeculectomy first and then tried to struggle through the lens extraction with a mushy, soft eye. That does not make any sense to me at all, but in case there was any confusion about it, you obviously want to do the cataract part first and then move on to the trabeculectomy.

Dr. Quigley: If you are going make a trabeculectomy, do the trabeculectomy flap first, which is a lot easier on a firm eye. Do the cataract operation, then finish the trabeculectomy. The point is well taken. The risks depend upon whether you have experience in the procedures. Let us assume we are talking about somebody who has done a few of the procedures. By the way, what is the risk of not doing the trabeculectomy in the well-controlled glaucoma patient that my colleagues do not want to operate on? The risks are two. There is a 65% rate of high spikes of pressure which are not controlled by the preoperative medications and which will require much more serious medication during the first postoperative week. Second, the data show that, far from doing better because you did a cataract operation, the medical control of patients 12 months after cataract surgery in a glaucoma patient requires more medication in a substantial number.

Dr. Zimmerman: Harry, let me just pin you down there. You are saying that the risk benefit ratio is better in a combined in someone who knows the procedure and has excellent experience and has done a number of them. That is better than leaving the patient on a beta blocker and doing just the cataract extraction?

Dr. Quigley: It is my guess that that is the case and that is how I am behaving, but there is not a clinical trial that indicates that.

Dr. Zimmerman: I do not disagree, but boy have we come a long way on that. Mike Kass?

Dr. Kass: I think we cannot totally gloss over the complications of combineds, and I do a lot of them too. I am not saying this to speak against it, but I think there are more complications. There is certainly more bleeding because you are going to do an iridectomy, which you probably do not do routinely in a cataract. There are more wound leaks including late leaks from blebs, late endophthalmitis, and I think there is probably a little bit more inflammation, more iridocyclitis. I have not seen good data, but I would guess that there is probably a bit more astigmatism, although I am sort of old fashioned enough that I think in somebody who has real glaucoma, astigmatism is not the end of the world.

I must say I disagree strongly with one thing that Harry said, which is that the pressure control is worse after cataract extraction. I think there are numerous studies showing that just taking the cataract out alone at a year, and probably some time thereafter, these people will have better control on average. That is why you cannot find an effect of the antimetabolites in that the control group is doing so well anyway. I think that there is a positive effect on pressure just from taking the cataract out. This is an old observation. It goes back 30 years. It holds just as true now with the phaco as I think it did with the old intracaps.

Dr. Zimmerman: Dr. Spaeth, you had a comment?

Dr. Spaeth: I think what Mike said is really important. Everything you add increases the likelihood of complications, including those PIs. Such a benign procedure in most cases, but we stopped doing peripheral iridectomies in cataract extractions because they do not need them. They do much better when they do not have them. So every additional step adds to the likelihood of a significant complication. As far as the final point that Mike made is concerned, one of the things that Thom is trying to get at here is that we are in the midst of a major evolution regarding surgical thinking and surgical techniques. There was a lovely paper at the last ARVO meeting on following patients for a long period of time following phacoemulsification, and it did not appear, I think it was five years out, that there was any change in intraocular pressure, mean preoperative intraocular pressures were something like 22 and the mean postoperative pressure three to five years later was 22. Using phacoemulsification small incision surgery, small lenses, our previous thinking may be wrong. That may not result in lower intraocular pressure.

Dr. Zimmerman: Harry?

Dr. Quigley: The paper I am referring to is a paper that Lorraine McQuigen wrote. This paper was published in about the mid 1980s and it summarized our experience at Wilmer in operating on patients with glaucoma who did not have a trabeculectomy performed. What Mike is referring to, about 30 years of experience, may be very important if you want to look at intracapsular cataract surgery and what its effect was and the wounds that were being done then. The surgery we are doing now, the way we are doing it now, in our experience of several hundred cases, did not improve the control of glaucoma patients who had field loss and were on medicines. If you look at series in which a cataract surgeon who mostly does cataract surgery says, "I operated on a few glaucoma patients and the control was better", I do not know the state of their glaucoma, and they may very well have had milder glaucoma. So maybe milder glaucoma gets better, but in my office, it does not.

Dr. Zimmerman: There are a number of papers and even one from our group, which showed that if you put it in the bag we found a benefit in glaucoma patients of all severity as far as pressure control is concerned. It was an average number and it was not terribly impressive, and it was not something you could live with, but it was something. Let us go to another side of it, which Harry mentioned. We expect in a pretty routine glaucoma patient that we would see filtering surgery somewhere in the 80 or 90% success range. With a combined, we are talking about, Harry, 40, 50% success or 50/60% success. What is the difference there?

Dr. Palmberg: Without any antimetabolite?

Dr. Zimmerman: Yes, no antimetabolite.

Dr. Quigley: The success rate is not quite as low as you are indicating, but it depends on what you mean by success. If we are talking about pressure success, that is one thing, and field success is another. We seem to have gone over the subject of taking a cataract out without talking about fields and the effect of it. I would just like to mention that we have just done a second study on what happens to the visual field when you take a cataract out. You may be surprised that the improvement in the mean sensitivity of the patient's field is not very great when you take out cataracts. Scott Smith has just reported that it is about a mean deviation improvement of 1.6 dB on the Humphrey. You might expect, well gee, it ought to be a lot more than that. Apparently it is not, and there are some interesting things I will talk about in the workshop later about the CPSD and what that does. If you judge it by pressure control, the success rate that we achieved was more like 67% range for a combined procedure. That is lower than it is with straight trabec, because you have a bigger procedure, more inflammation, you are doing more things, you are injuring the eye more. That is what I have been assuming are the reasons it does not work.

Dr. Zimmerman: Does that push you into Paul Palmberg's camp then? Paul, would you use mitomycin C?

Dr. Quigley: I would follow Paul anywhere, but what are you talking about specifically?

Dr. Zimmerman: Paul, would you use mitomycin C routinely in a combined, because of Harry's comments of more junk, more inflammation, more mess?

Dr. Palmberg: Sure, I think the indication is stronger, just as it is for complex filtering surgery. Otherwise there is going to be more scarring and you are going to have less success. And the risk-benefit ratio is certainly shifted in the favor of using it. Especially if you get it out of the sponge. And I think that is important. You are actually going to get to the point where, as we have it, 86% of the people are at 15 or less off all medicines after a year. That is almost as good as primary filters with mitomycin, which was 89. So it lets you separate, dissociate cataract and glaucoma in these patients and deal with both if you need to deal with both, just deal with a filter if you need to, and if there is not enough cataract, leave it alone. You can come back and take it out temporally, or if the cataract is the only problem at the time, take it out temporally, leave the conjunctiva alone up above. We have got a lot more flexibility to individualize to our patients now than we had before. It is wonderful to have these procedures and mitomycin available.

Dr. Zimmerman: I agree with you, but I just feel that there is some learning with regard to doing a combined procedure with mitomycin C because of Harry's points. If we are talking about the fact that they were controlled on the beta blocker, but that the patients would like a home run, now you are going to do the combined with mitomycin. I would like George Spaeth and Mike Kass in unison to talk about the increased complications of using mitomycin C in a situation where they could have been controlled with a beta blocker postoperatively.

Dr. Spaeth: Well, you have just said that there are going to be increased complications. Some of us are not so good at making fornix-based flaps as others, and one of the nice things about small incision surgery is that, instead of having to struggle with that huge limbus-based flap and an extracap or even a big incision, it is now relatively easy to do a limbus-based flap in conjunction with the surgery. Of course, one can also do what Don mentioned before. That is, I think a limbus-based flap is important with mitomycin because it decreases the likelihood of complications, so do your flap on one side and your cataract extraction on the other.

Dr. Kass: Throughout the entire meeting, we have been talking about mitomycin C as if everybody uses it the same. This is a toxic drug, and there are, I think, real dose response characteristics, especially to the toxicity, and I think the dose that Paul uses is much higher than the dose I use. If we look at papers like the one Joe Schulman published, showing where he was using 0.4 or 0.5 mg/ml for five minutes and getting very high rates of hypotony, we do not see that. We use much lower concentrations and shorter times. So, I think that in some places here you get a trade-off that you may get less toxicity, but maybe you will get fewer people with pressures of 10, and I tend to err on the side of being a little safer. In the combineds, I will use like 0.2 mg for two minutes and my feeling is, okay, if this turns out not to be enough I can always go back and re-operate on this if I have to. Most of the time it is sufficient, and there is another quadrant, whereas I think treating hypotony maculopathy does not have such good outcome. So I err on the side of being a little safer than Paul and I think my goals for my patients are a little less than his. I do not feel that I have to get a pressure of 10 to be very happy with my results.

Dr. Zimmerman: I think that is excellent, pointing out clearly the art both technically and the art philosophically of approaching and thinking about and deciding and actually doing a combined procedure. Dr. Spaeth, you had a comment?

Dr. Spaeth: Yes. I do not want to let this go by as an opportunity to second what Don Minckler said earlier about light toxicity. This is especially of concern in these patients because now we are using the axial illuminator. In most cases you should not use an axial illuminator. If you do, you have to cover the cornea, but use oblique illumination if you are just doing a straight, guarded filtration procedure. The axial illuminator is of no benefit, but here we are using the axial illuminator. And these patients do get damaged, and I wonder if that does not explain some of Harry's comment that they do not seem to have as much benefit as you would think when you take the cataract out.

Dr. Quigley: We are talking about mean sensitivity of the central 30 degrees; visual acuity wise, our patients wound up almost exactly the same.

Dr. Spaeth: But acuity is a very rough measure of what is happening to visual function.

Dr. Quigley: Most light damage and most phototoxicity, if you try to produce it experimentally, winds up by being in the foveal area and involving central vision, because the eye preferentially refracts everything toward the fovea.

Dr. Spaeth: Let me just follow up on that. I can recall one lady who did not want to have her disc photographs repeated because she insisted that the bright light had damaged her vision. I told her no Mrs. such and such, it did not damage your vision, you really need the disc photographs repeated. So we repeated the disc photographs and measured the acuity before the disc photographs very carefully, took standard disc photographs, measured acuity afterwards, and she had gone down one whole line. I said, well you know, you are still dazzled.

Dr. Quigley: George, when did you measure it after the fundus photographs? Was it the same day?

Dr. Spaeth: We measured it the same day, we measured it at a week and we measured at a month, and she had lost one line.

Dr. Quigley: Well, lest everybody here thinks that the laser safety standards which are put out would allow us to be doing fundus photography that would cause that to happen on a routine basis, it has been studied and it does not happen very often, obviously. But since you have got a case, that is fine, George. I think it is a scary thing to be saying and I think it deserves a detailed study, if you are serious about it.

Dr. Spaeth: I do not know whether that was a real cause and effect situation there, Harry, but I do know that patients who have maybe 50,000 neurons left in their macula notice changes that we do not notice in patients who still have a million neurons.

Dr. Zimmerman: And we see that in low tensions, which will tell us that they are getting worse, and they are getting worse, but we cannot find it. I think the point is well taken, that they should not lie under the microscope for an hour and a half with that bright light.

Dr. Palmberg: Use the red free on the microscopes that have them and put a little sponge on the cornea whenever you do not need to be seeing the rest of them.

Dr. Zimmerman: We are getting into the zone of summing up here, so let me ask the audience, how many people do combined procedures on the patients we have been talking about? All right, Paul Palmberg, that is quite a number out there. Can you give them, from your experience, a few of the key points of your technique on doing a combined procedure?

Dr. Palmberg: One, there is the article in the *North American Clinics of Ophthalmology* that has the details. Rather than depend on anything I could say in a short time, if you want to see the technique, look at all the points there. You need to have good exposure and, for that, stretching the pupil in one way or another is important. I like using Luther Frye's maneuver with a couple of Kugland hooks, just to stretch it out. We have talked about not losing the capsule and how to avoid that, and getting a good hydrodissection so you will be able to rotate. I think a lot of them had to do with phaco technique, but let me get beyond that to the filter. I think it is most important in any case done with mitomycin to have enough resistance at the time of surgery, tested by you in the operating room, that you are not going to have hypotony. If you do that you will not have flat chambers, you will not have problems with hypotony maculopathy very often. So I think that is something that can be avoided. I like the idea of having a wound on all my filters with some valve-like property, so that the pressure in the eye is about 5 or so, even before you put in stitches. That is more protection against getting hypotony later on. If you do all that, then doing combined procedures is going to give you very good results. If it were not for about the one half of one percent of patients getting endophthalmitis, I would probably still be doing combined procedures on virtually all glaucoma patients who needed a cataract taken out. But I backed off on the people who were well controlled with mild damage and only taking one drug because of that one half of one percent risk, and because some of the patients have uncomfortable blebs afterwards. So I just do a temporal phaco on these people and leave their conjunction for the future if they should need it.

Dr. Spaeth: Paul, as a person who was very much involved in the study that Dr. Quigley referred to, what are your comments, what are your thoughts about the black/white surgical controversy with regard to surgical results?

Dr. Palmberg: I guess a couple of things: one is that, in the 5-fluorouracil trial, of course none of those were primary filters, so I am not sure that it would help us to know about primary filters. I know that quite a few English ophthalmologists who moved to the Bahamas or the Caribean found that their surgery success rates went from 90% to about 50%. Judging from what I have seen of Caribean patients, in particular the success rate of primary filters is certainly less. I think Harry's point is well taken, that you have to control for age in that and a lot of it may have to do with these being much younger people at the time they undergo surgery.

Glaucoma: surgical challenges

Contents

Filtering surgery with antimetabolites

Paul Palmberg

Bascom Palmer Eye Institute, University of Miami School of Medicine, Miami, FL, USA

Abstract

The use of antimetabolites in complex filtering surgery is now routine, with mitomycin having been shown to be far superior in efficacy to 5-fluorouracil (5-FU). Mitomycin also markedly increases the success of combined cataract extraction and filtering surgery when an adequate dose is delivered, and its use should soon be routine as well. The risk-benefit relationship for the use of antimetabolites in primary filtering surgery remains to be determined by the study of longer-term results, and may differ for different patient groups (elderly versus young, white versus Hispanic versus Afro-American, compliant patients versus non-compliant, mild versus advanced glaucoma damage, state of the conjunctival vessels). It is clear that higher success rates are achieved with either five injections or intraoperative sponge administration of 5-FU, or sponge administration of mitomycin, and that lower mean tensions and less need for supplemental medication is noted with antimetabolite use. While complications appear to be increased somewhat by antimetabolite use, techniques to avoid or repair such complications are steadily reducing the risk side of the risk-benefit ratio, suggesting that some form of antimetabolite use will be routine in primary filtering surgery in the future as well.

The rationale for using antimetabolites in glaucoma filtering surgery

There is a wide spectrum of opinion among glaucoma specialists regarding the appropriate role of antimetabolites in filtering surgery. Upon reflection, this is not surprising since there is a divergence of opinion about what we are trying to accomplish with the surgery and about the likely long-term positive and negative results of using or failing to use antimetabolites. Clearly, both 5-fluorouracil (5-FU) and mitomycin C inhibit fibroblast proliferation in filtering blebs in humans, and they result in blebs that exhibit both greater filtration and somewhat greater vulnerability to leakage and infection[1-3]. Is this trade-off a good bargain in general in glaucoma surgery, or only in cases where the risk of failure is high?

We all agree, of course, that ideally filtering surgery would permanently lower the intraocular pressure to a level ('target pressure') that would avoid pressure-dependent damage during the remaining life of the patient, preferably without the need for supplemental medical therapy. The surgery would result in a minimum of such complications as cataract, endophthalmitis, hypotony maculopathy and bleb discomfort. Unfortunately, we have no way to determine prospectively what pres-

Address for correspondence: Paul Palmberg, MD, PhD, Bascom Palmer Eye Institute, University of Miami School of Medicine, P.O. Box 016880, Miami, FL 33101-6880, USA

Peril to the Nerve – Glaucoma and Clinical Neuro-Ophthalmology, pp. 171–177
Proceedings of the 45th Annual Symposium of the New Orleans Academy of
Ophthalmology, New Orleans, LA, USA, April 25-28, 1996
edited by Barry J. Leader and Jonathan C. Calkwood
© 1998 Kugler Publications, The Hague/The Netherlands

sure the ganglion cells of a particular patient can tolerate, nor which patient would suffer an important complication from the use of an antimetabolite. With regard to primary filtering surgery, we are only able to look at sparse aggregate data on the medium-term outcomes of previously treated patients, and to guess what would best serve the patient at hand over the remainder of their life. We will return to a consideration of the issues involved in the use of antimetabolites in primary filtering surgery after reviewing the more solid evidence regarding their utility in complex filtering surgery.

The use of antimetabolites in complex filtering surgery

Predictably, the consequences of the use of antimetabolites in filtering surgery are becoming clear first in the management of patients with the most difficult to treat and rapidly progressive cases. It has taken only a few years in a randomized, controlled clinical trial to show that the outcome of complex filtering surgery was better with the use of 5-FU than without it, with regard to control of pressure, need for supplemental medication or reoperation, and retention of vision[4]. The reason that it did not take long to arrive at a result was that the time to failure was so rapid in the control group, with half failing by 18 months. The success rates were: 5-FU 80% and control 60% at one year, 5-FU 56% and control 26% at three years, and 5-FU 48% and control 21% at five years.

Even while the 5-FU trial follow-up data were being collected, the results became obsolete, since the use of 5-FU had largely been replaced by the use of mitomycin C in complex filtering surgery, based on comparative trials[5,6]. In similar patients and by similar criteria, the success with mitomycin was about 85% at three years, and life-table analysis did not show the rapid fall off of success over time for mitomycin that was seen in the 5-FU trial[4,7].

A complete assessment of the outcome of surgery needs to take into account not only the effectiveness of the procedure, but also the side-effects. Even when that is done, the risk-benefit ratio in complex filtering surgery has also been found greatly to favor the use of antimetabolites. At three years after surgery in the 5-FU trial, the logMAR visual acuity had worsened by 0.29 in the 5-FU group and by 0.55 in the control group, corresponding to a drop in Snellen acuity of roughly 2.5 lines versus seven lines. The greater loss in visual acuity and greater need for reoperation in the control group far outweighed any of the side-effects of 5-FU use. The incidence of endophthalmitis was 2% in the 5-FU group and 1% in the control group, with little visual consequence, as the final visual acuity was 20/30 in two patients and 20/60 in the other. Bleb leaks developed in 9% of 5-FU patients and 2% of controls, but only one of the 5-FU group patients with a bleb leak became infected[4].

On the basis of the information available, nearly all glaucoma specialists strongly favor the use of mitomycin in complex filtering surgery. The consequences of not using it are so unfavorable in so short a time for the majority of patients that concerns about the possible late occurrence of side-effects in a few of the patients receiving it have been discounted. With a success rate of 85% for mitomycin at three years versus 56% for 5-FU, a reduction in failure of 29%, the benefit far outweighs the possible slight excess of endophthalmitis and hypotony maculopathy cases. I have observed 18 cases of endophthalmitis in more than 1100 mitomycin procedures of all types (1.7%), but without as complete a follow-up as that obtained in the 5-FU trial[8]. In the same patients, hypotony maculopathy oc-

Table 1. Combined cataract and glaucoma surgery with and without mitomycin

Technique	No.	Tension (mmHg)			Average medications used		Off medications	<16 mmHg
		pre-operatively	1 year	Δ	pre-operatively	1 year	%	%
ECCE filter	20	18.2	14.3	3.9	2.2	1.0	40	60
ECCE mitofilter	74	20.5	11.0	9.5	2.2	0.2	82	85
Phacofilter	36	21.0	17.1	3.9	2.0	0.7	56	N/A
Phaco mitofilter	28	18.9	10.7	8.2	2.0	0.14	89	86

The results of combined cataract and glaucoma filtering surgery are summarized in four prospective studies[10-13]

curred in 12 (1.1%), but was surgically reversed in all 11 operated on[9]. Concern remains, however, regarding the unknown risk of very late complications, possibly including scleral melting (not yet observed).

The use of mitomycin in combined cataract-glaucoma surgery

At the present time, data are accumulating which also strongly favor the use of mitomycin in combined cataract and glaucoma filtering surgery. Again, this is a group of patients in whom the results of surgery without an antimetabolite are rather unfavorable, while those with mitomycin are quite favorable (Table 1). The change in pressure achieved at one year in either extracapsular combined or phacotrabeculectomy without antimetabolites was only -3.9 mmHg, while with mitomycin, it was -9.5 mmHg with ECCE filter and -8.2 mmHg with phacofilter. Similarly, only 40% of patients one year after ECCE filter and 56% of patients one year after phacofilter without antimetabolites were off glaucoma medications, while 82% of mitomycin-ECCE filter and 89% of mitomycin-phacofilter patients were off medications[10-13]. The risk-benefit ratio also seems to be greatly in favor of using mitomycin, as the complication rates in combined procedures were not greatly increased at 1.4% for endophthalmitis and 0.4% for hypotony[8,9].

The use of mitomycin or 5-fluorouracil in primary filtering surgery

Controversy remains regarding the use of antimetabolites in primary filtering surgery. There is no doubt that the use of five injections of 5-FU[15], or the intra-operative use of mitomycin, will yield a much lower mean intraocular pressure at one to two years of follow-up, and a markedly lower percentage of patients requiring supplemental medical therapy. The consequences for retention of vision and visual field are, at present, only inferred from previous data suggesting the existence of a 'dose-dependent' relationship between intraocular pressure and risk of glaucoma progression[14-16]. It will probably take five to ten years to demonstrate a benefit and to document the magnitude of this benefit. Meanwhile, the use of such agents does increase the risks of encountering endophthalmitis and hypotony[8,9]. Advocates of the use of mitomycin or 5-FU in primary cases project from the information at hand that the risk-benefit ratio of antimetabolite use will be highly favorable, as in complex and combined cases. Opponents of the use of antimetabolites in primary filtering surgery believe that their current success is adequate, and fear increasing the complication rate. In between, some advocate the selective use of these agents in patients with higher intraocular pressures, advanced glaucoma damage, or for risk factors for failure, such as young age, Afro-American race or conjunctival hyperemia from intensive medical therapy. The use of antimetabolites markedly decreased the likely need for supplemental medical therapy. Their use would also be particularly advantageous in patients who could not be counted on to use add-on medical therapy, because of non-compliance or, especially in Third World countries, lack of ready access to medical care due to distance or poverty.

Which view is correct? As I am fond of saying, long-term therapy can only be guided by long-term results. In other chronic, slowly progressive conditions, such as high blood pressure and insulin-dependent diabetes, it took nearly a decade to demonstrate the clear-cut benefit of 'tighter control' and to define the 'dose-response' relationship between blood pressure and the risk of heart attack or stroke or between HgA_{1c} and the risk of progression of diabetic retinopathy, nephropathy and neuropathy. Side-effects of therapy were more noticeable than benefit early in the clinical course of those conditions as well. Having served on the monitoring committee of the Diabetes Control and Complications Trial, I had an opportunity to observe that the control group did better by most measures for the first two years, but the tight control group achieved a markedly better outcome thereafter, and overall[17]. In the case of glaucoma surgery, the data are not yet in, but we have strong clues favoring efforts to achieve lower target pressures.

The case for achieving low-normal pressures

In the last few years there has been a strong trend among glaucoma specialists to be more aggressive in lowering the intraocular pressures of our patients. The impetus for this shift in management strategy came first from the recognition that medical therapy, which had as its goal a lowering of pressure into the upper normal range, was failing to stabilize the disease in a large majority of patients. For example, in 1982, Hart and Becker[18] reported that 73% of patients cared for in the glaucoma center at their institution showed progressive visual field loss during a ten-year follow-up. The average intraocular pressure had been 20.4 mmHg[18]. In 1986, Mickelberg et al.[19] similarly reported that 76% of their patients showed progression during a mean follow-up of 7.6 years[19]. In 1987, Odberg reported that 71% of his patients progressed during a 5- to 18-year follow-up. He also provided the first evidence that there was a dose-response relationship between the intraocular pressure and visual field progression (Table 2). He found that only at low normal pressures was a substantial protection achieved[20]. I found in the literature confirmatory information regarding visual field stability as a function of mean pressure after filtering surgery, and this information was presented at the American Glaucoma Society in 1988. It was incorporated into the Preferred Practice Pattern for Primary Open-Angle Glaucoma of the American Academy of Ophthalmology (Table 3)[17]. However, all these studies were fairly small and no detailed 'dose-response' relationship with long-term prospective follow-up has yet been published. Ongoing clinical trials, such as the Advanced Glaucoma Intervention Study, the Comparison of Initial Glaucoma Treatments Study, the Glaucoma Laser Trial, and the Normal-Tension Glaucoma Trial, could yield the needed information, if the lower-normal pressure range is adequately represented in the results.

Table 2. Odberg's observation of a dose-response relationship between intraocular pressure and progression in advanced glaucoma[20]

Pressure level (mmHg)	No.	Field progression in 5-18 years (%)
All <16	9	33
10-20, mostly <16	17	47
10-20, mostly >15	11	82
Some >20	37	84
All >20	6	100

Table 3. The dose-response relationship between intraocular pressure and progression of field loss in surgical series[17]

Mean tension (mmHg)	Worse (%)	Years follow-up	Authors
14.4	6	5	Roth *et al.* (steroid)[17]
15.0	18	5	Kidd and O'Connor[17]
15.7	10	4+	Kolker[17]
16.0	35	3.5	Werner *et al.*[17]
17.3	35	4	Greve and Dake[17]
18.1	29	5	Rollins and Drance[17]
19.1	58	5	Roth *et al.* (no steroid)[17]

The study of Roth *et al.* included patients randomized either to receive or not receive topical steroids postoperatively. The patients who received topical steroids were observed to have more ischemic blebs, lower pressures, and more stable fields at the five-year examination.

The ability to achieve low-normal pressures with antimetabolite use in primary filtering surgery

The extension of the use of 5-FU to primary filtering procedures was reported by Whiteside-Michael *et al.* to markedly improve the pressure control achieved. Using a reduced dosing schedule of four to six injections over the first two weeks after surgery, they noted an 86% success rate (Ta <21 mmHg, off medication at two years) versus only 51% without 5-FU. The median pressures at two years were 17 mmHg without 5-FU and 12 mmHg with 5-FU[15]. In a similar study, we achieved considerably improved results at 18 months postoperatively (Table 4), increasing the percentage of patients controlled off medication (at a more stringent criteria of a pressure of 15 mmHg or less) from 35% to 81%[18]. With mitomycin in a separate study, 90% achieved a pressure of 15 mmHg or less off medication at one year. Median pressures at one year were 15 mmHg with no antimetabolites, 10 mmHg with 5-FU, and 11 mmHg with mitomycin.

Complications with the use of 5-fluorouracil or mitomycin in primary filtering surgery

While the use of antimetabolites in filtering surgery helps us achieve a high success rate and low mean intraocular pressure through the inhibition of fibrosis, the resulting thin and avascular blebs are also more vulnerable to developing leaks and infection, and provide little protection against the development of hypotony if the scleral flap resistance is inadequate. Encountering such problems, some spe-

Table 4. Results of primary trabeculectomy with and without 5-fluorouracil

	>20 mmHg (%)	Need medications (%)	IOP <16 mmHg off medications (%)
No 5-FU	17	33	35
Five injections of 5-FU	5	11	81
Mitomycin	7	7	88

The results for filtering surgery with and without 5-FU were in comparable, but non-randomized, patients, at 18 months' follow-up[21]. The mitomycin cases have not yet been reported, and are for 12 months' follow-up.

cialists have backed away from the use of antimetabolites in primary filtering surgery. Others have reassessed their operative technique and have found modifications that markedly reduce the incidence of complications, and have found more effective ways to treat complications.

The situation is analogous in many ways to the development of phacoemulsification surgery, in which step-wise modifications in technique have markedly reduced the risk and expanded the applicability of the procedure. The introduction of tunnel incisions and computer controlled vacuum and aspiration to better maintain the anterior chamber, continuous tear capsulorrhexus to prevent radial tears in the anterior capsule, hydrodissection, down-slope sculpting, nuclear cracking and chopping to accomplish lens disassembly with less risk of tearing the posterior capsule or zonules, capsule-friendly second instruments to protect the posterior capsule, intracapsular phaco to protect the corneal endothelium, and foldable lenses to minimize incision size and astigmatism, has yielded a procedure far superior to extracapsular extraction. Yet earlier on, before these developments took place, many prematurely wrote off phacoemulsification after losing a nuclear fragment or encountering corneal edema.

What are the problems and solutions in the case of the use of antimetabolites in filtering surgery? The major problems appear to be hypotony, especially hypotony maculopathy, leaking blebs and infected blebs. Previous concerns regarding corneal toxicity with 5-FU and mitomycin have proven unwarranted with regard to primary filtering surgery. Thus, the incidence of corneal epithelial defects with the use of 5-FU is very low when a reduced schedule of four to six injections is used, or the drug is delivered intraoperatively on a sponge. In the case of mitomycin, the drug has a very focal action and does not affect corneal endothelial cell counts when applied prior to the entry of the eye and followed by thorough rinsing.

In the case of hypotony, rates of as high as 10% with 5-FU and 25% with mitomycin have been reported, but can be held to about 1% with 5-FU and 2% with mitomycin when proper attention is given to creating an adequate scleral flap resistance at the time of surgery[15,16,22,23]. Details of how one may create a 'corneal safety valve incision' that sets a minimum intraocular pressure of 4-6 mmHg for an eye, and of techniques then to adjust the intraocular pressure to 8-12 mmHg by suturing of the scleral flap, and estimation of the pressure at equilibrium flow, are given in the chapter on the complications of filtering surgery. Even when hypotony is present and reduces the visual acuity, the vision can be restored by the use of the 'two sets of stitches' technique, also detailed there. With the use of these techniques, only one of the 1100 eyes which I have operated on with mitomycin has a persistent reduction in vision of as much as three lines due to hypotony and only a few more are reduced by a line or two. Other specialists have reduced the problem of hypotony by using well-guarded filtering ostia, multiple scleral flap sutures, intraoperative testing to be sure the scleral flap resistance is adequate, and/or reduced the time or concentration of mitomycin used.

The most serious consequence of 5-FU or mitomycin use to date has been the increased incidence of endophthalmitis. But, even this risk can be reduced to an acceptable level, as detailed in the chapter on late complications.

References

1. Blumenkranz M, Claflin A, Hajek AS: Selection of therapeutic agents for intraocular proliferative disease: cell culture evaluation. Arch Ophthalmol 102:598-604, 1984
2. Jampel HD: Effect of brief exposure to mitomycin C on viability and proliferation of cultured human Tenon's capsule fibroblasts. Ophthalmology 99:1471-1476, 1992
3. Gressel MG, Parrish RK II, Folberg R: 5-Fluorouracil and glaucoma filtering surgery. I. An animal model. Ophthalmology 91:384-393, 1984
4. The Fluorouracil Filtering Surgery Study Group: Five-year follow-up of the Fluorouracil Filtering Surgery Study. Am J Ophthalmol 121:349-366, 1996
5. Skuta GL, Beeson CC, Higginbotham EJ, Lichter PR, Musch DC, Bergstrom TJ et al: Intraoperative mitomycin versus postoperative 5-fluorouracil in high-risk glaucoma filtering surgery. Ophthalmology 99:438-444, 1992
6. Kitazawa Y, Kawase K, Matsushita H, Minobe M: Trabeculectomy with mitomycin: a comparative study with 5-fluorouracil. Arch Ophthalmol 109:1693-1698, 1991
7. Cheung JC, Murali S, Wright MM, Pederson JE: Mitomycin C filtering surgery: intermediate-term outcome study. Invest Ophthalmol Vis Sci 36:S87, 1995
8. Greenfield DS, Suner IJ, Miller MP, Kangas TA, Palmberg PF, Flynn HW: Endophthalmitis following filtering surgery with mitomycin. Arch Ophthalmol 114:943-949, 1996
9. Suner IJ, Greenfield DS, Miller MP, Nicolela MT, Palmberg PF: Hypotony maculopathy following filtering surgery with mitomycin C: rate of occurrence and treatment. Ophthalmology 104:207-215, 1997
10. Wong PC, Ruderman JM, Krupin T et al: 5-Fluorouracil after primary combined filtration surgery. Am J Ophthalmol 117:149-154, 1994
11. Joos KM, Bueche MJ, Palmberg PF et al: One year follow-up results of combined mitomycin C trabeculectomy and extracapsular cataract extraction. Ophthalmology 102:76-83, 1995
12. O'Grady JM, Juzych MS, Skin DH et al: Trabeculectomy, phacoemulsification, and posterior chamber lens implantation with and without 5-fluorouracil. Am J Ophthalmol 116:72-78, 1993
13. Palmberg P: Combined cataract and glaucoma surgery with mitomycin. Ophthalmol Clin N Am 8:365-381, 1995
14. The Diabetes Control and Complications Trial Research Group: The effect of intensive treatment of diabetes on the development and progression of long-term complications in insulin-dependent diabetes mellitus. New Engl J Med 329:977-986, 1993
15. Whiteside-Michael J, Liebmann JM, Ritch R: Initial 5-fluorouracil trabeculectomy in young patients. Ophthalmology 99:7-13, 1992
16. Kupin TH, Juzych MS, Shin DH, Khatana AK, Olivier MMG: Adjunctive mitomycin C in primary trabeculectomy in phakic eyes. Am J Ophthalmol 119:30-39, 1995
17. Palmberg P: The Rationale and Effectiveness of Glaucoma Therapy. Appendix 1. Preferred Practice Pattern for Primary Open-Angle Glaucoma. San Francisco, CA: American Academy of Ophthalmology, 1992
18. Hart WM, Becker B: The onset and evolution of glaucomatous visual field defects. Ophthalmology 89:268-279, 1982
19. Mickelberg FS, Schulzer M, Drance SM, Lau M: The rate of progression of scotomas in glaucoma. Am J Ophthalmol 101:1-6, 1986
20. Odberg T: Visual field prognosis in advanced glaucoma. Acta Ophthalmol (Kbh) 65 (Suppl) 182:27-29, 1987
21. Palmberg P: Scar wars. In: Ball SF, Franklin RM (eds) Glaucoma: Diagnosis and Therapy, pp 131-137. Amsterdam: Kugler Publ 1993
22. Geijssen HC, Greve EL: Mitomycin, suture lysis and hypotony. Int Ophthalmol 16:371-374, 1992
23. Zacharia PT, Deppermann SR, Schuman JS: Ocular hypotony after trabeculectomy with mitomycin C. Am J Ophthalmol 116:314-326, 1993

Early complications after glaucoma filtering surgery (the 'dirty dozen')

Harry A. Quigley

Glaucoma Service and Dana Center for Preventive Ophthalmology, Wilmer Institute, Johns Hopkins University School of Medicine, Baltimore, MD, USA

Retrobulbar hemorrhage

The rate of this complication is unknown but is probably lower than 1:1000. While it does not often threaten vision, it is frequently severe enough to cause postponement of the surgery. Peribulbar anesthesia may affect the rate of this problem and topical anesthesia for trabeculectomy may be feasible.

Systemic health problem

While it is considered uncommon to experience illness from local anesthesia, in the one study documenting serious health risk in the perioperative period, as many as one per 1000 persons suffer an adverse reaction. These include heart attacks, strokes, aspiration, malignant hyperthermia, acute allergic drug reactions, and other problems.

Early endophthalmitis

The rate of infection immediately after filtering surgery has not been estimated. Using the rate of endophthalmitis during the first week after cataract surgery, the chance of bacterial infection is in the range of 1:5000.

Flat anterior chamber (serous choroidal detachment)

It is unique to glaucoma surgery that problems occur related to the fact that a wound has been left open to the intraocular cavity. The problems can be categorized as those due to leaks at the conjunctival wound closure, those due to overfiltration through the scleral flap of trabeculectomy, and the (uncommon) cyclodialysis cleft. With the use of tight flap sutures and either suturelysis or

Address for correspondence: Harry A. Quigley, MD, Wilmer 120, Johns Hopkins Hospital, 600 N Wolfe Street, Baltimore, MD 21287, USA

Peril to the Nerve – Glaucoma and Clinical Neuro-Ophthalmology, pp. 179–181
Proceedings of the 45th Annual Symposium of the New Orleans Academy of
Ophthalmology, New Orleans, LA, USA, April 25-28, 1996
edited by Barry J. Leader and Jonathan C. Calkwood

releasable sutures, these problems have been minimized. The majority of choroidal detachments resolve spontaneously.

Hemorrhagic choroidal detachment

This is the postoperative equivalent of expulsive hemorrhage and derives from low intraocular pressure and motion in the eyewall. Evidence for this mechanism is the fact that risk factors for the problem include high myopia and aphakic/pseudophakic status, especially vitrectomized eyes. The clinical picture includes severe and continuing pain with sudden onset of major vision loss. Eye pressure can be low or high and the anterior chamber is sometimes flat. The best management has not been determined (*i.e.*, the timing of drainage – or even whether all such eyes should undergo drainage). A high proportion of these eyes will lose substantial vision, most often related to proliferative vitreoretinopathy.

Hypotony maculopathy

Since the use of mitomycin C (and to a lesser extent, 5-fluorouracil), a new complication has emerged. Soon after surgery, an appearance similar to that of proliferative vitreoretinopathy develops. Associated with serous retinal elevation and folds in the choroid, it is only partly related to the intraocular pressures below 5 mmHg that are characteristic of this state. A toxic effect on the chorioretinal structures is suspected. The actual incidence of this problem has not been accurately estimated (although it may be as many as 5% of eyes treated with mitomycin), nor is it known whether it is dose-related. Some have advocated the prevention of exposure of the sclera to mitomycin (placing the sponge on the conjunctiva only).

Hyphema

As many as 10% of eyes have some degree of blood in the anterior chamber after filtering surgery. In many cases, the sudden decrease in intraocular pressure after suturelysis or removal of releasable sutures will cause the initiation of bleeding from small vessels in the wound area. Most of these will resolve spontaneously.

Dellen

As many as 10% of eyes after filtering surgery will develop a bleb which height leads to an insufficient resurfacing of the cornea in front of the elevation. These frequently lead to a foreign body sensation and require artificial tears, ointments, or patching. In a few cases, the bleb must be revised to a lower height to allow comfort.

Tight flap with high pressure

Since the use of suturelysis and releasable sutures is associated with tying the scleral flap tightly shut, there may be a very high intraocular pressure early after surgery. Typically, this is resolved by cutting or releasing the sutures. When subconjunctival hemorrhage or poor patient cooperation blocks suturelysis or suture release, this is not possible. These eyes must be either managed medically until suture loosening is possible, or must undergo reoperation.

Malignant glaucoma

The development of aqueous humor blockade posterior to the iris/lens diaphragm is quite uncommon, but the picture of a flat anterior chamber with high pressure still occurs.

Management includes assurance that a patent iridotomy is present, followed by use of osmotic agents and cycloplegics, medical pressure lowering, and ultimately vitrectomy.

Superficial punctate keratitis

The use of 5-fluorouracil by subconjunctival injection almost routinely leads to a superficial punctate keratitis during the first to third weeks after surgery. While the slit-lamp appearance of the cornea is not dramatically abnormal, the loss of corneal clarity is sufficient to reduce vision to 20/200 and is very disturbing to patients (and surgeons). It clears spontaneously, but is resistant to patching.

Astigmatism

A frequent finding after surgery is the development of a plus cylindrical correction in the axis of the trabeculectomy scleral flap. This is particularly bothersome to the patient who has not required glasses prior to surgery. The cylinder slowly resolves during the months following surgery. No satisfactory explanation (or preventive measure) has been provided, as it does not remit when tension on the scleral flap is released by suturelysis. Perhaps cautery to the sclera during surgery produces the change in corneal shape.

Late complications after glaucoma filtering surgery

Paul Palmberg

Bascom Palmer Eye Institute, University of Miami School of Medicine, Miami, FL, USA

Abstract

The introduction of adjunctive antimetabolites in filtering surgery has greatly boosted the success of such procedures, from 26-85% at three years in complex filtering procedures, and from 79-92% in primary filtering procedures at two years, by the usual criteria of obtaining pressures in the normal range, with supplemental medical therapy as required. If more stringent criteria, more likely to yield the maximum reduction in risk of future field loss, are used, such as obtaining a pressure in the mid-normal range without supplemental medical therapy, the success rate with complex filters rises from 20-80% at one year and in primary filters from 35-81% with 5-FU and 90% with mitomycin at 18 months.

Along with increased efficacy, the use of antimetabolites increases the risk of encountering leaking, painful or infected blebs, and promotes the development of hypotony when inadequate scleral resistance is created at surgery. Nevertheless, the risk/benefit ratio is clearly far in favor of the use of antimetabolites in complex or combined surgery, and may be in favor of their use in primary filtering surgery. In the case of primary filtering surgery, longer-term follow-up will be needed to determine the effect of the intraocular pressures obtained on long-term visual field stability in order to specify the benefit of antimetabolite use, and long-term surveillance for complications and their effect on vision will be needed to determine the risk.

Advances in our ability to avoid or repair complications of filtering surgery may shift the risk/benefit ratio by reducing either failure rates or complication rates. Among the techniques discussed in this presentation are YAG laser treatment of the internal ostium or needle elevation of the scleral flap in patients with failing filters, medical treatment of Tenon's cysts, compression sutures, autologous blood injection and other techniques for dealing with leaking or painful blebs, and the use of a corneal safety valve incision to reduce the risk of hypotony maculopathy and the two sets of stitches technique to repair it. Also discussed are the advantages of bleb location under the upper eyelid, and of using a 100 μm or greater spot for laser suture lysis in order to reduce bleb complications.

Introduction

The complications which we will address are failing blebs, leaking blebs, painful blebs, hypotony and endophthalmitis.

Failing blebs

Bleb failure in filtering surgery can be external or internal. External obstruction is caused by vascularization or scarring of Tenon's capsule and conjunctiva, and

Address for correspondence: Paul Palmberg, MD, PhD, Bascom Palmer Eye Institute, University of Miami School of Medicine, P.O. Box 016880, Miami, FL 33101-6880, USA

Peril to the Nerve – Glaucoma and Clinical Neuro-Ophthalmology, pp. 183–193
Proceedings of the 45th Annual Symposium of the New Orleans Academy of
Ophthalmology, New Orleans, LA, USA, April 25-28, 1996
edited by Barry J. Leader and Jonathan C. Calkwood
© 1998 Kugler Publications, The Hague/The Netherlands

by fibrosis of the episclera around the scleral flap. Internal obstruction is caused by blockage of the ostium by the iris, vitreous (after vigorous massage), or a membrane of cells derived from the iris pigment epithelium, corneal endothelium or sclera.

Evaluation of a failing bleb to determine the site or sites of increased resistance should, therefore, include slit-lamp examination to detect a Tenon's cyst inside the conjunctiva as a tense dome with discrete borders (a 'balloon within a balloon'). Inspection of the scleral flap sutures is accomplished by compression of the overlying conjunctiva and Tenon's with a Ritch or Hoskins suture lysis lens. Gonioscopy can check the patency of the internal ostium and whether or not the scleral flap has a proper separation from the outer end of the ostium, leaving a gap for flow.

A Tenon's cyst may be treated by reinstitution of medical therapy for up to six months to allow for evolution of the bleb to a lower pressure, as advocated by Sherwood et al.[1] and by Scott and Quigley[2]. Costa et al.[3] have shown that this strategy was successful in nine of ten patients, with the mean tension falling from 25 mmHg before reinstitution of medical therapy to 20 mmHg at one month, and that, as the blebs evolved, the mean fell to 17 mmHg by three months and 14 mmHg by six months. Needling is indicated when added medical therapy does not lower the pressure to a level at which one would be willing to observe the patient.

Needling may be performed at the slit-lamp after applying Iopidine (Alcon, Fort Worth, TX) for vasoconstriction, proparacaine for anesthesia, cleansing the lids with povidone iodide soap, and placing a lid speculum. A 30-gauge needle, placed on a 1-ml syringe and bent in a bayonette shape, using a blade breaker, makes an ideal tool for needling.

When Tenon's cyst formation is not the problem, or not the only problem with bleb function, scleral flap sutures may be cut with the sharp edge of the needle tip. The scleral flap then may be elevated by passing the needle tip in under it, tearing side to side and lifting. It is important to see the scleral flap edge clearly enough to allow passage of the needle tip through the scleral wound, as only along the wound is the tissue weak enough to tear, avascular and free of nerve endings. Visualizing the edge of the scleral flap is made easier by compressing the overlying conjunctiva and Tenon's with a Ritch or Hoskins suture lysis lens held in the other hand. The iris or a cellular membrane may be dislodged from the internal ostium by passing the needle tip under the scleral flap and into the anterior chamber, and twisting the tip to each side. Alternatively, the iris may be pulled out of the ostium by passing a 30-gauge needle through a paracentesis and stroking the iris surface adjacent to the ostium[4].

Alternatively, the Nd:YAG laser may be used to cut the iris or a cellular membrane that is obstructing the internal ostium. The laser is applied at 4-8 mJ through a gonioprism to the ostium itself and to the junction of the wall of the ostium and the overlying scleral flap. The endpoint of this treatment is visualization of the opening of a 'cave' beyond the ostium (the space under the scleral flap), as well as a softening of the eye and expansion of the bleb.

Leaking blebs

The blebs obtained with 5-fluorouracil or mitomycin usually appear ischemic and thin. There has been a good deal of concern about the possible occurrence of late-onset leaking blebs. While such leaks fortunately are not common, they should be closed in order to reduce the risk of infection.

Several treatments are possible. The most conservative treatment is to apply an 18-mm therapeutic soft contact lens for one to two weeks, partially tamponading the leak while the conjunctival epithelium has an opportunity to heal over the hole[5]. Since flow through the hole is likely to impede the motion of cells to cover it, the administration of aqueous suppressants during this time is probably helpful. However, in our experience, this treatment only succeeded in one of five cases. A treatment that was fairly successful with leaking blebs in the past, in the pre-antimetabolite era, the application of 10% trichloroacetic acid on the wooden end of a cotton applicator stick to the leaking site (followed by thorough rising), was unsuccessful in six cases. Direct suturing of the leaking site is thought unwise, reasoning that the passage of even a vascular needle would create new holes in these very thin blebs. Somewhat more successful was the use of peribleb or intrableb injection of about 0.1 ml of autologous blood[6-8]. However, this succeeded in only four of ten cases for leak, and in another case, treated for hypotony without a leak, precipitated a corneal graft rejection and reactivated a toxoplasmic choreoretinitis in the macula[10]. The use of blood also has a disturbing propensity to result in regurgitation of blood from the bleb into the anterior chamber, and even into the vitreous cavity. Such a reflux of blood into the eye can be impeded by first placing a viscoelastic substance into the anterior chamber. We have recently noted that better success in sealing a leak and less tendency to reflux can be obtained by the simple expedient of bringing the tip of our specially bent 30-gauge needle right up behind the hole in the bleb (from within the bleb), and slowly injecting the blood through the hole until clotting occurs. When less drastic methods fail, a fairly definitive treatment is bleb excision with advancement of conjunctiva from behind, although this requires a trip to the operating room and carries a considerable risk of bleb failure. Another surgical option is the recently reported use of free conjunctival grafts[11].

We have devised a new treatment for leaking blebs, in which a 9-0 nylon suture is anchored in the peripheral cornea with a 1-mm long bite parallel to and 1 mm from the limbus, the suture is draped back over the bleb near the leak site, a 3-4 mm bite of conjunctiva and Tenon's is taken behind the bleb, the suture is draped back over the bleb on the other side of the hole, the suture is tied tightly, and the knot is rotated into the cornea (Fig. 1). The suture compresses Tenon's capsule within the bleb, decreasing flow through it, bringing to mind the concept expressed by Scott and Quigley that compression of Tenon's capsule by pressure within a Tenon's cyst reduces the hydrolic conductivity of the tissue[1]. The procedure was successful in closing leaks in 73% of patients, with healing taking place within one to four weeks, during which time the patients received Polytrim qid and Pred Forte qid and the leak site was Seidel tested weekly[10].

Painful blebs

Grajewski *et al.*[12] were the first to observe that the upper lid can capture air as it moves over a filtering bleb, producing a bubble of tear fluid (Fig. 2a). When the bubble pops, it can produce a burning sensation. Hodapp named this condition 'bubble dysesthesia'[12]. I noticed that it seemed to occur in blebs which extend along the limbus to the nasal or temporal side of the 12 o'clock position, forming a 'kidney-basin' shaped trough which was the site of air capture. Drawing from our observation that bleb compression sutures used for leaking blebs frequently caused a permanent lowering of the bleb profile and the production of 'white sus-

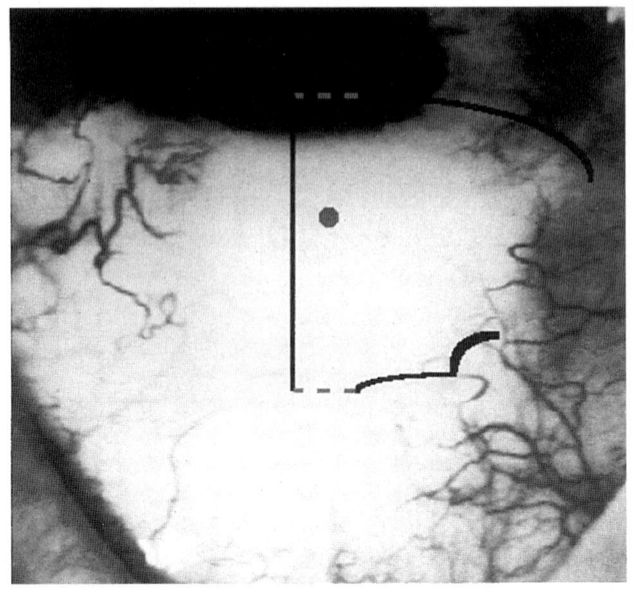

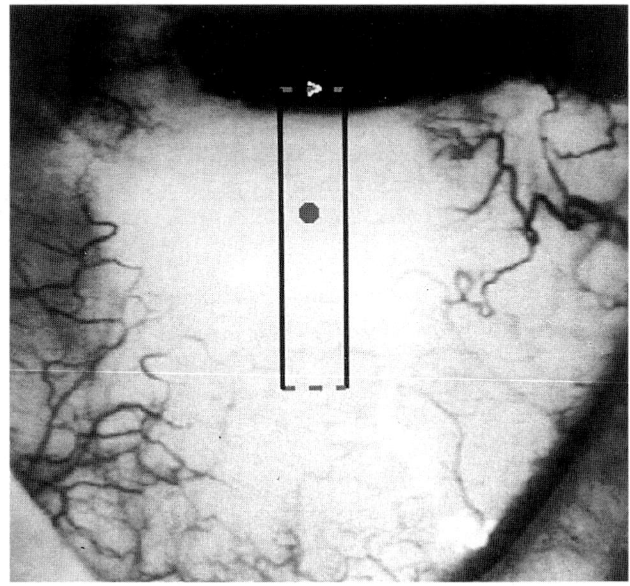

Fig. 1. Compression stitch: *a.* A 9-0 nylon stitch is passed in the peripheral cornea, laid back over the bleb on one side of the leak, and then a bite taken of conjunctiva and Tenon's, but not episclera. *b.* The knot is then tied tightly, and the trimmed knot is turned into the peripheral cornea.

pender' stress lines in the Tenon's underlying where the suture had been, I thought it likely that compression stitches placed over such blebs could prove therapeutic. Indeed, we found that 83% of 29 eyes were markedly improved by the effect of having a compression stitch in position for one to four weeks (Figs. 2b-d)[11].

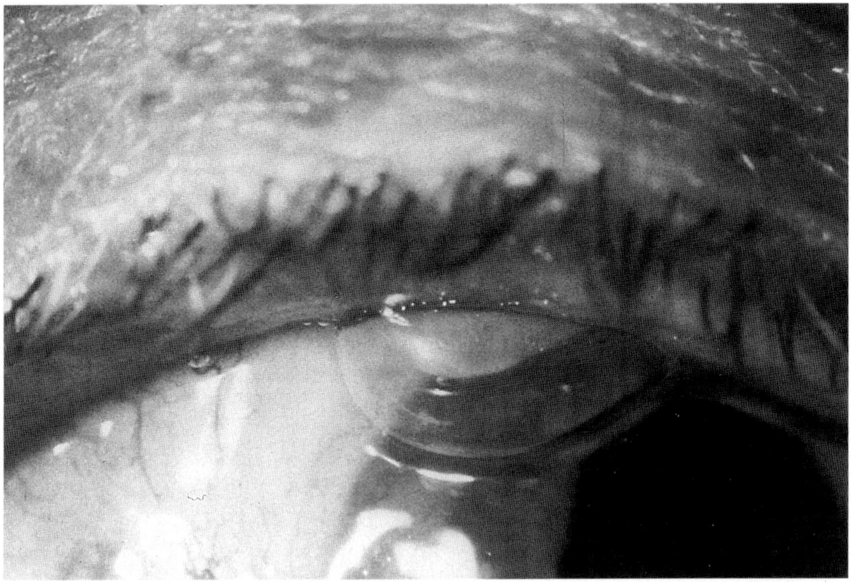

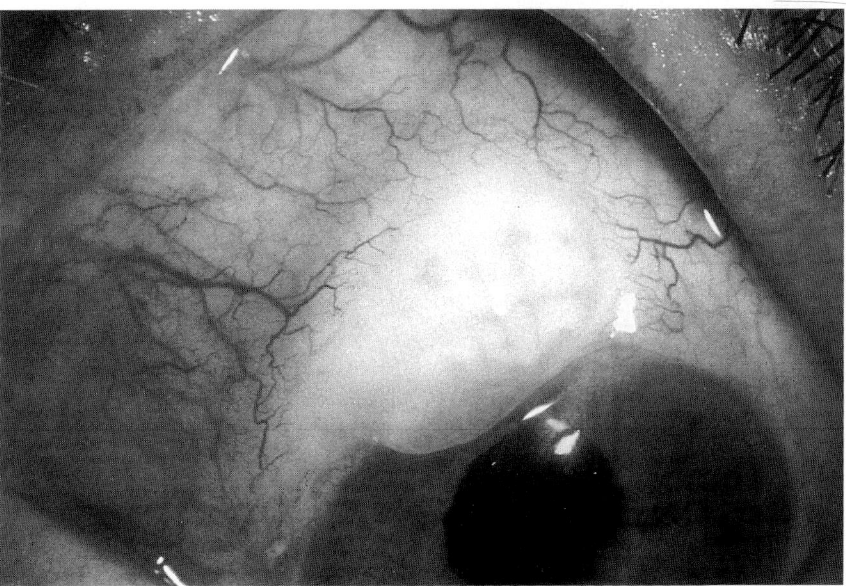

Fig. 2. Bubble dysesthesia and the use of compression sutures. *a.* A bubble is formed where air is captured by the upper lid as it passes over a kidney-basin shaped bleb. *b.* The bleb in this case.

Hypotony

One concern about the use of mitomycin in filtering surgery is the risk of causing reduced vision from hypotony. Such reduction in vision occurs in two forms: *1.* a milder form in which the vision is reduced by the presence of irregular or vari-

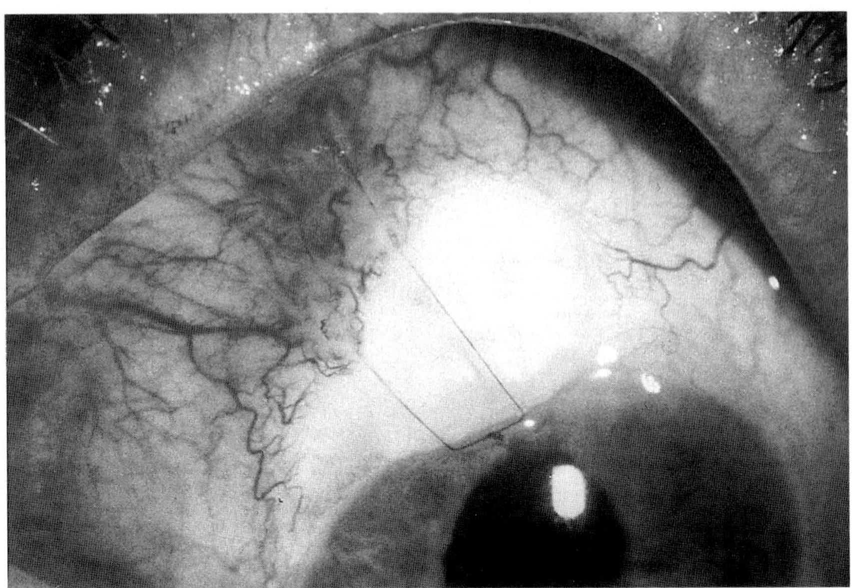

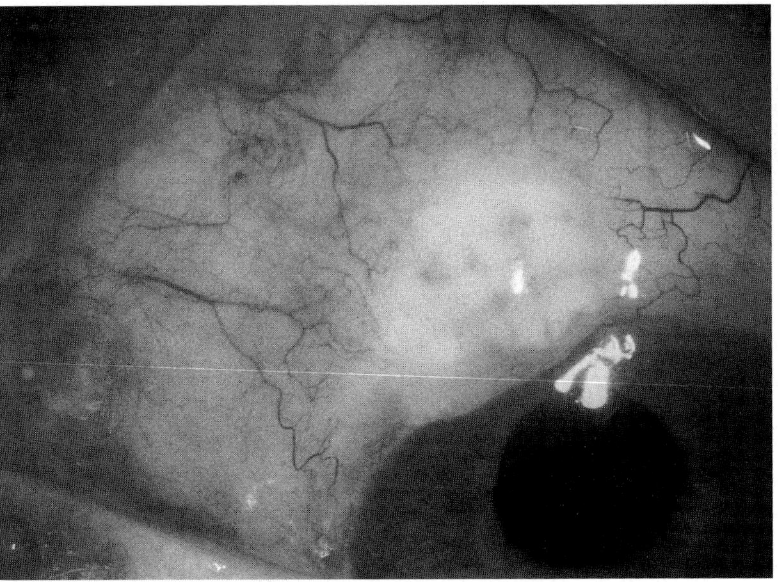

Fig. 2. Bubble dysesthesia and the use of compression sutures. *c.* Compression stitch in place. *d.* Bleb appearance after four weeks and after removal of compression stitch. The bleb profile is permanently reduced in height.

able astigmatism; and *2.* a more severe form in which the vision is reduced by the presence of choreoretinal folds, which condition Gass has named hypotony maculopathy[13].

Although hypotony maculopathy was recognized as early as 1955 by Della-

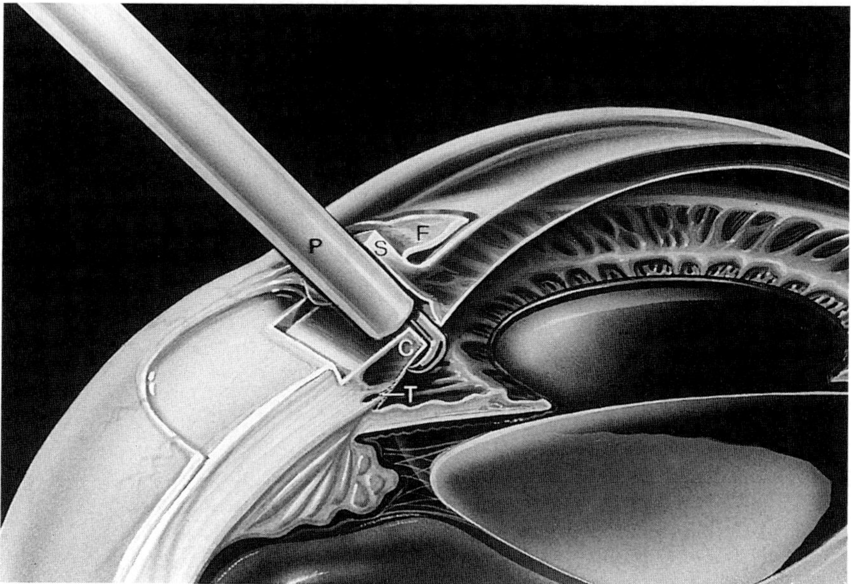

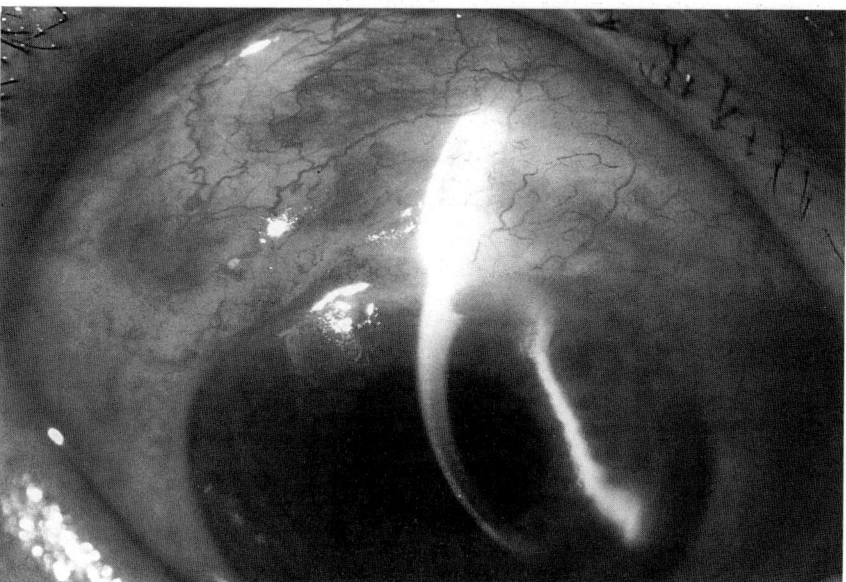

Fig. 3. The corneal safety valve incision. *a.* A 2.5-mm wide scleral flap of one-half depth and 1 mm in length is outlined, and then a 1-mm tunnel is undermined into clear cornea in front of the base of the scleral flap. Two 0.75-mm side-by-side punch bites are removed from the posterior lip of an entry at the anterior end of the tunnel. *b.* The slit-lamp appearance of the safety valve incision.

porta[14], it rarely occurred with even full-thickness filtering surgery, was unheard of with trabeculectomy in the preantimetabolite era, and was rare even with 5-FU filtering surgery. With mitomycin use, however, the incidence of hypotony

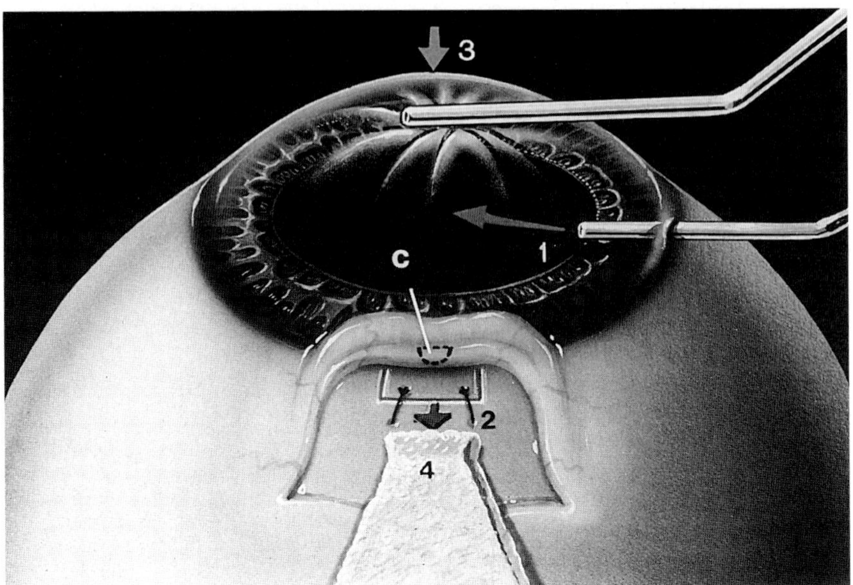

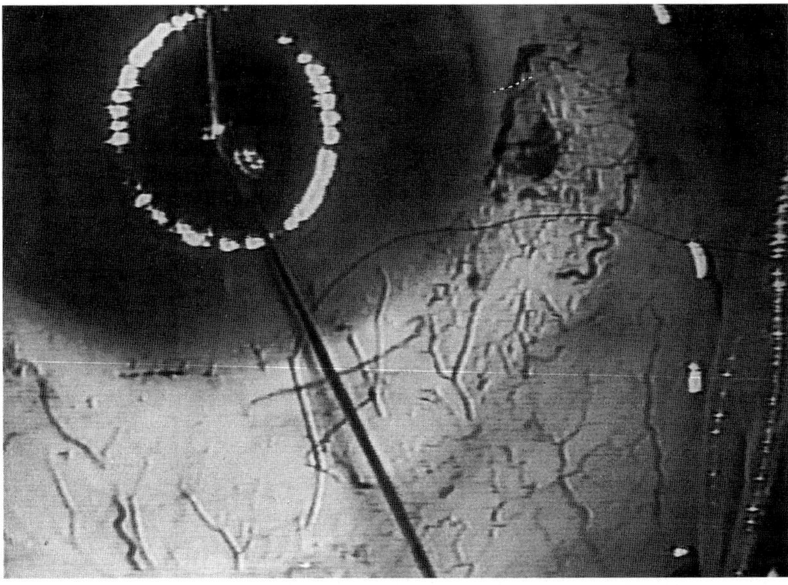

Fig. 4. The use of a 30-gauge cannula to estimate the intraocular pressure at equilibrium flow. *a.* Balanced salt solution is placed in the anterior chamber through a paracentesis, the flow is observed until it reaches equilibrium, and then the cannula is used to feel how much force is needed to depress the central cornea, a crude but sufficient form of applanation tonometry. *b.* Use of the cannula in the operating room.

maculopathy has been reported to be 3-24% in primary filtering surgery and 2-5% in complex filtering surgery[15-20].

Gass hypothesized that the choreoretinal folds in hypotony maculopathy were caused by a contraction of the underlying elastic sclera that occurred when the eye-wall was no longer stretched by a positive intraocular pressure. In line with this hypothesis, we have observed an increased risk of hypotony maculopathy in the young (in whom the sclera is more elastic), in myopes (in whom the sclera is thinner), and in patients in whom the preoperative pressure was particularly high (in whom the sclera was under more tension).

In order to try to reduce the risk of occurrence of flat chambers and hypotony maculopathy, I introduced a 'corneal safety valve incision' into my filtering procedures involving antimetabolites in 1988. My concern was that, at the time of laser suture lysis or the eventual dissolution of the nylon sutures in the scleral flap, such eyes might otherwise suffer hypotony due to lack of resistance to flow out from under the scleral flap and through the conjunctiva-Tenon's layers, since scarring had been inhibited by antimetabolite exposure.

The corneal safety valve incision is a 1-mm tunnel anterior to the base of the scleral flap (Figs. 3a and b). A vertical entry is made into the anterior chamber at the anterior margin of the tunnel, and two side-by-side bites made in the posterior lip of that entry with a 0.75 mm Kelly's Descemet punch. The remaining 0.25-mm tunnel acts as a valve. It does not open until the pressure in the anterior chamber is about 4-6 mmHg, as estimated by pushing on the center of the cornea with a 30-gauge cannula (Figs. 4a and b). Thus, as balanced salt solution is placed in the anterior chamber through a paracentesis, the chamber deepens before flow through the tunnel begins. The valved incision creates a third resistance to aqueous outflow, and helps to reduce the risk of hypotony. With its use, we encountered 11 cases of hypotony maculopathy in over 1100 mitomycin filtering procedures, a lower proportion than reported by others using more conventional trabeculectomy incisions.

When hypotony maculopathy did occur, we found that we could repair it quite effectively with a new technique of reoperation, in which the intraocular pressure was temporarily adjusted to about 20-25 mmHg in order to put the sclera on stretch and flatten the choroid and retina. Eleven of my own patients and five referred by others have been successfully repaired.

The goal of the 'two sets of sutures' technique is both to flatten the choreoretinal folds and to reset the intraocular pressure at the target pressure. To do so, first one set of stitches is placed in the scleral flap with sufficient tension to adjust the intraocular pressure to the target pressure at equilibrium flow, using a 30-gauge cannula to estimate the pressure, as outlined earlier. Then, a second set of stitches is placed, using greater tension on the stitches to achieve an estimated pressure of 20-25 mmHg at equilibrium flow. The patient is seen a few hours postoperatively to check that the pressure is in the desired range, and then the next day and weekly for one to four weeks, until the retina is flat and vision is restored. Laser suture lysis of the second set then adjusts the intraocular pressure to the target pressure.

Endophthalmitis

The filtering blebs obtained through the use of either 5-FU or mitomycin are usually ischemic and tend to be thin-walled due to inhibition of fibrosis. They are more prone to develop leaks and endophthalmitis than blebs obtained with trabeculectomy without antimetabolite use. Some 1% of superior limbal blebs and 3% of inferior limbal blebs in 5-FU filters became infected within a few years. With mitomycin, the risk became 1.8% above and 13% below, leading us to abandon inferior blebs. Higginbotham *et al.*[21] and Caronia *et al.*[22] have reported similar results and drawn the same conclusion.

Some 18 of over 1100 mitomycin filters have become infected, with useful vision being lost in four eyes, and good vision being retained in about half. The infections occurred from a few months to three years postoperatively. In about half the cases, laser suture lysis or needling appeared to play a role. After suture lysis with a 50-μm spot, and using a suture lysis lens, burns in the conjunctiva are frequently seen. A dimple forms at that spot, with an adhesion of Tenon's to sclera that may later, as the bleb increases in size and thins, tear a hole in the bleb. I have observed that, in the thin, transparent blebs obtained with mitomycin, the substitution of a 100-μm spot size for suture lysis is effective, even though the energy density is only one-fourth as great, and at 0.3-0.7 W at 0.02 seconds avoids bleb burns.

The organisms isolated at vitrectomy were typical of bleb infections, including *Staph. epidermidis*, *Haemophilus influenza* and Streptococcus species. While our patients underwent pars plana vitrectomy with intravitreal injection of gentamicin, vancomycin and dexamethasone, the rapidity of treatment is important. In a patient care setting where vitrectomy could not be done swiftly, it would probably be better just to give intravitreal antibiotics than to transport the patient elsewhere for initial care. Rapidity of treatment is also facilitated by instructing all patients on the warning signs of endophthalmitis, the urgency of rapid treatment, and giving them a specific place to go for treatment and a 24-hour phone number for reaching the surgeon.

I believe, on the basis of five years of experience, that all mitomycin blebs should be placed in the 12 o'clock position, where they will be fully covered by the upper eyelid, and not superonasally or superotemporally, as has been advocated for trabeculectomy in the past. The success rate with mitomycin filters is sufficient, 92% in primary filters and 85% in complex filters, that one need not be overly concerned to provide an opportunity for repeat filters, and the increased risk of infection or leak in blebs that protrude out from under the lid is now the more important consideration. Such placement avoids rubbing of the lid margin over the bleb and thus keeps meibomian glands affected by posterior blepharitis from contaminating the bleb. Further, I favor the use of tunnel incisions, 2.5 mm in width and 1.5 mm behind the limbus, in order to avoid any dissection of Tenon's insertion. An intact Tenon's layer leads to the creation of ischemic, but not transparent, blebs in mitomycin-treated eyes, and probably greater resistance to bleb leak or infection.

References

1. Sherwood MB, Spaeth GL, Simmons ST, Nichols DA, Walsh AM, Steinmann WC, Wilson RP: Cysts of Tenon's capsule following filtration surgery: medical management. Arch Ophthalmol 105:1517-1523, 1987
2. Scott DR, Quigley HA: Medical management of a high bleb phase after trabeculectomies. Ophthalmology 95:1169-1173, 1988
3. Costa, VP, Correa MM, Kara-Jose, N: Needling versus medical treatment in encapsulated blebs: a randomized, prospective study [Abstract]. Paper presented at the Brazilian Congress Against Blindness, Sao Paulo, September, 1996
4. Greenfield DS, Miller MP, Suner IJ, Palmberg PF: Needle elevation of the scleral flap for failing filtration blebs after trabeculectomy with mitomycin C. Am J Ophthalmol 122:195-204, 1996
5. Blok MD, Kok JH, Van Mil C et al: Use of megasoft bandage lens for treatment of complications after trabeculectomy. Am J Ophthalmol 110:264-268, 1990

6. Wise JB: Treatment of chronic postfiltration hypotony by intrableb injection of autologous blood. Arch Ophthalmol 111:827-830, 1993
7. Nuyts RM, Greve EL, Geijssen HC, Langerhorst CT: Treatment of hypotonous maculopathy after trabeculectomy with mitomycin C. Am J Ophthalmol 118:322-331, 1994
8. Smith MF, Magauran RG, Betchkal J, Doyle JW: Treatment of postfiltration bleb leaks with autologous blood. Ophthalmology 102:868-871, 1995
9. Chen PP, Palmberg PF, Davis JL, Culbertson WW: Corneal graft rejection and recurrent toxoplasmosis after intrableb autologous blood injection [Letter]. Arch Ophthalmol 114:633, 1996
10. Wilson MR, Kotas-Neumann R: Free conjunctival patch for repair of persistent late bleb leak. Am J Ophthalmol 117:569-574, 1994
11. Palmberg PF, Zacchei AC, Mendosa A, Robinson J: Compression sutures: a new treatment for leaking or painful filtering blebs. Abstract 2032, ARVO 1996
12. Grajewski A, Hodapp E, Huang A: Bubble dysesthesia. Paper presented at the American Glaucoma Society, February 1995, Key West, FL
13. Gass JDM: Hypotony maculopathy. In: Bellows JG (ed), Comtemporary Ophthalmology, pp 343-366. Baltimore, MD: Williams & Wilkins 1972
14. Dellaporta A: Fundus changes in postoperative hypotony. Am J Ophthalmol 40:781-785, 1955
15. Neelakantan A, Krishnan N, Sridhar RB et al: Effect of the concentration and duration of application of mitomycin C in trabeculectomy. Ophthalmic Surg 25:612-615, 1994
16. Costa VP, Wilson RP, Moster MR et al: Hypotony maculopathy following the use of topical mitomycin C in glaucoma filtration surgery. Ophthalmic Surg 24:389-394, 1993
17. Zacharia PT, Depperman SR, Schuman JS: Ocular hypotony after trabeculectomy with mitomycin C. Am J Ophthalmol 116:314-326, 1993
18. Zacharia PR, Depperman SR, Schuman JS: Ocular hypotony after trabeculectomy with mitomycin C. Am J Ophthalmol 116:314-326, 1993
19. Kitazawa Y, Suemori-Matsushita H, Yamamoto T, Kawase K: Low-dose and high-dose mitomycin trabeculectomy as an initial surgery in primary open-angle glaucoma. Ophthalmology 100:1624-1628, 1993
20. Wise JB: Treatment of chronic postfiltration hypotony by intrableb injection of autologous blood. Arch Ophthalmol 111:827-830, 1993
21. Higginbotham EJ, Stevens RK, Musch DC et al: Bleb-related endophthalmitis after trabeculectomy with mitomycin C. Ophthalmology 103:650-656, 1996
22. Caronia RM, Liebmann JM, Friedman R, Cohen H, Ritch R: Trabeculectomy at the inferior limbus. Arch Ophthalmol 114:387-391, 1996

Glaucoma drainage devices: promise and problems

Don Minckler

Department of Ophthalmology, University of Southern California School of Medicine, Los Angeles, CA, USA

Introduction

Glaucoma drainage devices (GDDs) have become a commonly used option for the treatment of complicated glaucomas[1-3]. Although no accurate utilization data are available, manufacturers suggest that between 3000 and 4000 of these devices are being utilized per year in the United States (Federal Drug Administration [FDA] Ophthalmic Devices Panel meeting, Jan 22, 1996, Gaithersburg, MD). Many more are utilized per year around the world, especially the Molteno implant, still the 'gold standard' device to which all other GDDs have been compared by clinical users (Fig. 1). GDDs currently commercially available in the US have been marketed with the FDA's permission by virtue of their 'substantial equivalence' to the Krupin-Denver implant (the predicate US device), but none has been 'FDA approved'[4]. A subcommittee of the American National Standards Institute (ANSI), in cooperation with the American Academy of Ophthalmology, interested users and manufacturers and the FDA is currently evolving standards for GDDs, including specific clinical protocols for establishing the safety and efficacy of new devices. The FDA will evaluate and possibly change the classification of GDDs from Class III to Class II in the near future, probably by the end of 1996.

Features common to all implants currently in use in the United States include explant location at the equator of the globe, explant construction from materials (polypropylene, polymethyl methacrylate, or silicone rubber) to which fibroblasts cannot tightly adhere, and a silicone rubber drainage tube with an internal diameter of 300 μm. Differences between devices include variations in design, explant surface area and shape and the presence or absence of valves or flow restrictors[5-12].

Pathophysiology

Numerous clinical and histological observations in humans indicate that once placed on the eye, the explant portion of a GDD rapidly provokes the formation of a fibrous capsule around itself and the connecting tube over the subsequent postoperative period (Figs. 2 and 3)[6]. Continual remodeling of the fibrous capsule

Address for correspondence: Professor Don S. Minckler, MD, Department of Ophthalmology, University of Southern California School of Medicine, Richard K. Eamer Medical Plaza, Los Angeles, CA 90033-466, USA

Peril to the Nerve – Glaucoma and Clinical Neuro-Ophthalmology, pp. 195–205
Proceedings of the 45th Annual Symposium of the New Orleans Academy of
Ophthalmology, New Orleans, LA, USA, April 25-28, 1996
edited by Barry J. Leader and Jonathan C. Calkwood
© *1998 Kugler Publications, The Hague/The Netherlands*

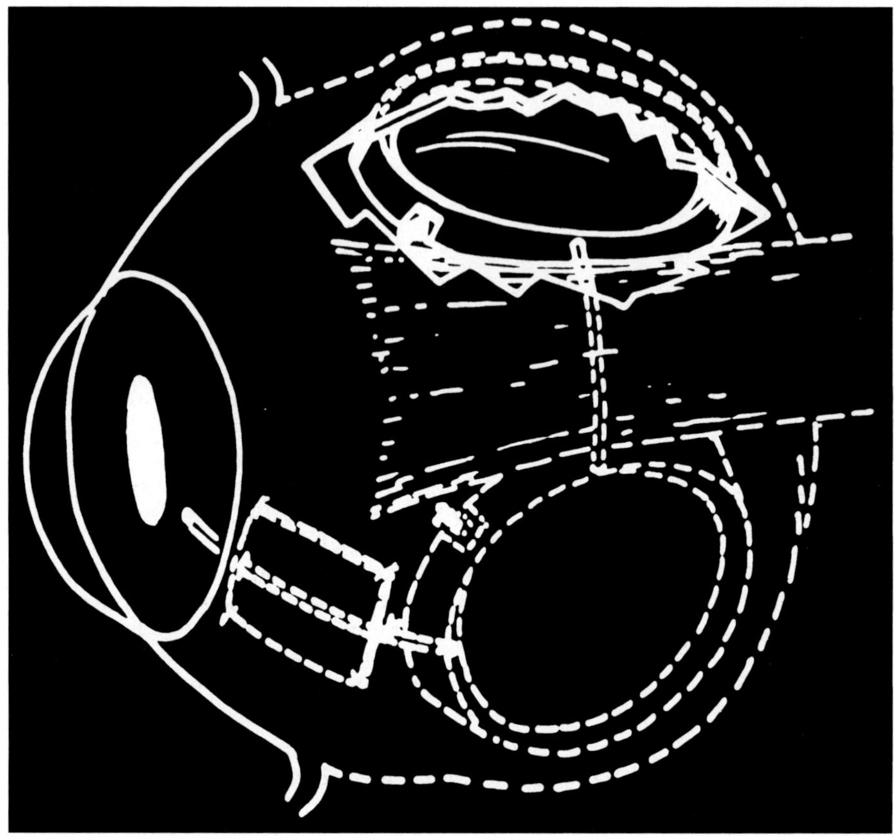

Fig. 1. Diagram illustrating a double-plate Molteno glaucoma drainage device in position with a cut-away view of the secondary plate and its capsule. A scleral patch is in place over the drain tube and a 'temporary' ligature is present at the posterior edge of the scleral patch graft.

around the explant, including degeneration of the inner lining and elaboration of new collagen bundles in the mid portions of the wall, continue thereafter at variable rates. These processes are part of the expected inflammatory response to the flow of aqueous into periocular tissues and most likely reach a balance between tissue loss and new tissue formation in successful cases. Similar changes no doubt occur in the boundary layer of ordinary filtering blebs after trabeculectomy. If the inflammatory response becomes excessive in either standard blebs or around GDDs, filtration will fail.

Experimental studies have demonstrated that aqueous crosses the capsule wall into periocular intercellular spaces by simple passive diffusion[16]. Escaping aqueous is then picked up by lymphatics or capillaries and returned to the blood stream. In contrast to perilimbal filtration, conjunctival microcysts are seldom seen with GDDs, suggesting that transconjunctival movement of aqueous is relatively less common than after trabeculectomy.

Following ligature release or tube insertion in the course of a two-stage implant installation, a filtering bleb is usually immediately apparent over the explant portion of the device as aqueous fills the potential space between the explant and the capsule. The capsule formed is always easily separated from overlying Tenon's

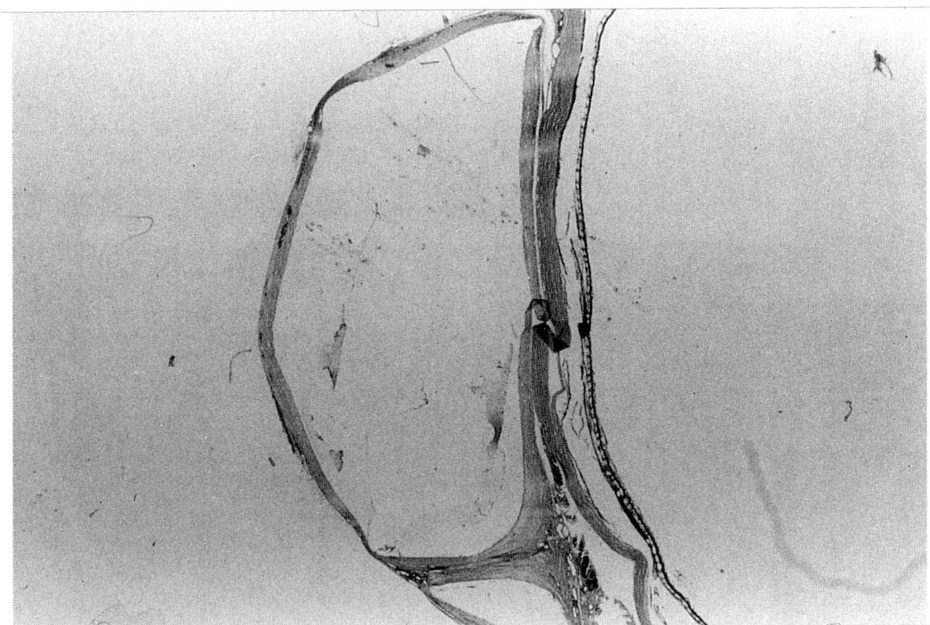

Fig. 2. Photomicrograph of monkey eye with mature capsule overlying a single-plate Molteno GDD. The GDD has been lost in processing. A tongue of fibrous tissue has extended through a suture hole, fastening the two walls of the capsule together. (Masson's trichrome × 15.)

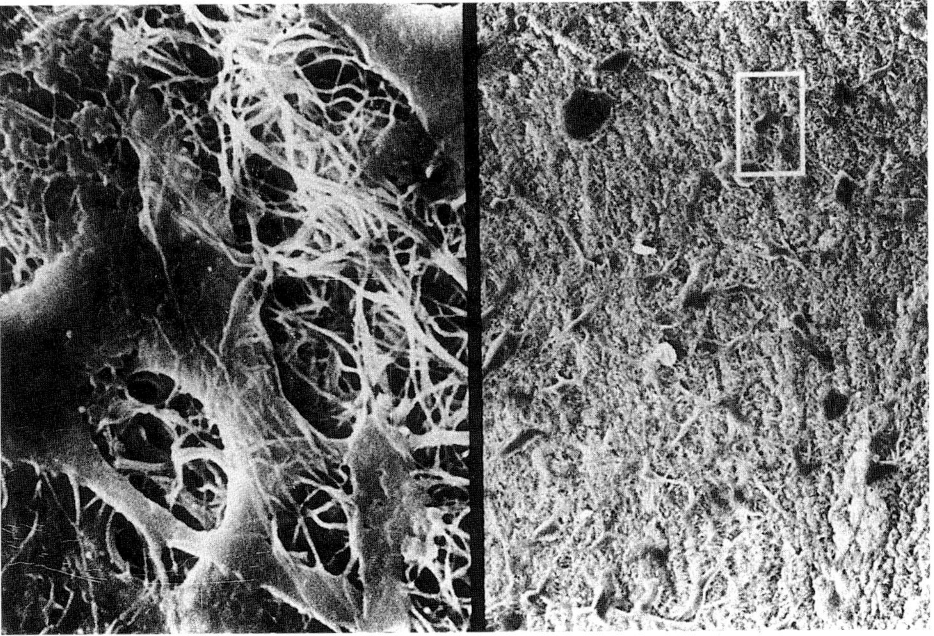

Fig. 3. Scanning electron micrograph at low and higher magnification of the inner surface of the filtration bleb from 'failed' Molteno GDD in a human eye, removed in the process of surgical revision. In the higher magnification photograph, the inner surface is an open collagen mesh with a sparse population of probable fibroblasts.

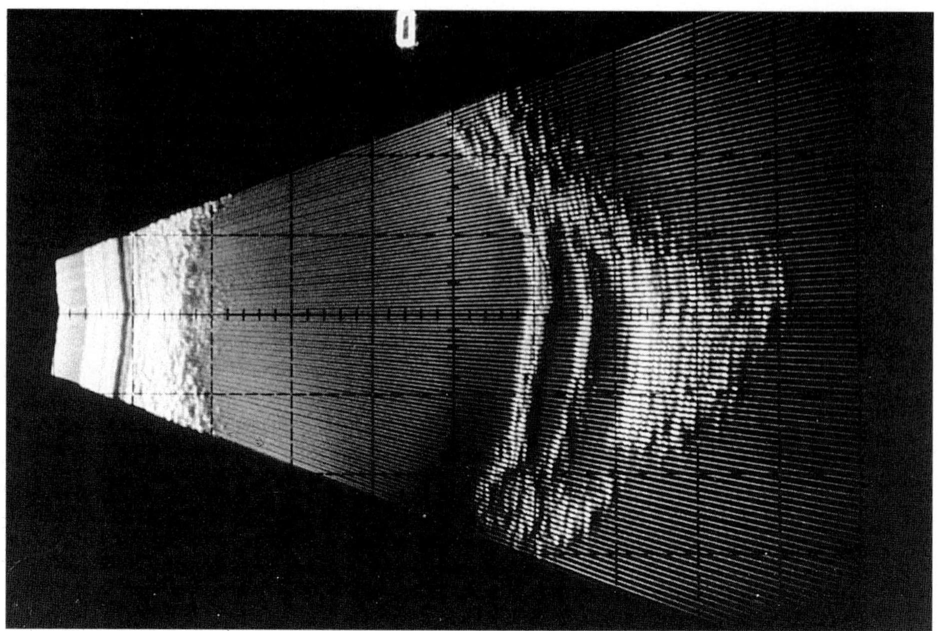

Fig. 4. B-scan ultrasound of a functioning bleb around a Baerveldt GDD in a human eye. The plate is represented by the middle echo, surrounded by echo lucent fluid on both sides. The characteristic flattening of the adjacent eye wall is apparent.

fascia and can be dissected as an intact layer from underlying episcleral tissues. Except for transient leak around the tube at the site of scleral penetration, aqueous flow out of the eye occurs via the tube lumen.

A variable inflammatory reaction, provoked by aqueous flow follows beginning tube function and drainage of aqueous into the periocular compartment, whether or not a capsule is present around the explant. The inflammatory reaction is commonly associated with a rise in intraocular pressure (IOP) (hypertensive phase) which may last for weeks[6]. The usual clinical course postoperatively parallels that following standard filtering surgery, with waning of inflammation and stable decrease in IOP by four to six weeks after beginning function. IOP levels seldom stabilize below the mid-teens with GDDs, even with the addition of aqueous suppressing medication such as topical beta blockers[6].

The drain tube itself offers no resistance to flow between the anterior chamber or vitreous cavity and the bleb space at flow rates many times those expected normally.[16] As fibroblasts cannot establish a tight bond to the explant material, the flow of aqueous creates a pool of fluid next to the plate. Ultrasound studies in monkey and man and experimental marker studies suggest that all surfaces of the bleb around the explant function to drain fluid (Fig. 4)[6,7]. The explant, bound to the episclera only at its anterior edge, literally 'floats' in a pool of aqueous.

In monkey and man, the inner lining of the bleb around the explant remains an open mesh of collagen fibers without an epithelial or fibroblastic lining except in pathological situations such as epithelial ingrowth (Fig. 3)[17]. Fluid movement across this boundary capsule has been shown in monkey and rabbits to be directly related to pressure, and to the surface area of the bleb, and inversely related to bleb capsule thickness. The ability of fluid to move across the bleb wall [hydraulic conductivity (μl/min/mm^2/mmHg)] is the same regardless of bleb surface area[18,19].

Studies in monkeys and rabbits have demonstrated that the capsule around the explant is histologically similar in experimental eyes with functioning drainage devices to the capsule in control eyes where aqueous flow never occurs[16]. Physiological flow studies in monkeys suggested that aqueous flow into the bleb capsule may actually improve capsule permeability over time, perhaps by a 'washout' effect. No experimental or clinical studies to date have determined whether or not permitting immediate aqueous flow as with 'valved' implants alters the biology of the fibrous capsule which always forms around the explant.

The maturation of filtering blebs around explant material in rabbits may regularly include the development of a fibrous inner bleb wall lining, possibly explaining the relatively short duration of IOP lowering after glaucoma drain installation in that species[19]. Such differences between primates and other species obviously limit the validity of long-term experimental studies in non-primates.

In summary, available experimental and pathological studies of glaucoma drainage implants indicate that these devices function by promoting simple passive diffusion of aqueous across the capsular boundary around the explant portion of the device into the intercellular orbital compartment. Collection and removal of aqueous from the periocular intercellular space presumably occurs via venous capillaries or lymphatics. The lumened tube provides a relatively non-occludable conduit for aqueous movement from anterior chamber or vitreous cavities into the bleb.

Indications for clinical use of GDDs

At present, the most reasonable indications for GDDs include 'complicated' glaucoma histories with failure of medical or laser treatment and failure of standard surgical procedures (trabeculectomy or full thickness filtering surgery) including antifibrotic agents (5-fluorouracil or mitomycin). Associated surface disease such as extreme dry eye or pemphigoid also are reasonable indications for considering a GDD. If visual potential is poor (less than 20/200) and comfort is the primary clinical goal, cyclodestructive procedures such as transscleral Nd:YAG or diode laser or cyclocryotherapy are probably preferable. Other specific clinical problems in which GDDs seem reasonable include neovascular glaucomas not responding to panretinal photocoagulation, epithelial ingrowth beyond excisional surgery, traumatized eyes with conjunctival or scleral injury precluding standard filtering surgery or a requirement for contact lens use. Congenital glaucoma not amenable to standard surgery (goniotomy or trabeculotomy) is also a relative indication for consideration of a GDD. If anatomic anomalies preclude standard goniotomy or trabeculotomy as in some examples of Axenfeld's, Reiger's, Peter's or aniridia, GDDs may be an acceptable primary therapy. Trabeculectomy with antifibrotic agents is being utilized in children with good short-term success, but is of concern with regard to a high risk of late infection if avascular blebs develop.

Surface area and technique considerations

It is desirable to provide a sufficiently large explant to maximize aqueous drainage in hopes of achieving a normalization of IOP and minimize the need for supplemental medications. The largest currently available ready-made implant (one side surface area) is the Baerveldt 425 mm^2 device which can be installed through a single quadrant incision and extended under adjacent rectus muscles. Similar or even larger surface areas can be attained with the Schocket procedure with a wide, 360° encircling element, necessitating, however, damage to all four quadrants of conjunctiva[20,21]. A 'modified' Schocket procedure can be an effective method for IOP control if a pre-existing buckle is available[22].

Large, wide implants such as the 350 mm^2 Baerveldt and the previously available 500 mm^2 Baerveldt which extend under adjacent rectus muscles have been associated with a high risk of muscle impairment and strabismus, especially when installed upper nasally[23]. Strabismus associated with larger implants probably can result from bulk effects (high, vaulting blebs or globe displacement) or from direct impairment of rectus or oblique function (stretching, fibrous adhesions). Recently, the various sized Baerveldt implants have been 'perforated' to allow fibrous cross adhesions between the upper and lower portions of the capsule in hopes of reducing the vaulting and bulk effect of the otherwise large bleb.

Managing postoperative hypotony with non-valved GDDs

Two-stage drainage device installations, and temporary partial or complete ligature of the drain tube are all methods to minimize hypotony following drainage device installation. Many reports, published and anecdotal, have testified to the hazards of installing an unrestricted drain into a glaucomatous eye. Besides immediate hypotony and its attendant complications, shallowing or flattening of the anterior chamber and sandwiching of the drain tube between iris, or lens and endothelium may produce significant corneal damage.

The ideal interval between the first and second stages of a two-stage installation of a glaucoma drain tube is probably three to five weeks. After this interval, a distinct fibrous capsule will be present and the risk of hypotony following tube installation (without any ligature) will be minimal. A two-stage installation with several weeks interval between stages is especially desirable in infants and in adults with badly battered eyes to prevent hypotony and its complications.

Leak around the standard silicone rubber tube as it crosses the limbal tissues may be minimized by using a 23- or 25-gauge needle to make the tract. The smaller the tract, the more difficult tube installation may be. The larger the tract, the more likely temporary (and unpredictable) leakage will occur. Many eyes will develop a temporary anterior filtering bleb due to leak around the tube or anterior migration of fluid leaking through the tube if not completely occluded. Cutting the tube with a sharp bevel is especially helpful before installation into a tight needle tract. Testing the integrity of tube closure with balanced salt infusion before installation of the ligated tube into the eye is helpful to ensure complete closure. There is always some risk that an absorbable ligature will stretch or be displaced and that some leak through the tube may occur before desired postoperatively.

Several clever methods of temporarily occluding a drain tube, such as with the Molteno, Baerveldt, or Schocket devices have been reported. These vary from simple occlusion with an absorbable suture to differing 'rip cord' suture techniques, which provide reasonably practical methods of opening the drain tube at the most desirable time postoperatively without major surgical intervention. Prolene sutures can be used to occlude the anterior chamber portion of the drain tube and broken subsequently by laser. Repair of lacerated tubes or extension of inadvertently shortened tubes may be accomplished by constructing a tube graft utilizing slightly larger diameter tubing (Stortz #N5941 3 [ID 0.64 mm] placed as a segment over the standard tubing (Stortz #N5941 1 [ID 0.30 mm]). (For summary, see: Mills RP, Implantation of Glaucoma Drainage Devices, AAO, Skills Transfer Course Manual 1995-6.)

In general, resumption of antiglaucoma medications (beta blockers and carbonic anhydrase inhibitors) will be necessary pending tube opening. Modifications of the installation utilizing tube slits anterior to an occluding ligature or larger than necessary needle tracts for tube installation into the anterior chamber may also provide temporary IOP relief pending ligature release. Partial ligature of the tube has also been recommended. These temporizing methods, however, have variable and unpredictable duration of function.

A paracentesis should always be placed during surgery in a location which can easily be reached at the slit-lamp postoperatively to permit venting or reformation of the chamber if necessary. If viscoelastics are used during surgery with complete tube closure, they should be removed to minimize postoperative pressure rise.

Valves and flow restrictors

The complexity and practical problems (two-stage installation, hypotony risks) associated with use of non-valved devices such as the Molteno and Baerveldt implants have generated enthusiasm for incorporating hypotony preventing 'valves' or 'flow restrictors' in GDDs. In theory, such a modification should eliminate the risk of hypotony and greatly simplify their clinical utilization.

Devices with valves include the Krupin disc, the Ahmed valve, the White Shunt Pump and the Joseph implant[13]. The OptiMed device includes a flow restrictor. All these devices, with the exception of the White Shunt Pump, which has a unique molded tube, utilize the same silicone rubber tube (ID 0.3 mm) to connect the fluid spaces inside the eye to the explant.

To date, reported clinical studies of these 'valved' devices all include postoperative hypotony as a complication, presumably due to leak around the tube or failure of the valve or flow restrictor to provide adequate immediate resistance. Some reports on valved devices have included larger percentages of clinically significant hypotony postoperatively than with non-valved, temporarily ligatured devices[12].

In vitro studies using micromanometric measuring equipment and physiological flow rates (@ 2 μl/minute) have demonstrated that once opened by perfusion with balanced salt or plasma, valve closure with Krupin and Ahmed devices does not occur (Fig. 5)[13]. In bench studies comparing the Krupin disc, Ahmed and OptiMed devices, only the OptiMed flow restrictor consistently maintained resistance to flow after the infusion pump was stopped. These same studies also included verification of advertised 'opening and closing pressures' for these two devices in air, probably not useful clinically because the 'valves' are routinely perfused with balanced salt before insertion into living eyes.

During *in vivo* studies at 24 hours postoperatively in rabbits, measurements with the same micromanometric system demonstrated that the tissue reaction around the explant portion of Krupin, Ahmed, Baerveldt, Molteno, and OptiMed devices contributed to measured resistance[13]. At 24 hours postoperatively in the rabbit, disruption of the conjunctival wound resulted in rapid drop in IOP to zero regardless of the specific device installed. In these same experimental studies, virtually no effect of the ridge on the 'ridged Molteno' could be demonstrated.

Considering the findings during *in vitro* and *in vivo* measurements and the con-

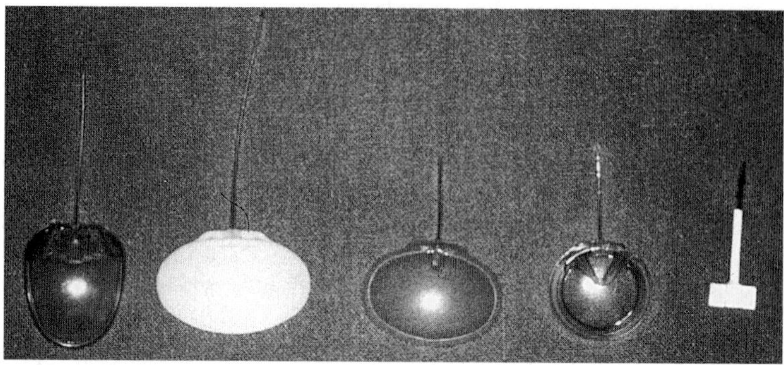

Fig. 5. Photograph of five currently available GDDs; from left to right Ahmed, Baerveldt, Krupin disc, Molteno (single plate), and OptiMed. (Reproduced from Prata *et al.*[13], by courtesy of the Editors of *Ophthalmology* [Fig 1].)

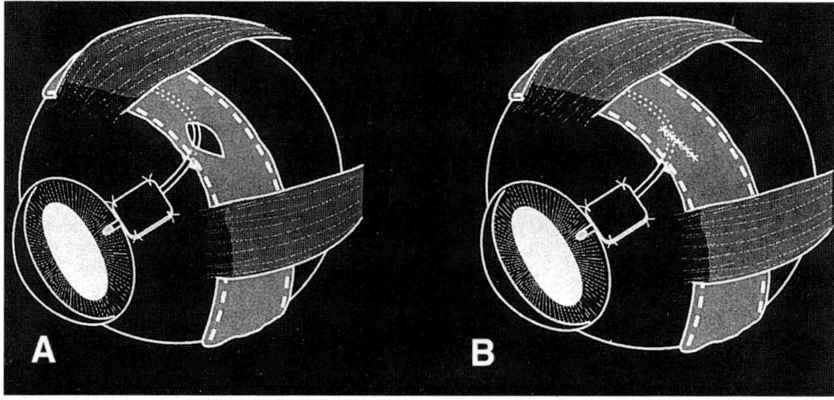

Fig. 6. Diagram illustrating a 'modified' Schocket procedure in which a segment of tubing is used to connect the anterior or vitreous chambers to a pre-existing buckle capsule. (Reproduced from Sidoti *et al.*[22], by courtesy of the Editors of *Ophthalmology* [Fig. 1].)

tinuing clinical problem of hypotony with 'valved' implants, skepticism that valves or flow restrictors are yet sufficiently evolved to solve the hypotony problem is justified. In any case, beyond the first many days after capsule formation, valves or flow restrictors in these systems may have no useful function, since resistance resides in the capsule around the explant.

Combined retina and cornea procedures, pars plana installation

In complex, combined disease problems where IOP control is or is likely to become poor, consideration of a GDD may be justified as an alternative to other types of filtering surgery or cyclodestruction. A first-stage GDD with episcleral placement of the explant and possible later tube installation may be done at the same time as retinal or corneal surgery is undertaken. Such a two-stage drain installation is a relatively safe method of providing a 'backup' IOP control system. Drain implants may function well, even in eyes containing silicone oil[24]. Pars plana

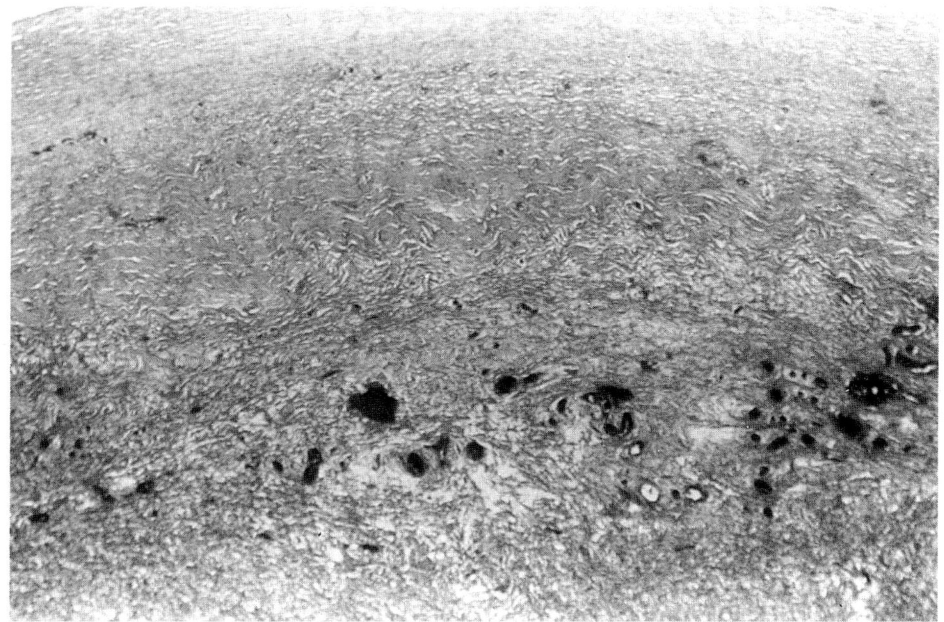

Fig. 7. Photomicrograph of markedly thickened capsule over a Molteno GDD removed in the process of surgical revision after clinical failure. The capsule wall is several times thicker than expected normally and the collagen more dense. (Hematoxylin and eosin, original magnification × 120.)

tube installation in previously vitrectomized and lensectomized eyes is often advantageous, especially if the anterior chamber is shallow or there are extensive peripheral anterior synechiae. In cases with a pre-existing buckle, a segment of tubing may be used to connect the anterior chamber or vitreous cavities to the capsule around the buckle (Fig. 6).

The use of GDDs for IOP control in complex cases of combined cataract and glaucoma is of potential interest but has not been carefully studied.

GDDs and penetrating keratoplasty

Graft rejection may be aggravated or accelerated by any type of filtering surgery including GDDs. Although the mechanism of such an effect remains unproven, the speculation has been that filtering surgery may increase exposure of the graft to the host defense mechanisms. Cyclodestructive procedures are an obvious alternative to filtering surgery for IOP control in post-keratoplasty eyes.

Complications unique to GDDs

Glaucoma drainage devices may be associated with all of the complications of standard filtering surgery, especially clinical failure due to excessive fibrosis around the filtering bleb (Fig. 7). The most obvious and important complication

Grand Rounds III

Topics: trabeculectomy in patients with early cataract, Holmium lasers, new drugs, topical CAIs, ALT: 180° versus 360°, TPA, cyclodestruction, bleb massage

Moderator: Clifford Hendricks

Clifford Hendricks, MD: *The patient is a 72-year-old with a vision of 20/30 minus and 1-1/2 plus nuclear sclerosis and cortical spoking with glaucoma that requires surgery. Would you do a trabeculectomy alone or anticipate cataract progression and do a combined procedure?*

Paul Palmberg, MD: I think obviously you would have to talk to this person. There is a 20/30 cataract that when you turn the lights up in the room is still 20/30 or 20/40. Then there is a 20/30 cataract, if it is a posterior subcapsular, that might fall off to 20/80 or 20/200. So first of all, you have to know what effect this is having on the person's vision and whether they are having glare symptoms or problems. But let us say it is not enough that you would have done this as a cataract otherwise. I have been doing filtering procedures on this kind of patient because I do not think that you are going to have any trouble doing the cataract later on if you have to. It will not mess up your filter because you could do a temporal phaco later. And many of these will not progress. Particularly, more recently, I have been doing my filters with the safety valve incision, the chamber is deep before there is any flow out of the eye, so I do not need an iridectomy unless the patient has blepharospasm or some other problem. My impression is that I get a lot less cataract and a lot less cataract progression with that. I would be more inclined to try to not have to do an iridectomy in this case, and to have normal flow of aqueous over that lens to keep feeding it properly.

Michael A. Kass, MD: I think there are a number of other things you would want to consider: the vision in the other eye, how much field loss there is in this eye. This person might be 20/30 if the cataract was out, anyway. I would talk to the patient. If they are not really disabled with it, I would do the same. I would do the filter and maybe this person will go on for five or ten years, or the rest of their natural days, and not need the cataract. I do not think you should routinely assume that cataracts will necessarily accelerate because you do the filter.

George L. Spaeth, MD: That is old data, I think. I think you are right, Mike. With better techniques, less hypotony, fewer flat chambers, the incidence of cataract getting worse rapidly is much lower. The one last thought though is that you of course want to make sure the patient does not develop posterior synechiae, so they

Peril to the Nerve – Glaucoma and Clinical Neuro-Ophthalmology, pp. 207–213
Proceedings of the 45th Annual Symposium of the New Orleans Academy of
Ophthalmology, New Orleans, LA, USA, April 25-28, 1996
edited by Barry J. Leader and Jonathan C. Calkwood
© *1998 Kugler Publications, The Hague/The Netherlands*

have to be well dilated. Otherwise, the cataract extraction at a later date is going to be difficult. So, that patient needs to be on real good cycloplegia and for a long period of time.

Dr. Hendricks: *Next question, whatever happened to the Holmium laser?*

Dr. Spaeth: Since we have one, I will answer that question. It has some very nice indications. A patient who is pseudophakic and in whom you need a low pressure, is an excellent candidate for Holmium laser sclerostomy. They work well and are relatively easy to do. For that particular indication, it is almost worthwhile in itself.

Dr. Kass: I took that course some years ago. I am sure many other people here in the audience did. The thing that struck me is that there are some problems with this. One is it is a full thickness filter and we have just gone to this elaborate mechanism of trying to move away from that. The other thing is that it makes it more difficult, not impossible, but more difficult, to use antimetabolites in the way that you would like, but this can be gotten around. And the third thing that influenced me against this is that, if you look at the published results, they are not as good as those we get by operating. Something not only has to be simpler, it should be better as well. And at least, from what I can tell from the published results, we do better with standard means.

Dr. Palmberg: Yes, about 50% was the published result in the kind of aphakic patient, and that was with two operations. So as far as I could tell in our area, the only indication was it was something that could be done in the office. From a capitated managed care standpoint, it saved money not putting people in the hospital. But a very good surgeon in our area had a success rate of about 50% without antimetabolites and had 10% complications including such things as the iris coming up and sticking in the hole, so that the enthusiasm in our area in Florida has plummeted for the use of the machine.

Dr. Spaeth: I am not disagreeing with what you are saying. I think the indications are very tight, but occasional patients are handled very well, very easily. In a pseudophakic patient who has conjunctiva in which you can just slip that probe in easily, it works very well.

Dr. Hendricks: *Next question. I have noted that patients either have a great response to Trusopt or none at all. Do you agree?*

Dr. Kass: No.

Dr. Hendricks: *No? I guess then, what is your experience with Trusopt?*

Dr. Kass: I think it is like most other drugs. I think people respond, you get this gradation of response. Generally speaking, I have been pretty happy with this drug. It certainly makes life a lot easier for the patients in terms of putting people on a carbonic anhydrase inhibitor. It is now a relatively easy thing to do. It used to be such a chore, by the time you went through all the possible side-effects with them and everything, it was a major deal. Now I think you can put people on this drug and expect reasonable response in a fair number of people. I have not seen this all or none phenomenon. I think you get the kind of typical range of response that you do from most other meds.

Dr. Spaeth: You cannot, however, think that this drug is going to be free of side-effects. It has the same side-effects as the systemic carbonic anhydrase inhibitors. They get GI upsets, they get fatigue, they lose weight, they get hoarse, which is a new one, that did not seem to bother the other folks so much. But certainly, a significant percentage of them get hoarse. It is a potent medication with potent side-effects.

Dr. Palmberg: It can probably replace Neptazane 25 or 50 twice a day. It can probably replace Diamox 125 four times a day, something of that order. It is not going to make the patient acidotic, so if somebody is on a gram of Diamox a day, you are not as likely to get good control. You might, but it does not have that second phase of effect of carbonic anhydrase inhibitors. Nevertheless, I love it as a second drug. I think, as Thom Zimmerman suggested, it probably can be used twice a day when combined with a beta blocker. Outside of the bad taste in the mouth in people who have to be taught about nasolacrimal obstruction, or else about closing their eyes gently for five minutes, except for that problem and the very rare patient with diarrhea or some systemic problem with it, it has been a very well-tolerated drug. I think it is more preferable to adding pilocarpine as a second drug. So I am much more inclined to add it and to try to get the pressure down into the mid normal range, instead of floating around 18 to 20 in a glaucoma patient. I feel safer and I do not think it creates problems for the majority of patients.

Dr. Hendricks: *Do you consider this then just strictly a second-line drug?*

Dr. Palmberg: Well, if a patient cannot take a beta blocker, I have used it as a first-line drug. But I think we need to know about it for a longer period of time before I would feel quite as safe as I do with the beta blockers.

Dr. Kass: One interesting thing is I tried to switch over every patient who was on systemic CAIs. I thought I would see hundreds of grateful patients who told me they did not realize how terrible they felt, and this was not true. When you think about it, the reason is that everybody who felt terrible had already stopped the drug. What you had left were the survivors, and some patients told me that they preferred taking the pills to the drops. I think it just showed that a number of people over the years, Lichter and others, have shown that only about half the people at best can tolerate long-term systemic CAI therapy. What you had was probably the other 30 or 35% who were still on it in your office and they were not having problems with it. I was amazed, one, by the number of people who could not tell the difference, and two, by how many people had much lower pressures on Trusopt than they had on Diamox, and of course, you know what the answer to that is.

Dr. Spaeth: One last thought with regard to your question, though, and that is, I am not sure that we should continue this concept of "first-line drug". The question is, is it the first drug for this particular patient? And that means pilocarpine with some people, and epinephrine compounds with other people, it means dorzolamide with others, and phospholine iodide with others. There is no standardized patient, there is no first-line drug. They are all sometimes the best drug for the particular patient you are considering.

Dr. Hendricks: *Good. Next question. ALT 180 versus 360, and do you routinely use half a percent or one percent apraclonidine for prophylaxis?*

Dr. Spaeth: If the question is, do I do 180 or 360, I do 360 in all patients, except in those in whom I think there is a significant risk of damage due to a pressure rise. Patients whose pressures are high, who have far advanced optic nerve damage, who have a trabecular meshwork which is not likely to respond well to increased debris or inflammation, those patients will get 180. But they are rare. So I would say, probably 95% of the argon laser trabeculoplasties I do are 360 degrees. I use aproclonidine in all those patients in whom I am concerned about a pressure spike. I do not use it routinely.

Dr. Kass: I will give the opposite answer then to all those questions. I do 180 routinely, and if I get a partial response that is not quite what I want, I will then go back a month or two or whatever later and do the other 180, but if I get the response I want from the 180, I will just stop there and see what happens, and I use aproclonidine 0.5% routinely in patients. I do not see any reason not to use it, since I think it is not as easy to predict who is going to get a pressure rise, and I think it is helpful and the drug in single use seems to be remarkably safe. So, I use it routinely before all the trabeculoplasties.

Dr. Palmberg: Yes, I use it before all of them and I do 360 degrees. I do not know of any reason not to do it. And when you use the 0.5% bottle, you can treat so many patients with that one bottle that there is really no cost saving by avoiding it.

Dr. Hendricks: *What is your experience and recommendations with postoperative TPA injections in trabeculectomies and seton devices?*

Dr. Kass: Using TPA (tissue plasminogen activator) will dissolve fibrin clots. I have used it on a few occasions. I do not remember who was giving the talk. I guess it was Dr. Quigley this morning talking about somebody with a high pressure and you gonioscope them and you see that the ostium is plugged. You wait a day or two and it is still plugged, or you get this horrendous fibrin mass in the anterior chamber and you think it is going to cause the filter to fail. You can give intracameral TPA and people have used various doses. I think the dose I have used is 5 µg. Although some people use much higher doses, I think it is better to give a smaller dose and wait and see what happens. I think occasionally this is effective. I think it is the kind of thing that you would do once a year, even if you did a lot of filters. I just do not have a reason to do it often.

Dr. Spaeth: It is also effective in dissolving clots and in producing lovely fresh bleeding. It is not without complications.

Dr. Palmberg: But if you have got somebody who has a lot of blood plugging the ostium and you put them back on medical therapy to see if you could tide it over and it has not gotten better, it is really wonderful. In those three or four cases in which I have used it, it was really nice to have had it.

Dr. Kass: Let me just make the point. I think that the re-bleeding is somewhat dose-dependent. Some of the retina people have published using like 25 µg. I think that if you use smaller doses, you will get a lower incidence of bleeding, not zero but lower. That is a real concern, that you can get rid of blood and give them more blood. If you have ever done this, the fibrin you sometimes see is just gone, it melts, it is an amazing-looking thing.

Dr. Hendricks: *What do you feel about laser cyclodestruction as an acceptable option in the treatment of a young black male who is post multiple failed filtering procedures, including trab with mitomycin and Molteno implant. He has progression of field loss, elevated intraocular pressure, visual acuity 20/25? If not, what is your best option?*

Dr. Palmberg: I would find a place to put another tube in, because I have not yet seen the patient in whom I would do a cyclodestructive procedure on a seeing eye. I guess if I had put four drainage tubes in taking every quadrant (I am making a hypothetical case), then maybe I would do it.

Dr. Spaeth: I am not quite as rigid as that. Cyclodestruction procedures can work well, but they are by definition destructive. It makes much better sense to do everything you can to try to control the glaucoma by increasing outflow, before you start killing the parts that are essential to the wellbeing of the eye.

Dr. Kass: I would agree with George. I think if you had done all these things in this patient, it might be something you would do. There are a couple of real worries: phthisis, cataract, but particularly, I think, macular edema in somebody with good vision. So I think that cyclodestructive procedures are almost always your last choice in somebody who has good vision.

Dr. Palmberg: This is not an 80-year-old aphake with a pressure of 23 where you need a little bit of lowering, in which case maybe it is a much better option. This is a young black person whose pressure probably is 40 or 50 and, to destroy enough ciliary body in that patient to get the pressure down in a useful fashion without having it go into phthisis later, I think, is not really likely to be successful. That was the reason why I would be so aggressive, if you will, trying to get flow out of the eye instead.

Dr. Spaeth: But you could change the description of the case and, in my opinion, make the cyclodestructive procedure the treatment of choice. Let us say that this was a 20-year-old black or white, Asian, it does not matter, individual who has a huge globe following congenital glaucoma with a thin, thin sclera and has had retinal detachment, is pseudophakic, and has a very fragile eye. The pressure has been 40 for two years. This patient is in the 50, 60, 70% category for getting a suprachoroidal expulsive hemorrhage. You just do not want to open that eye. You do not want that eye hypotonus. Those patients can do very well for a long period of time with cyclodestructive procedures, such as a very carefully graded, well-titrated cyclophotocoagulation. The procedure should definitely not be jettisoned. It has good indications.

Dr. Kass: I think it is also fair to say that, while I do not think any of the members of this panel are particularly enthusiastic about cyclodestructive procedures, there are good, careful researchers who think much more highly about them than we do. You may not be getting a totally balanced presentation here.

Dr. Hendricks: *In incipient bleb failure, when do you recommend massage of the globe, if in fact you believe this is effective, what is the proper technique for doing so?*

Dr. Palmberg: I used to do a fair amount of massage because Mike, who was my teacher, showed me how to do it, and so probably should comment on it. Now that we are using antimetabolites, there are not very many people who seem to need it. What I do when I do have somebody who needs it, is to close their eye, get them to look straight ahead, and, after washing their hands, to push their cornea directly in as if they were putting their finger into a bowling ball, not rubbing from side to side, pushing in, holding it, going 1001, 1002, for about ten presses. I have them do it in the office; *a.* to make sure they can do it; and *b.* to make sure it actually lowers the pressure. Because if it does not lower the pressure in the office, you might as well forget about it. If it lowers it five or ten points, then I have them do it with the idea that perhaps we are stretching the bleb, and that during the time between the massages, perhaps it will be lower after a while.

Dr. Hendricks: *And when would you start this?*

Dr. Palmberg: I guess when I think the bleb is contracting and I am not going to be able to make it better by either laser suture lysis or needling to elevate the scleral flap, just basic failure of the conjunctiva and Tenon's.

Dr. Spaeth: Paul was talking earlier about the term mitomycin trabeculectomy and was saying that there is no such thing as a mitomycin trabeculectomy because everybody uses mitomycin differently. Massage fits into that same category. I think all of us at Wills use a specific routine. You must do it in at least 50%, probably 75% or more, of patients who have guarded filtration procedures. The afternoon of the surgery or the next morning, you take an applicator and push right over one of the radial grooves and you see the fluid come up and you get a nice elevation of the bleb. You gonioscope the patient first to make sure there is no problem. But if there is no problem, then what you have done is to take a little fibrin out or a little blood, and you have encouraged the filtration. It is absolutely benign, and it works to improve the pressure control. You see the pressure go from something like 24 down to 12, and you see a high bleb. In a routine case, you can do this for maybe a day or two. In a patient who has had an antimetabolite, maybe up to a week. Long-term digital ocular compression has not, to my knowledge, been demonstrated to change the clinical course of any patient. We did a study in which we tried looking at the patients over a period of time. The first thing was if you measured the pressure at the time that the 'massage' was being given with a pneumotonometer, the pressure went up to about 120 to 140 mmHg for 10 or 20 seconds. What is that doing to an already fragile lamina? A little scary. The pressure comes down in most people if they have a bleb that is working, but you measure it an hour later and, in about 90% of the patients, the pressure is back up to exactly where it was before. So I am not a fan of massage because I think there are some patients who get damaged. There is a potential for damage and, long term, I am not sure that it works.

Dr. Kass: Let me just say that I think the maneuver George described is also very good if you either lyse sutures or release them. Sometimes you do that and you do not quite get the effect you want, so you just push on it a little bit and all of a sudden it pops open and that is a very nice thing to do.

Dr. Hendricks: *I would like to thank our panelists this morning.*

Medical and surgical management of neovascular and uveitic glaucoma

Don Minckler

Department of Ophthalmology, University of Southern California School of Medicine, Los Angeles, CA, USA

Neovascular and open-angle glaucoma in diabetes

Neovascular and uveitic glaucomas remain among the most difficult glaucoma management problems. Perhaps the most important 'ocular insight' in recent decades has been that retinal ischemia, manifested by capillary non-perfusion using fluorescein angiography, can identify eyes at risk for neovascular proliferations, including neovascular glaucoma. This now well verified concept has permitted a dramatic shift in the historical clinical algorithm from 'reaction' to 'proactive' preventive focal or panretinal photocoagulation (PRP)[1].

The relative risk of neovascular glaucoma (NVG) remains high among diabetics who have been insulin-dependent for ten to 15 years. The other two major underlying etiologies for NVG include branch or central retinal vein occlusions and obstructive carotid artery disease[1].

Currently, controversy persists as to whether or not chronic open-angle glaucoma occurs with an increased rate among diabetics, and whether or not diabetes is actually a risk factor for open-angle glaucoma[2]. Traditional wisdom has been that the two disorders, diabetes and chronic open-angle glaucoma, are associated, and that diabetes is a risk factor for open-angle glaucoma, at least in individuals beyond 40 years of age. Standard teaching has advised looking for diabetes among newly diagnosed open-angle glaucoma patients or conversely to expect a high incidence of open-angle glaucoma among newly diagnosed diabetics. Newer studies, however, are challenging these views.

During the recently completed Baltimore Eye Survey, some 5308 individuals of both black and white races were surveyed[2]. Diabetes was identified by history and the method of treatment tabulated as 'insulin-dependent or non-insulin-dependent'. Diabetes was highly prevalent in the population studied with 10.6% of white subjects and 17.2% of black subjects having the disease, respectively. Diabetes was not statistically significantly associated with open-angle glaucoma in this cross-sectional, population-based prevalence survey conducted between 1985 and 1988. The authors do admit a 'trend' indicating that diabetes and elevated intraocular

Address for correspondence: Professor Don S. Minckler, MD, Department of Ophthalmology, University of Southern California School of Medicine, Doheny Eye Institute, 1450 San Pablo Street, Los Angeles, CA 90033-4666, USA

Peril to the Nerve – Glaucoma and Clinical Neuro-Ophthalmology, pp. 215–219
Proceedings of the 45th Annual Symposium of the New Orleans Academy of
Ophthalmology, New Orleans, LA, USA, April 25-28, 1996
edited by Barry J. Leader and Jonathan C. Calkwood
© 1998 Kugler Publications, The Hague/The Netherlands

pressure (IOP) are associated, but the statistical significance was marginal. This study may have underestimated the actual incidence of diabetes because blood sugars were not done either to confirm the diagnosis or as part of routine screening. Also, in the calculations of risk for diabetes among screened patients, no correction could be made for presumed increased mortality among diabetics. The authors noted that diabetes is generally regarded as 'underdiagnosed'.

Whether or not diabetes itself is truly a risk factor for open-angle glaucoma, other disorders associated with diabetes including elevated blood pressure and systemic hypertension do appear to be holding up as risk factors for open-angle glaucoma[3]. Recent studies from The Netherlands have estimated the prevalence of open-angle glaucoma among their population[4]. In the first 3062 individuals studied, 1.1% were determined to have open-angle glaucoma using IOP, disc examination and perimetry.

Pathophysiology of neovascular glaucoma

Neovascular glaucoma has long been thought to be triggered in diabetes, and in other forms of retinal vascular disease, by the diffusion of some substance from ischemic retina into the anterior segment. Neovascularization is often initially noted around peripheral iridectomies and the pupil margin, areas obviously likely to be exposed to relatively high concentrations of a provocative substance emanating from the retina. A recent update on the status of the long sought 'evil humor' indicates that identification of the responsible factor or factors is progressing[5]. The product of ischemic retina primarily responsible for neovascular proliferation is thought to be an angiogenic protein, 'vascular endothelial growth factor' (VEGF) also known as 'vascular permeability factor' (VPF).

Clinically, NVG may become apparent as slowly or rapidly developing fine capillaries on the pupillary margin or iris surface before IOP is elevated. Alternatively, NVG may suddenly appear as an acute glaucoma with pain and corneal edema simulating acute angle closure. According to Ohnishi *et al.*, fluorescein gonioscopy will often demonstrate angle vessels before they appear near the pupil, in some cases in pre-proliferative diabetic retinopathy[6]. It is a mistake to proceed with laser trabeculoplasty (LTP) without excluding diabetic retinopathy and NVG, thinking one is dealing with ordinary open-angle glaucoma, non-responsive to medication. LTP can provoke a dramatic acceleration of angle vessel growth and precipitate an IOP crisis, somewhat akin to fertilizer!

Histopathology of the iris in eyes removed for intractable NVG generally reveals remarkable angle closure, due to contraction of a fibrovascular membrane on the iris surface. The neovascular membrane often vaults a false angle. Ectropion uveae is the classic clinical finding that correlates with contraction of an anterior iris membrane. Presumably a population of myofibroblasts, which contain contractile cytoplasmic elements, actually ratchets the iris anteriorly and progressively closes the angle. Myofibroblasts are probably only transiently present during the contraction phase and are not identifiable in end-stage specimens.

Pupillary block is not generally present in rubeosis iridis with NVG and laser iridectomy is seldom indicated. Often the iris is pulled so far anteriorly that ciliary processes may be easily visualized through the pupil, which is lifted off the lens surface.

The natural course of events in untreated NVG leads rapidly over a few months to intractable glaucoma and loss of vision due to cataract, optic nerve injury, corneal opacity and pain. In eyes with intractable NVG which survive longer than was formerly possible because of more effective treatment of elevated IOP, new vessels may envelope the lens, cover the ciliary body and extensively invade the anterior vitreous.

Approximately 60% of patients will develop retinopathy after 15 years' duration of insulin-dependent diabetes mellitus (IDDM). Neovascularization of the anterior segment (rubeosis iridis) will develop in about 5% of diabetics without proliferative retinopathy, but in as many as 45-65% of patients with untreated proliferative retinopathy. Lensectomy and vitrectomy increase the risk of rubeosis and NVG[1].

During the Diabetes Control and Complications Trial (DCCT), about 24% of patients in the standard treatment group developed neovascularization of the disc or elsewhere over nine years of follow-up. The intensively treated group had a much lower incidence of neovascularization over the same period of about 8%[8].

Panretinal photocoagulation will induce remission of vessels and improvement in IOP control in many cases, especially if treatment is relatively early in the course of angle involvement. In our experience, benefits to IOP control correlate with clinical remission of angle vessels and usually are apparent in favorable cases within two to four weeks of PRP. An angle closed by PAS will not re-open after PRP, but the progression of angle closure may be stopped and angle function may be remarkably improved as inflammation and active vessel proliferation subside.

Medical treatment of neovascular glaucoma

Miotics should be stopped because they are vasoactive and tend to irritate already inflamed eyes. Apraclonidine can be useful and has seemed less irritating than miotic agents. Aqueous suppression with beta blockers and topical or systemic carbonic anhydrase inhibitors seems reasonable, at least for short periods of time while waiting for PRP to have its effect. If vessel remission does not follow within weeks of adequate PRP, surgical intervention is indicated to control IOP.

Trabeculectomy may be successful after PRP has induced remission of neovascularization, but has a poor success rate in untreated NVG. Most now recommend 5-FU or mitomycin C as adjuncts to trabeculectomy in cases with NVG, even if PRP has been completed. Long-term studies of trabeculectomy with antifibrotic agents in NVG are lacking.

In end-stage eyes with NVG, topical atropine and steroids will often increase comfort. Some patients with NVG tolerate remarkably high levels of IOP without corneal edema or pain.

Laser treatment of neovascular glaucoma

Direct treatment of angle vessels is seldom performed and was never proven to be useful. Although a rationale can be cited for treatment of vessels vaulting the spur to supply vascular arcades on the meshwork, there is also obvious risk of doing additional damage to the outflow apparatus.

Clinical controversies: my toughest cases – what would you do?

Moderator: George L. Spaeth

George L. Spaeth, MD: This will be a little bit different from what I had planned because unfortunately we do not have three of our excellent panel here: Quigley and Zimmerman and Minckler, who bring important different positions. But the three of us will do the best we can and I will probably speak a little bit more than I otherwise would have. First, a housekeeping thought. The published text will, of course, have all our presentations, and some of them will be in a great deal more detail than we were able to give them. I have in the back a very sketchy handout of the gonioscopic grading system which I described, but that will be given in detail in the text. It is the sort of thing that you need to have there with you when you are doing it at the start, and then after two or three days it is second nature.

The last thought has to do with this particular assignment, which were my toughest cases. The first thing I want to do is to define what tough case means. For instance, consider a one-eyed patient with traction retinal detachments, diabetic proliferative vitreous disease, and a neovascular glaucoma, dense cataract, and 20/400 in the only eye. That is a tough case.

Then there is also the tough case in which everything that you have in the way of information is gray, or you do not have enough information and you do not know how to get it. Frequently, I am disturbed by the fact that I have a patient whose long-term outlook I am not at all concerned about. They are going to do just fine. But I really do not know what to do. Do I treat, or do I not treat? There are all kinds of little details, and I spend 15 minutes, half an hour, discussing all these options with them and they are very disturbed, because the decision-making in those cases can be very tough. I think it is important to distinguish between different types of toughness.

In many of the patients who have desperate problems, the decision-making is very easy. They are tough for the patient, but they are not really tough for us. When we have a case in which the decision-making is difficult and there is a lot of uncertainty involved, I think we have to be very careful not to transfer that uncertainty over to the patient.

Consider first a 74-year-old Caucasian woman who comes to see you because she is having trouble with her vision. She has moderate rheumatoid arthritis for which she takes aspirin. She has had a deep vein thrombosis in the left leg, and is currently on Coumadin. Otherwise, her general health is fairly good. She first learned she had glaucoma approximately three years previously and she has been taking Timoptic 0.50% twice daily in both eyes since that time. An argon laser trabeculoplasty was done in both eyes a year ago. She is unaware of what her intraocular pressure has been as her doctor has not told her. She is of Russian Jewish extraction and has little knowledge of many members of her family as she immigrated to the United States many years ago. However, her grandmother became

Peril to the Nerve – Glaucoma and Clinical Neuro-Ophthalmology, pp. 221–227
Proceedings of the 45th Annual Symposium of the New Orleans Academy of
Ophthalmology, New Orleans, LA, USA, April 25-28, 1996
edited by Barry J. Leader and Jonathan C. Calkwood

blind when she was an old lady. The patient can no longer read and is mildly unhappy because she likes to cook and is having difficulty seeing well enough to make the meals the way she wants, and to enjoy what she has cooked. However, she is relatively content with her visual status. Visual acuity is 20/100, best corrected, in both eyes. Intraocular pressure is 38 mmHg in the right eye and 28 mmHg in the left eye on Timoptic 0.50% twice daily. There is a right afferent pupillary defect. Her anterior chambers are shallow. The lenses show nuclear and cortical opacities that are believed to account for about 20/100 visual reduction, which was what her visual acuity was. The angle of the right eye in my system would be (b)c10r with 2+ iris bowing, and scattered peripheral anterior synechiae that close approximately 30% of the angle. The angle of the left eye is slightly deeper, but with the same isolated peripheral anterior synechiae. There is 2+ pigmentation of the posterior trabecular meshwork in both eyes. There is concern that dilating the pupils may induce an angle closure. It is not possible to get a detailed view of the fundus, but the right optic nerve appears to have no remaining rim superiorly, temporally, or inferiorly, and the left optic nerve appears to have lost its rim inferiorly with a thin rim remaining temporally. The visual field of the right eye shows a total superior altitudinal defect with almost complete inferonasal loss as well. In the left eye, there is a moderately dense superior visual field defect of an arcuate nature. What other information do you need before you can decide upon a plan of action? There are lots of issues here, but let me just turn to Paul, you are looking in this direction, would you like to start?

Paul Palmberg, MD: Is there any peripupillary iris transillumination that would suggest pseudoexfoliation rubbing pigment epithelium off that might give you an angle-closure glaucoma with intermittent angle closure, because she had 2+ pigmentation?

Dr. Spaeth: Yes, there is localized peripupillary atrophy. What do you think has caused those peripheral anterior synechiae, these little volcano-like peripheral anterior synechiae that extend 360 degrees around the angle?

Michael A. Kass, MD: I think it was the LTP.

Dr. Spaeth: So your initial thought would be to dilate this patient, and how would you go about that? But before we get to that, let us just give a little more information. You note that the patient has had no episodes of blurred vision and no headaches. You observe a dense Sampolesi line inferiorly. You conclude that the peripheral synechiae are probably due to the previous argon laser trabeculoplasties and the narrowing of the anterior chamber angle that is typical of the exfoliation syndrome. The lenses do not look sufficiently large that a phacomorphic-type of mechanism is believed likely, but you cannot see the fundus adequately to evaluate the macula. The pressure was 38 and 28. Very specifically, do you go right ahead and dilate the pupils? Do you get their pressure controlled first? Do you do a peripheral iridotomy first? What is your exact and very concrete plan of action? Mike?

Dr. Kass: I would probably dilate one pupil in the office. I would use a weak agent. I would probably try to pre-treat the patient's IOP with Iopidine and perhaps a drop of Trusopt, assuming that there is no allergy to sulpha. I would dilate using a very weak agent, like one drop of half percent Mydriacyl in one eye only. I assume that would allow me to get a look at the disc, the macula, and the periphery, all of which are important here, because people with exfoliation can have a variety of problems. I would reverse this and keep the patient around until the pupil came back down to normal size. I would not just say "oh great, the pressure did not go up above 38" and let her walk out immediately. I would want to reverse the dilation and make sure she stayed around until I felt that her risk of getting into trouble was no greater now than it had been when she walked in the door.

Dr. Palmberg: Everything exactly the same, except when you dilate somebody with pseudoexfoliation, you may throw out an awful lot of pigment, especially if they had been on a miotic. Such a big pigment storm might cause a pressure that was so high you would really need to attend to it that day.

Dr. Spaeth: My approach would have been a little bit different, though I think we are dealing with the same information. This is a patient who has a superior altitudinal defect, very advanced, pressure of 38 to start with. I would be concerned that dilation, even if I gave the patient Iopidine, might very well in this patient with exfoliation syndrome, result in a big pressure rise. Her nerve might not tolerate that. So my approach would have been more conservative, in that I would have put the patient on some type of agent.

Dr. Palmberg: Iopidine and Trusopt?

Dr. Spaeth: Something like Trusopt would be a very good agent. I would proceed with a peripheral iridotomy first. I think the likelihood that this patient is going to develop an angle closure as well as a pigment release at the time of dilatation, is real, and you can at least minimize that, if not eliminate it, by doing a peripheral iridotomy. So my approach would have been to do an iridotomy first and then follow up with what they have suggested. Let us continue, because we now get to the next stage. The patient ends up being dilated with or without an iridotomy. At the time you dilate the patient, what you see is that indeed the disc of the right eye shows almost total excavation. The macula looks normal. The cataract looks as though indeed it is dense enough to account for the reduced acuity; but, you notice something about the lens of this patient which is disturbing to you, in the right eye. The right eye is the patient's worst eye from the point of view of the patient's function. In the left eye, you notice very similar findings. The cataract is almost as dense, but the cupping is much less advanced. What is it that you may be quite disturbed about when you now have a chance to look at this patient with a dilated pupil, something I did not mention?

Dr. Kass: The patient may very well have phacodonesis. You may be looking at somebody whose zonular support is less than optimal, and if you are thinking about doing something surgically in the near future, either for the cataract or the glaucoma, or both, this is obviously of considerable concern.

Dr. Spaeth: Exactly. Now, this patient then is put on medical therapy. As I say, I would do a PI. Over the next months, you follow the patient on Trusopt. The patient has an excellent response to Trusopt and a mild beta blocker, and the pressure stays around 20, maybe a little higher than you think is ideal, but certainly a big drop from 38. And about four or five months later the patient says, "You know, I really cannot do what I need, and I have got to see better". What do you suggest?

Dr. Kass: It seems to me, before you get to the surgery, that your two major problems are what to do about her anticoagulation and what social-family problems might exist. We have all had patients who, for instance, cannot have surgery because they cannot do something with a sick spouse or child.

Dr. Spaeth: Critically important and often overlooked. They are dying to have the surgery but they have alternate obligations. Let us say now that you have addressed that. What do you do about the anticoagulation? What surgery do you recommend on which eye?

Dr. Palmberg: I would operate on the left eye because the right eye does not have enough visual field for her to do the things she wants to do. That is the eye that could make her function if she did not have the cataract.

Dr. Spaeth: But Dr. Palmberg, my left eye is my better eye. If I lose that, I am in the soup and my right eye is terrible. That is the one I need to see better with.

Dr. Palmberg: Yes. We would have to have a discussion to explain why it was that we could not make that one better with enough visual field for her to do the things that she would like to do. I would do a phaco-filter on the left eye. I would not stop the anticoagulation. I think I would leave out the iridectomy so I would not be touching iris, and I have done this many times without trouble. In a few people, I have stopped the Coumadin and had them have another deep vein thrombosis or pulmonary embolus. I have kicked myself all over the place for having stopped the anticoagulation. And I think with the techniques we have now, we do not have many problems with bleeding, even in people on Coumadin. Although I would like to make sure they are in the therapeutic range and not the supertherapeutic range beforehand. And I would want to talk to their internist.

Dr. Spaeth: Would you stop the aspirin that the patient's taking for her arthritis and if so, how long before the surgery?

Dr. Palmberg: It is an interesting combination, somebody being on aspirin and Coumadin. In terms of anticoagulation there, there is no terrible risk to the patient by stopping it. I might ask her how much the arthritis pain has been bothering her. If it is not bothering her much, then stop it and maybe go to Tylenol for pain even though it will not help with inflammation, for five or six days, but I would not be very concerned.

Dr. Spaeth: Mike, how would you proceed?

Dr. Kass: I would do it a little differently. I would try to stop the aspirin, but I would do it for a longer period of time. Basically you have to resynthesize platelets in order to replace the effect. I would try to substitute a non-steroidal agent which would presumably help the patient with her pain and stiffness. About the Coumadin, I would talk to the patient's doctor. There are a fair number of patients who are on Coumadin and you call up their doctors and they say, "oh, sure, we can stop it. I am not sure why I still have it" kind of thing. So I would talk to the internists and let them decide about that. You can do it on Coumadin. My preference would be to have her off of it if it is possible to do so. And the third option is to switch them to heparin, but I am not sure that is worth all the bother and the hospitalization. As far as which procedure...

Dr. Spaeth: Before you move on to that, how many of you routinely ask your patients before surgery if they are taking an aspirin compound? Virtually everybody. Do you by any chance also give them a list of the 483,000 compounds that contain aspirin? Because it is amazing how many agents have aspirin in them. Furthermore, one of the other things that I have found is that ever since the Harvard Health Study, a very significant proportion of people are self-medicating themselves with aspirin and they think of it like a vitamin. You have to ask specifically, "Are you taking aspirin?" I have not gotten to the point where Paul is about doing filtering procedures without iridotomies or iridectomies. And I have been burned on patients who were taking aspirin who get recurrent, persistent hyphemas. The idea of not doing iridectomy might be a solution, but you have to be very careful because there is going to be some bleeding around the area of the flap. Mike's point about how long it takes for the aspirin effect to dissipate is an important one, too.

Dr. Palmberg: About nine days, is it not, for the complete turnover of the platelets?

Dr. Spaeth: We use two weeks as it works in well with what you are usually doing. Now on to the next situation, which is what procedure you do? Mike, you were starting on that.

Dr. Kass: I am not so sure I would give up on this lady's right eye. You went through her field and, I am sorry, I thought you described a superior defect, that the inferior field was intact.

Dr. Spaeth: That is correct.

Dr. Palmberg: No, inferonasal is gone.

Dr. Kass: Inferior nasal was also gone?

Dr. Spaeth: The inferior field is good.

Dr. Kass: If the inferior field is intact and she PAMS well, I would not object to doing the right eye first, particularly if the patient is adamant about this. Some people just simply do not want you to operate on their good eye first. Although I think there are occasions when you should do that. In this case, if she had an intact inferior field, it would also depend on how bad the zonules look to me, because that might very well influence what kind of result I thought I might obtain. If the lens was really loose to the point where you thought for sure you were going to wind up having to do a probable vitrectomy or sew in a PCIOL, it might influence which eye I did. If it were only a little bit loose, I think I would probably do a cataract extraction/trabeculectomy with an antimetabolite in her right eye.

Dr. Spaeth: This to me is I think one of the very difficult situations as far as decision-making is concerned, where you think that something is pretty clear and the patient thinks something is pretty clear the other way around. My preference would have been to do what Paul said, and that is to try to convince her that she is probably better off having the left eye operated on because the right eye is going to be tough surgery, and the likelihood of getting a good result less. But having said that, you then have a huge burden to make sure you get her through that surgery in the left eye without problem, because that is her better eye. So, I would suggest the left eye, but if she says 'no', I would do the right eye. Now, indeed Mike, this is a really difficult looking surgical situation because that lens is very shaky. Paul, you think maybe you can get the patient through, how would you change your technique to make it as unlikely as possible that you rupture the zonules? It is not the posterior capsule, it is the zonules. How can you make sure that you are least likely to rupture the zonules, and would you use a foldable lens? If so, which? And would you put the lens in the bag or in the sulcus, assuming that you were able to get through the surgery without rupturing the zonules?

Dr. Palmberg: I think it really depends a lot on the degree of phacodonesis. If it is something you can barely detect, but you feel that the zonules are all intact, the lens is not tilting back in some way with patient movement, then I think you can do it. You have to have the world's best hydrodissection that separates between the cortex and the capsule exactly with no hydration of the cortex. You have to get in underneath, as Fine talks about, lift the capsule, and get one wave around. I push very gently on the nucleus to get that fluid back out of the bag. If you get a wonderful cleavage plane there, then later when you are taking the cortex out you will not pull the whole bag out with it, because it will already be free. You are going to make a larger capsulotomy so that on the rotation of the nucleus it is not so tough to do, but you certainly do not want to get that capsulotomy out into the zonules. You are probably going to make a 6, 6-1/2, 7 mm capsulorhexis. I also use prayer and supplication.

Dr. Spaeth: Was this a patient in whom you perhaps would bowl rather than make a cruciate incision so that you do not have to rotate the lens, and if you decided to rotate the nucleus, would you do it with a two-handed technique or would you do it with a one-handed technique, what would you be careful of while you were rotating it?

Dr. Palmberg: I would definitely be using both the phaco tip and a Drysdale spatula for the rotations, so that I would be keeping the nucleus very well centered all the time that I was trying to slip it around inside the bag. I would not want to have the additional stress on the zonules of pushing the lens in one direction. I would still probably do a cracking technique, and I would get extremely deep. I am taking nucleus and epinucleus at the same time when I crack, so that I am going to be able to deconstruct this lens centrally and have very little left to have to pull out by aspiration afterwards. Because that is where you get in trouble in these cases. It is not usually during the phaco; it is during the aspiration of the remaining cortex, especially if you have left an epinuclear plate.

Dr. Spaeth: Would either of you consider an extracapsular cataract extraction on that patient?

Dr. Kass: Sure, if the lens looked very loose, sure I would.

Dr. Palmberg: If you do not think you can do phaco on it because there are actually some broken zonules, I guess so. However, I went from thinking that phaco was contraindicated in these cases to thinking it was highly indicated, as opposed to extracapsular, because at some point in an ECCE you are putting a lot of stress on the zonules. I certainly have broken zonules and lost vitreous in those cases, and I feel safer now doing phaco. Another consideration is if you do not do a lot of phaco, this is a case for somebody else to do. This is not a case that you need unless you are just awfully good at sneaking in and out of these eyes.

Dr. Spaeth: My thoughts are along the lines of what you said. But if you decide that this is a patient for an extracap, that is one of the places where it is essential not to 'express the nucleus'. You cannot do it. You have to pull this nucleus out, and you can do that by hooking it with some kind of needle, some people use a cryo; there are a variety of different ways of doing it. But you cannot push that nucleus out. It has to be pulled out without any posterior pressure on the zonules.

Dr. Palmberg: Some Viscoat underneath the nucleus to lift it up and use a spatula.

Dr. Kass: The other thing is of course the lens. If you really think this bag is loose, I think this is a good case to put the lens in the sulcus and probably not to use a foldable lens for this, but to use a larger one-piece lens. Make a larger incision, and put it in the sulcus so that you are not depending on this zonular support too much.

Dr. Palmberg: There are foldable lenses with haptics long enough that you could put them in the sulcus, and that is what I would do.

Dr. Spaeth: The reason why I chose this particular case is because it is not rare. Bob Ritch and others have stressed how common the exfoliation syndrome is. It may be the most common type of glaucoma we see. It is something you really have to look for. The relationship between the amount of exfoliative change and the propensity for the zonules to tear is not good. All the patients with the exfoliation syndrome are predisposed.

We have reached the end of our conference time.

Neuro-Ophthalmology

Contents

Optic neuritis

Norman J. Schatz

University of Miami, Bascom Palmer Eye Institute, Miami, FL, USA

Optic neuritis manifests as a loss of visual of acute to subacute onset, associated with variable degrees of visual loss. Pain often occurs in and about the orbit, exaggerated with eye movements. Characteristically, visual acuity, color vision, and central visual field loss occur, but a variety of patterns of visual field defects are encountered.

The differential diagnosis must include: pituitary apoplexy, vasculitis, contiguous sinus disease, sarcoidosis, and infiltrative optic neuropathy.

The Optic Neuritis Treatment Trial (ONTT) enrolled 457 patients aged between 20 and 50 years, between 1985 and 1991. The average age was 32 years, and 77% were females. The data collected have been a cornerstone influence in our clinical approach. Multiple sclerosis will develop within two years of an attack of optic neuritis in approximately 20% and within 15 years in 45–80% of patients.

Optic neuritis is frequently the first manifestation of multiple sclerosis. At time of onset, even without other signs or symptoms of demyelination, MRI of the brain often demonstrates other white-matter lesions.

Of the predictive factors, the most valuable is the MRI scan. In the ONTT, brain MRI images in 418 patients with optic neuritis showed that 40.9% had no MRI lesions, 10.8% had Grade I lesions, and 9.1% Grade II (I and II categories were non-specific for demyelination).

Of the Grade IV scans with predominantly diagnostic periventricular or ovoid lesions, only 21% had a clinical diagnosis of no multiple sclerosis, 42% possible multiple sclerosis, 67% probable, and 76% definite multiple sclerosis.

Of the 457 patients entered in the ONTT at 15 clinics, the diagnoses were: no multiple sclerosis in 66.9%; possible multiple sclerosis, 19.9%; probable multiple sclerosis, 7.6%; and definite multiple sclerosis, 5.6% (Table 1).

Grades 0 and I were considered normal or non-specific. Of 418 patients MRI classified, 40.9% were Grade 0 (normal), 10.8% Grade I, 9.1% Grade II, 6% Grade III, and 32% Grade IV. In patients with no clinical evidence of multiple sclerosis, Grade 0 findings compared to Grade IV MRI findings showed no difference in age, gender or pain, but Grade IV MRI occurred more frequently with poorer visual acuity, absence of disc edema, and absence of history of preceding viral infections.

The majority of the abnormal MRI scans had at least four lesions (13% had punctate change only, 19% one lesion ≥3 mm only, 12% two lesions, 4% three le-

Address for correspondence: Norman J. Schatz, MD, Mercy Neuroscience Institute, Suite 209, 3661 South Miami Avenue, Miami, FL 33133, USA

Peril to the Nerve – Glaucoma and Clinical Neuro-Ophthalmology, pp. 231–234
Proceedings of the 45th Annual Symposium of the New Orleans Academy of
Ophthalmology, New Orleans, LA, USA, April 25-28, 1996
edited by Barry J. Leader and Jonathan C. Calkwood
© 1998 Kugler Publications, The Hague/The Netherlands

Table 1. Distribution of positive MRI scans in the ONTT

Diagnosis on entry	Cases 457/MRI 418	MRI classification		Normal scan
No multiple sclerosis	66.9% (280)	Grade IV	21.3%	53%
Possible multiple sclerosis	19.9% (83)		42.0%	22.2%
Probable multiple sclerosis	7.6% (32)		67.6%	8.8%
Definite multiple sclerosis	5.6% (23)		76.9%	11.5%

sions, and 53% four or more lesions). Gadolinium enhancement was not evaluated for 'activity' of disease in isolated optic neuritis.

The significance of MRI abnormalities of the optic nerve, or of enhancing characteristics of the nerve, regarding future prognosis, are even less clear. The ONTT study has categorized MRI change in detail to determine the prognostic importance of type, location, and number of lesions.

Should all optic neuritis patients have routine MRI scans? The early diagnosis of multiple sclerosis may provide the possibility of preventive measures, at least in the future. For example, the studies on β-interferon, myelin basic protein, immune suppression, and i.v. methylprednisolone, suggest that chronic relapsing multiple sclerosis may be favorably influenced by therapeutic measures.

In the ONTT, high-dose i.v. steroids demonstrated a dramatic restraining effect on the development of other neurological events, although this effect on the development of multiple sclerosis wore off after two years.

The evidence of the ONTT suggests the following guidelines, MRI scans designed to demonstrate MS-like signal abnormalities will be performed, treatment with an intravenous regimen will be advised for all patients with Grade III and IV scans or severe impairment of acuity, especially with retrobulbar disease.

Visual field defects were analyzed, as can be seen in Table 2. Showing diffuse field loss occurred in 48.2% of patients, and localized defects in 51.8%. Of the localized deficits, altitudinal defects (15%), quadrant defects (13.1%), cecocentral scotoma (8.3%), and hemianopias (4.2%) were encountered. All defects tended to improve over time. 68.8% of patients had visual field defects in the fellow eye at baseline (Table 3). These defects tended to return to normal at the six-month follow-up in 50% of patients so involved, independent of treatment.

The effect of i.v. corticosteroids on acute optic neuritis and the subsequent development of multiple sclerosis revealed that among the 389 patients in the ONTT who did not have MS at the entry of the Study, 10 (75%) of 134 intravenously treated patients developed one such neurologic event within two years compared to 21 (16.7%) of the 126 in the placebo group. This beneficial effect lessened after the first two years.

Conclusions from the Optic Neuritis Treatment Trial

1. Prednisone not only did not improve visual outcome, it was also associated with an increased rate of new attacks of optic neuritis.
2. When vision was <20/200, i.v. methylprednisolone followed by oral prednisone (11 days) produced a faster recovery of visual function, but outcomes at six months and one year were unaffected.
3. Untreated visual acuity improved to 20/20 in 59% of eyes, and to better than 20/50 in 94% of eyes.

Table 2. Affected eye: distribution of visual field defects*

	Baseline No. (%) (n=448)		*6 months* No. (%) (n=431)		*1 year* No. (%) (n=401)	
Normal	0		220	(51.0)	224	(55.9)
Diffuse	216	(48.2)	85	(19.7)	84	(20.9)
Localized	232	(51.8)	126	(29.2)	93	(23.2)
altitudinal	67	(15.0)	3	(0.7)	1	(0.2)
three quadrant	32	(7.1)	1	(0.2)	0	
quadrant	27	(6.0)	11	(2.6)	11	(2.7)
centrocecal	20	(4.5)	3	(0.7)	4	(1.0)
hemianopic	19	(4.2)	9	(2.1)	5	(1.2)
central	17	(3.8)	10	(2.3)	7	(1.7)
arcuate	16	(3.6)	9	(2.1)	8	(2.0)
peripheral rim	15	(3.3)	22	(5.1)	17	(4.2)
enlarged blind spot	7	(1.6)	6	(1.4)	4	(1.0)
double arcuate	5	(1.1)	2	(0.5)	3	(0.7)
vertical step	3	(0.7)	24	(5.6)	16	(4.0)
nasal step	3	(0.7)	7	(1.6)	4	(1.0)
paracentral	1	(0.2)	16	(3.7)	9	(2.2)
multiple foci	0		3	(0.7)	4	(1.0)

*Humphrey automated static perimetry. (Reproduced from Keltner *et al.*, by courtesy of the *Archives of Ophthalmology*.)

Table 3. Fellow eye: distribution of visual field defects*

	Baseline No. (%) (n=448)		*6 months* No. (%) (n=431)		*1 year* No. (%) (n=401)	
Normal	140	(31.3)	228	(66.8)	275	(68.6)
Diffuse	84	(18.8)	55	(12.8)	49	(12.2)
Localized	224	(50.0)	88	(20.4)	77	(19.2)
peripheral rim	101	(22.5)	33	(7.7)	22	(5.5)
paracentral	30	(6.7)	16	(3.7)	15	(3.7)
vertical step	28	(6.3)	15	(3.5)	16	(4.0)
arcuate	17	(3.8)	5	(1.2)	2	(0.5)
nasal step	14	(3.1)	4	(0.9)	3	(0.7)
multiple foci	8	(1.8)	6	(1.4)	4	(1.0)
quadrant	8	(1.8)	3	(0.7)	6	(1.5)
double arcuate	6	(1.3)	1	(0.2)	0	
hemianopic	5	(1.1)	1	(0.2)	1	(0.2)
enlarged blind spot	3	(0.7)	1	(0.2)	3	(0.7)
central	3	(0.7)	1	(0.2)	2	(0.5)
centrocecal	1	(0.2)	1	(0.2)	2	(0.5)
altitudinal	0		1	(0.2)	0	
three quadrant	0		0		1	(0.2)

*Humphrey automated static perimetry. (Reproduced from Keltner *et al.*, by courtesy of the *Archives of Ophthalmology*.)

4. Patients with visual acuities <20/200 had a slightly worse visual prognosis, but 91% were 20/40 or better after six months.
5. Ninety-two percent of patients had ocular pain during acute visual loss.
6. Laboratory studies were of no value, although 15 patients had ANA titer >1:320, but these showed no difference in clinical course.

Atypical optic neuritis must be considered when the onset is simultaneous in both eyes, the disease is chronic, steroid-dependent, or associated risk factors exist.

Vasculitis may rarely account for an acute form of optic neuritis. The patients have often had a previous diagnosis of systemic vasculitis (systemic lupus erythematosus, Sjögren's rheumatoid arthritis or radiation exposure). MRI may be helpful in demonstrating the disruption of the blood-brain barrier, as evidenced by optic nerve enhancement. Systemic signs of disease are often helpful, as well as signs of steroid dependence and confirmatory laboratory studies.

Sarcoidosis, as a cause of retrobulbar optic neuritis, should be entertained in all cases of bilateral optic neuropathy, and in unilateral disease when visual loss is profound and does not remit, or when steroid dependency occurs. Skin tests for anergy, gallium uptake, serum ACE levels, and pulmonary function tests, may be helpful in supporting the diagnosis of sarcoid.

Optic neuritis is a commonly encountered clinical problem for which a rational approach to diagnosis and treatment is evolving. MRI has made a major impact on our knowledge, and we are indebted to the ONTT for the data it has generated.

Bibliography

Beck RW, Arrington J, Murtagh FR et al: Brain magnetic resonance imaging in acute optic neuritis: experience of the Optic Neuritis Treatment Trial. Arch Neurol 50:841-846, 1993

Beck RW, Cleary PA: Optic Neuritis Treatment Trial: one-year follow-up results. Arch Ophthalmol 111:773-775, 1993

Beck RW, Cleary PA, Anderson MM et al: A randomized, controlled trial of corticosteroids in the treatment of acute optic neuritis. N Engl J Med 326:581-588, 1992

Beck RW, Cleary PA, Backlund JC: The course of visual recovery after optic neuritis: experience of the Optic Neuritis Treatment Trial. Ophthalmology 101:1771-1778, 1994

Beck RW, Cleary PA, Trobe JD et al: The effect of corticosteroids for acute optic neuritis on the subsequent development of multiple sclerosis. N Engl J Med 329:1764-1769, 1993

Beck RW, Kupersmith MJ, Cleary PA, Katz B: Fellow eye abnormalities in acute unilateral optic neuritis: experience of the Optic Neuritis Treatment Trial. Ophthalmology 100:691-698, 1993

Chrousos GA, Kattah JC, Beck RW et al: Side effects of glucocorticoid treatment: experience of the Optic Neuritis Treatment Trial. JAMA 269:2110-2112, 1993

Editorial: High-dose corticosteroid regiment retards development of multiple sclerosis in Optic Neuritis Treatment Trial. Arch Ophthalmol 112:35, 1994

Glaser JS: Optic neuritis and ischemic optic neuropathy: what we thought we already knew. [Editorial] Arch Ophthalmol 109:1666-1667, 1992

Katz D, Taubenberger JK, Cannella B et al: Correlation between magnetic resonance imaging findings and lesion development in chronic, active multiple sclerosis. Ann Neurol 34:661-669, 1993

Keltner JL, Johnson CA, Spurr JO, Beck RW: Visual field profile of optic neuritis: one-year follow-up in the Optic Neuritis Treatment Trial. Arch Ophthalmol 112:946-953, 1994

Miller DH: Magnetic resonance imaging in monitoring the treatment of multiple sclerosis. Ann Neurol 36:591-591, 1994

Morrissey SP, Borruat FX, Miller DH et al: Bilateral simultaneous optic neuropathy in adults: clinical, imaging, serological, and genetic studies. J Neurol Neurosurg Psychiat 58:70-74, 1995

Rizzo JF, Lessell S: Optic neuritis and ischemic optic neuropathy: overlapping clinical profiles. Arch Ophthalmol 109:1668-1672, 1992

The ischemic optic neuropathies: what's new?

Joel S. Glaser

Mercy Neuroscience Institute and Departments of Ophthalmology, Neurology, and Neurosurgery, University of Miami School of Medicine, Bascom Palmer Eye Institute, Miami, FL, USA

Introduction

Infarction of the optic disc, and rarely of the retrobulbar portion of the optic nerve, is a poorly understood but well-recognized, and unfortunately all too common, cause of sudden loss of vision, especially in the presenescent and elderly population. Surely primary, or *common* ischemic optic neuropathy (ION) is the most frequent basis of disc swelling in adulthood beyond 50 years. By 'ischemic', we also include other diverse etiological subsets only infrequently associated with ION, including severe hypertensive episodes, juvenile and adult insulin-dependent diabetes, acute blood loss or hypotension, collagen arteritis, radionecrosis, contiguous to inflammation, etc. But where such more specific mechanisms are evident, the clinical situation with regard to therapies and outcome differs substantially in several ways from the typical idiopathic, or perhaps 'arteriosclerotic', ION. It is this *common* type that is first discussed.

Common ('arteriosclerosis', non-arteritic)

In contrast to inflammatory or demyelinative retrobulbar optic neuritis, ION characteristically involves the prelaminar portion of the optic nerve with a rather constant ophthalmoscopic appearance of disc swelling; thus, the frequent prefix 'anterior' (AION) (Fig. 1). In fact, absence of disc swelling in the presence of acute monocular loss of vision makes a diagnosis of 'simple' ischemic infarction untenable. The rare exception to this rule is a form of retrobulbar ION associated with cranial arteritis (see below). Otherwise, abrupt visual loss in the elderly patient, but with a *normal* disc, should bring to mind the possibility of a rapidly expanding basal tumor, such as pre-existing pituitary tumor, or of carcinomatous infiltration of the optic nerve sheaths.

Common ION may be characterized as follows[1,2]: peak incidence is at age 60 to 70 years, but on rare occasions may occur earlier. Onset of altitudinal[3] or other field defects (Fig. 2) is sudden and usually, but not invariably, involves the central fixational area with reduced acuity that may range from normal to nil, but tends to

Address for correspondence: Joel S. Glaser, MD, Mercy Neuroscience Institute, Suite 209, 3661 South Miami Avenue, Miami, FL 33133, USA

Peril to the Nerve – Glaucoma and Clinical Neuro-Ophthalmology, pp. 235–248
Proceedings of the 45th Annual Symposium of the New Orleans Academy of
Ophthalmology, New Orleans, LA, USA, April 25-28, 1996
edited by Barry J. Leader and Jonathan C. Calkwood
© 1998 Kugler Publications, The Hague/The Netherlands

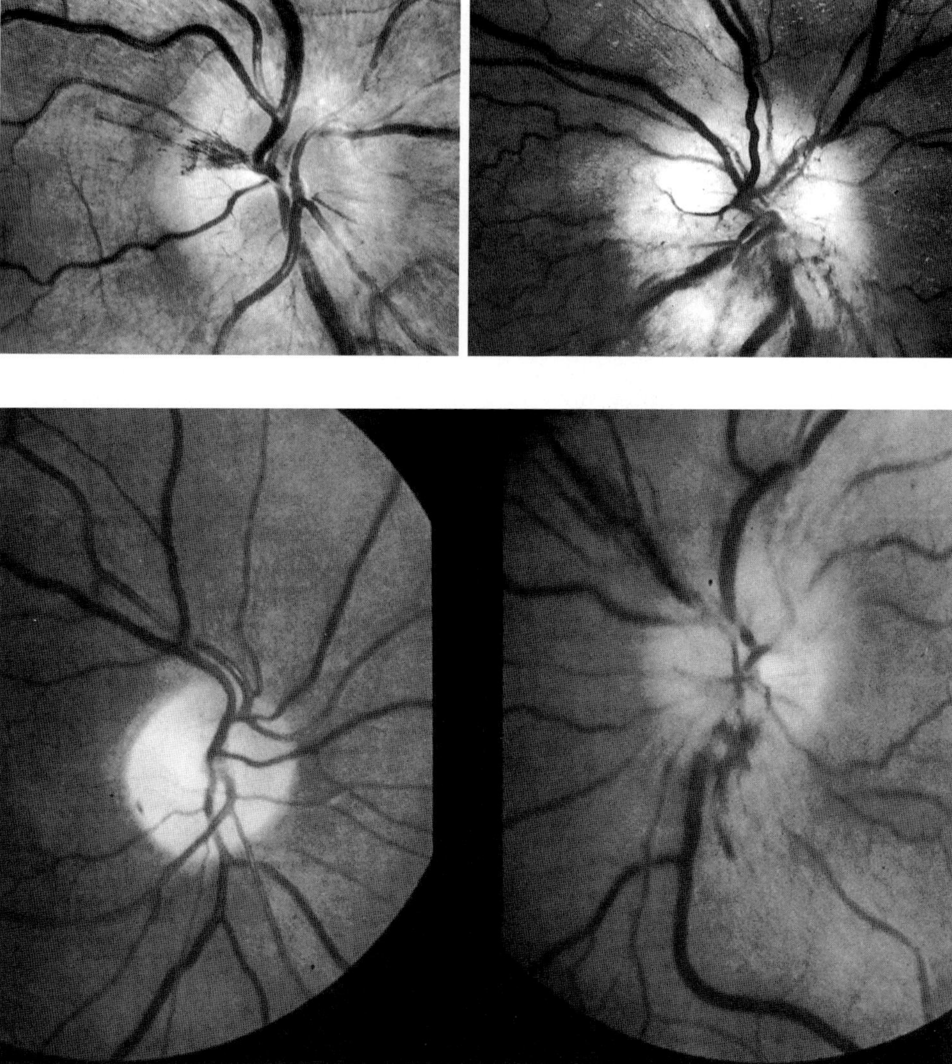

Fig. 1. Top. Left: acute right disc swelling with minimal hemorrhage in common anterior ischemic optic neuropathy. Right: another patient with more florid edema and hemorrhage. Note absence of cups in both discs. *Bottom.* Elderly patient with a history of visual loss in the right eye (left, disc shows optic atrophy), and now acute visual loss in the left eye with swollen, hemorrhagic disc (right). Combination of right optic atrophy and left swollen disc is 'pseudo-Foster-Kennedy syndrome'.

be more severely reduced in the arteritic form of ION. The visual deficit is typically maximal at onset, but deterioration may progress for a few days to several weeks[2,4]; recurrent disc infarcts in the same eye must be considered relatively rare[5,6]. In a review[7] of the same eye recurrences, the period between episodes lasted from ten days to nine years. Unlike infarction with cranial arteritis, premonitory ocular symptoms do not occur, and significant eye or brow discomfort, or headache, is exceptional, unlike optic neuritis, where orbital ache or pain on eye

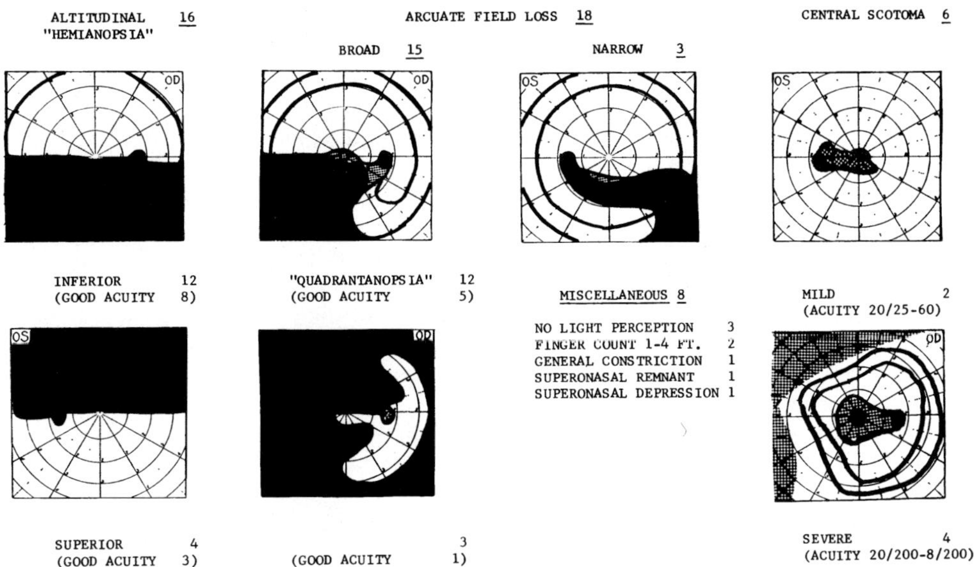

Fig. 2. Visual field defects in non-arteritic ischemic optic neuropathy; 48 eyes of 34 patients. (Reproduced from Boghen and Glaser[1], by courtesy of *Brain*.)

movement is a prominent symptom[8]. Many patients indeed note the visual deficit upon awakening, but this is not a fast rule. Indeed, Hayreh *et al.*[9] have suggested that, in the presence of other possible risk factors, exaggerated fall in nocturnal systemic blood pressure may predispose to nerve infarction.

The optic disc is swollen to some degree (Fig. 1), usually in a sector with small flame hemorrhages, and edema typically extends only a short distance beyond the border of the disc. A rare pre-symptomatic phase of disc swelling may be observed[10], *e.g.*, when a patient presents with characteristic ION with visual loss in one eye, and disc edema is surprisingly found in the contralateral fundus, but with good visual function; after a brief delay, disc edema progresses and vision declines. Perhaps this odd situation is related to chronic or subacute nerve ischemia with obstipation of axoplasm flow, but without frank major nerve fiber infarction.

Clinical and experiment studies[11] infer that ION is precipitated by insufficiency in posterior ciliary artery circulation and that branches of the peripapillary choroidal arterial system occlude, with consequent infarction of retinal nerve fiber bundles in the disc substance anterior to the lamina cribrosa. Olver *et al.*[12], and subsequently Onda *et al.*[13], have studied the morphology of the microvasculature of the retrolaminar area of the human optic nerve, and describe an elliptical anastomosis ('circle of Zinn-Haller') of branches of the medial and lateral para-optic short posterior ciliary arteries. This ellipse is divided into superior and inferior portions by the entry points of these branches into the eye, providing a potential 'altitudinal' blood supply to the retrolaminar optic nerve, which the authors suggest may play a role in the pathogenesis of the altitudinal pattern of visual field defects found so frequently in ION. The role of carotid embolic or occlusive disease is considered below.

Some small case studies[14] imply that chronic raised intraocular tension may play a role in ION, but in a larger series[15], no evidence was found to support this hypothesis. This author[16] has examined two patients who suffered progressive ION immediately following transient pressure elevations induced by topical corticosteroid therapy for conjunctivitis, occurring in otherwise healthy adults with no known preceding ocular or systemic risk factors.

The visual field defects in ION are variable, but usually take the form of arcuate scotomas or 'altitudinal hemianopias' of the superior or inferior half-fields (Fig. 2). These altitudinal or nasal pseudo-quadrantic defects are dense and easily discovered by hand- or finger-counting confrontational field techniques. The localizing value of the position of the 'vertex' of quadrantic and wedge-shaped defects has been emphasized by Alfred Kestenbaum: when the wedge originates at, or points toward, the blind spot, the defect is due to disease at the nerve head or just behind. The differential diagnosis of such *arcuate* scotomas, *i.e.*, with curvilinear or radial borders originating at the blind spot, includes: branch retinal artery occlusion, glaucoma, ischemic optic neuropathy, optic neuritis, hyaline bodies (drusen) of the optic disc, congenital optic pit, juxtapapillary inflammation and, very rarely, chiasmal interference. Central scotomas are the predominant field defects in about one-sixth[1] to one-fourth[3] of cases of common ION.

Optic atrophy ensues as disc edema resolves (Fig. 1), and some small loss of disc tissue may be evident, with increased cup size, but rarely is glaucomatous excavation precisely mimicked[17]. The ophthalmoscopic criteria that permit a retrospective diagnosis of optic atrophy of ischemic origin include arterial attenuation[18], although Frisen and Claesson[19] have quantitatively demonstrated a reduction in central retinal artery caliber of 17-24% in non-ischemic, descending optic atrophy due to retrobulbar nerve, or chiasm lesions.

Following ischemic infarction of one disc, there is great likelihood of second eye involvement, generally believed to occur sequentially in some 30-40%. Beri *et al.*[20] provide the following figures for ten-year cumulative incidence rates: for 190 patients 45-64 years of age, 55.3%; 154 patients 65 years or older, 34.4%; for 43 patients under age 45, 75.9%; for 43 patients with diabetes mellitus, 72.2%; for 107 patients with arterial hypertension, 42.2%; and for 44 patients with diabetes and hypertension, 60.6%.

In common ION, *simultaneous* bilateral disc infarction is practically unknown, and an underlying systemic disease such as cranial arteritis or severe renovascular hypertension must be suspected. The occurrence of *consecutive* disc infarction with fresh disc swelling in one eye, when coupled with contralateral previous optic atrophy, mimics the ophthalmoscopic combination popularized as the 'Foster Kennedy syndrome'[21] (Fig. 1), but there are obvious functional differences that separate acute disc infarction from papilledema of raised pressure (Table 1). Ironically, then, the celebrated 'diagnostic sign' of Kennedy is most typical of alternating, consecutive ION, and is exceedingly infrequent as a putative sign of intracranial frontal fossa masses.

While the precise roles of diabetes and hypertension are not known, certainly the prevalence of these systemic disorders is significantly greater in ION patients than in comparable age-matched groups[22]; correlations with these diseases seem greater in patients under age 45 years. Likewise, the association of cerebral and cardiac vascular disease[23] seems circumstantial. Ipsilateral carotid artery disease *per se* does not seem to be a risk factor[24]. Indeed, in a study of magnetic resonance (MR) brain images in ION patients[25], there did not appear to be an increased incidence of subcortical white matter lesions, *i.e.*, infarcts due to cerebral vascular disease. Therefore, that simple ION may be taken for a harbinger of future vascular events is moot. Giuffre[26] has reported that serum cholesterol, triglycerides and glucose

Table 1. Clinical characteristics of optic neuritis, papilledema and ischemic optic neuropathy

	Optic neuritis	*Papilledema*	*Ischemic neuropathy*
Symptoms			
Visual	Rapidly progressive loss of central vision; acuity rarely spared	No visual loss; ± transient obscurations	Acute field defect, commonly altitudinal; acuity variable
Other	Tender globe, pain on motion; orbit or brow ache	Headache, nausea, vomiting; other focal neurologic signs	Usually none; cranial arteritis to be ruled out
Bilateral	Rarely in adults; may alternate in MS; frequent in children, especially papillitis	Always bilateral, with extremely rare exceptions; may be asymmetric	Typically unilateral in acute stage; second eye involved subsequently with picture of "Foster-Kennedy" syndrome
Signs			
Pupil	No anisocoria; diminished light reaction on side of neuritis	No anisocoria; normal reactions unless asymmetric atrophy	No anisocoria; diminished light reaction on side of disc infarct
Acuity	Usually diminished	Normal acuity	Acuity variable; severe loss (incl. NLP) common in arteritis
Fundus	Retrobulbar: normal; Papillitis: variable degree of disc swelling, with few flame hemorrhages; cells in vitreous variable	Variable degrees of disc swelling, hemorrhages, cytoid infarcts	Usually pallid segmental disc edema with few flame hemorrhages
Visual prognosis	Vision usually returns to normal or functional levels	Good, with relief of cause of increased intracranial pressure	Poor prognosis for return; second eye ultimately involved in one third of idiopathic cases

are elevated in ION, and others[27] found a correlation of elevated concentrations of IgG anticardiolipin antibody in patients with arteritic ION, but not in common ION. Furthermore, the role of tobacco smoking has also been questioned[28].

A series of funduscopic analyses has addressed the question of cup-to-disc ratio as a possible morphological factor in the pathogenesis of common ION, culminating in the paper of Beck *et al.*[29]. By observing the disc appearance of the normal fellow eyes of ION patients, it is apparent that the optic cup is smaller or absent at a significant rate in common ION (but not smaller in arteritic ION); furthermore, one study[30] suggests that both the horizontal disc diameter and disc area are smaller in ION fellow eyes than in controls ($p<0.05$). Possibly, ischemic axons in the 'crowded' setting of a small scleral canal are predisposed to infarction. However, as patients with common ION may show variably sized contralateral physiological cups, and patients with arteritic ION may show contralateral cupless discs, no strong diagnostic distinction should be placed on the state of fellow-eye cup-to-disc ratio.

No medical therapies have proved effective in restoring vision in acute ION, although systemic corticosteroid usage could theoretically lessen the focal impact of edema and, therefore, short-term trials are not unreasonable. The untoward effects of corticosteroids on diabetes, hypertension and general well-being must be taken into account. Preliminary studies[31] indicate no useful effect of aspirin on the visual outcome of common ION. Although spontaneous significant recovery of vision is generally thought to be relatively rare, Movsas *et al.*[2] have documented that, of 116 eyes with an acuity of 20/60 or worse, 21% improved by three or more lines, and of 126 eyes with an acuity better than 20/60, 23% improved by three or more lines. Optic nerve sheath fenestration with drainage of perineural subarachnoid cerebrospinal fluid has been thoroughly investigated and, although Sergott *et al.*[32] reported good results, subsequent carefully controlled studies[33,34] show no benefit of surgery and, indeed, spontaneous recuperation of three or more lines of acuity may occur in as many as 43% of involved eyes.

Cranial (giant cell) arteritis

An arteritic form of ischemic optic neuropathy occurs with onset in a slightly older age group[1], usually with devastating visual loss. As pointed out by Wagner and Hollenhorst, arteritis may result in a *retrobulbar* form of nerve infarction, or may produce a picture similar to central retinal artery occlusion[35]. These authors also noted an appreciable incidence of fleeting premonitory visual symptoms similar to the amaurosis fugax from carotid atheromatous emboli. Such episodes may be precipitated by changes from the supine to upright head position and suggest impending nerve infarction; bed-rest with lowering of the head to flat or dependent levels is an important maneuver. (Of course, immediate hospitalization for intensive corticosteroid therapy is indicated.)

Very few cases of biopsy-proved cranial arteritis occur under age 50 years[36], but in the population age 50 years and over, annual *incidence* rates for cranial arteritis (CA) are estimated at 17.4[37] to 28.6[38] per 100,000; age-specific *prevalence* rate between ages 60 and 69 is 33/100,000, and over age 80, 844/100,000[35]. Most large series report a female:male preponderance of about 3:1.

Visual loss with arteritis ION tends to be more profound than with common ION[1,39]; levels of finger-counting to no perception of light are not uncommon. At times, the optic disc is characterized by a suggestive milk-pale edema that may extend some considerable distance into the retina, and central retinal artery occlusion with 'cherry-red spot' also occurs. Retinal nerve fiber layer infarcts may take the form of 'cotton-wool spots', usually accompanied by disc swelling[40]. As already mentioned, bilateral simultaneous ION implies CA as systemic background, and both therapy and laboratory investigations are bent towards that diagnosis. In one series[19] of 50 cases of arteritic ION, 19 of the 20 bilateral patients had both eyes involved by the time of initial visits. When second eye infarction occurs in CA, it does so within days to weeks, longer intervals being exceptional. The prognostic value of this point bears emphasis: if the second eye is not yet involved, and the patients are under adequate systemic corticosteroid therapy, the likelihood of bilateral visual loss becomes more remote with each passing week.

Other signs of orbital hypoxia include evidence of anterior segment ischemia: hyperemia of the conjunctival and episcleral vessels, mild-to-moderate corneal edema, lowered intraocular tension, anterior chamber cellular reaction, iris rubeosis, and rapidly progressive cataract. Irregular streaks and patches of chorioretinal pigmental disturbances secondary to *choroidal ischemia* may appear weeks after visual loss, and considerable disc cupping may ensue, at times mimicking simple glaucoma[41]. Diplopia is infrequent, probably reflecting diffuse ischemia of extraocular muscles[42], but symptomatic ophthalmoplegia of any degree may be obscured by the more dramatic complaint of severe visual loss. New onset of headache or of scalp tenderness, especially if coupled with chewing 'claudication', should be considered cranial arteritis until proved otherwise.

Ocular pneumotonography, which measures the ocular pulsation induced by perfusion pressure in choroidal (posterior ciliary) and ophthalmic arteries, has been used[43] to distinguish common from arteritic ION. In patients with arteritic ION, ocular pulse amplitude was only 4% of pulse amplitude of patients with arteritis but without ION, and only 6% of pulse amplitude of patients with non-arteritis ION. Moreover, half arteritis-ION patients showed pulsation loss in the non-infarcted contralateral eye. Return of pulse amplitudes to a normal range can occur rapidly upon systemic corticosteroid therapy, although in some cases the pulse does not revert to normal levels. Bosley *et al.*[44] suggest that ocular pneumoplethysmography (OPG-Gee), measuring ocular pulse amplitude that reflects the volume changes in the globe with each cardiac cycle, provides a diagnostic accuracy of 94% for CA, rivalling the accuracy of erythrocyte sedimentation rate determination or even temporal artery biopsy. Siatkowski *et al.*[45] found timed fluorescein fundus angiography useful in differentiating arteritic from non-arteritic ION, with delays in choroidal filling patterns, especially when dye appearance is delayed beyond 18 seconds.

It is critical to discover, where possible, those instances of ION due to cranial arteritis, because prompt steroid therapy may be effective in restoring some degree of vision[46-48], averting similar visual deficit in the other eye, and improving long-term systemic morbidity and mortality, although the Mayo series showed no statistically significant effect of arteritis on survivorship rates[35]. Patients with cranial arteritis may complain of weakness, weight loss, and fever. Myalgia of the large muscle masses of the shoulders, neck, thighs, and buttocks is common. These symptoms constitute *polymyalgia rheumatica*, which really cannot be clinically or histologically distinguished from cranial arteritis[49]. Other common complaints include pain in the jaw muscles precipitated by eating or talking (masseter 'claudication'), chronic suboccipital headache (mistakenly attributed to cervical osteo-arthritis, so common in this age group), and pain or tenderness of the scalp of the forehead or temples. A palpable, often non-pulsatile, temporal artery should be sought as a likely biopsy site.

The Westergren erythrocyte sedimentation rate (ESR) is the most consistently helpful laboratory test in the confirmation of the diagnosis of arteritis. Cullen[50], in comparing arteritis versus 'arteriosclerotic' (common, idiopathic) ischemic optic neuropathy, found only three of 19 patients in the latter group with ESR greater than 30 mm/hour (mean 26 mm), while only three of 25 patients with biopsy-positive arteritis had ESRs of 50 mm and below (mean 84 mm; 70 mm or above in 80%). Cullen also pointed out the rare occurrence of arteritis with normal ESR. In a series of 31 patients with temporal arteritis with severe visual impairment, Palm[51] reported the mean of the highest ESR values to be 96 mm with a range of 50-145 mm. Hamrin[52] found mean ESR values of 106 mm (51 biopsy-positive patients) and 99 mm (42 biopsy-negative patients); for the entire series of 93 cases, mean ESR was 103 ± 26.5 mm/hour (range 47-155 mm).

It is clear from the papers of Boyd and Hoffbrand[53] and Milne and Williamson[54] that ESR increases with age and is 'elevated' (*i.e.*, greater than 20 mm/hour) in apparently healthy elderly subjects. In at least 50% of persons with an ESR greater than 50 mm, no obvious reason was found[48]. Taking 20 mm/hour as the upper limit of normal, bacteriuria, ischemic heart disease, chronic respiratory symptoms show no association with a raised ESR. Miller and Green[55] provided the following rule for calculation of the maximum normal ESR at a given age: in men (age in years)/2; in women (age in years +10)/2. We are in agreement with the above authors and personally utilize 40-45 mm/hour (Westergren) as the upper limit of normal for the ESR in the elderly.

The affirmation provided by a positive artery biopsy is helpful when instituting long-term corticosteroid therapy in an elderly patient, but a negative biopsy in no way militates against a diagnosis of arteritis. Klein *et al.*[56] have established the presence of 'skip lesions' in temporal artery biopsies from patients with unequivocal cranial arteritis. They also point out that a temporal artery that is normal to palpation may show histological signs of inflammation and that patients with 'skip lesions' do not have a more benign form of the disease. Therefore, it may be argued that arterial biopsy is superfluous, since diagnosis or treatment is not altered by the results, especially in the full-blown case of cranial arteritis, accompanied by significant ESR elevation, with or without symptoms of polymyalgia rheumatica. Others[57] contend that multiple biopsies should be considered, especially in the 'occult' form of CA, *i.e.*, no systemic signs or symptoms, and normal or minimally elevated ESR.

In the appropriately aged patient with systemic or cranial signs or symptoms, and normal or (usually) elevated sedimentation rate, systemic corticosteroid therapy (*e.g.*, oral prednisone 80-100 mg daily; intravenous methylprednisolone 250 mg every six hours) should be instituted immediately upon presumed diagnosis. To reiterate: *in the patient with suspected arteritis, therapy should not be delayed for the results of ESR or biopsy.* Symptomatic response to steroids, excluding vision, may be dramatic within 24 hours, with relief of headache and malaise. Recovery of vision is considered rare[40-42,58] in both the retrobulbar and ocular forms of arteritic ION. However, Liu *et al.*[59] reported an overall improvement rate of 34% after intensive corticosteroid treatment.

Prolonged therapy should be dictated by symptomatic response to steroids and depression of the sedimentation rate. It is suggested that high dosage be maintained for approximately four weeks, then tapered so long as the patient remains symptom-free and the ESR is below 40 mm/hour (see above). The course of active arteritis is variable, and inflammation may continue despite adequate corticosteroid doses. It has been suggested that serum interleukin-6 concentration[60] may be a more precise indicator of successful suppression of tissue inflammation, but does not fully reflect the clinical status. Of course, complications of prolonged steroid usage are well known and include gastric ulcers, myopathy and weakness (which may be confused with persistent polymyalgia), osteoporosis, and recrudescence of tuberculosis.

Diabetes mellitus

It is presently unclear whether a direct relationship exists between diabetes and acquired optic neuropathies, other than as an apparent risk factor for common ION (see above). A genetically determined, early onset, progressive optic atrophy may be associated with juvenile diabetes, but the incidence in diabetes of retrobulbar neuritis or papillitis is probably no higher than in the non-diabetic population.

Skillern and Lockhart[61] collected 14 cases of 'optic neuritis' in poorly controlled diabetics. Apparently, slowly progressive loss of vision was a common symptom (as opposed to the frequently apoplectic onset of ischemic optic neuropathy), and visual fields showed central scotomas or peripheral contraction. No mention was made of altitudinal defects, and only two patients demonstrated diabetic retinopathy. Of greater importance is the report by Lubow and Makley[62] of teen-aged patients with long-standing juvenile diabetes who presented with hemorrhagic swelling of one or both optic discs, mimicking papilledema of increased intracranial pressure. Barr *et al.*[63] reported a series of 21 eyes in 12 juvenile diabetics, and outlined a clinical profile consisting of symptoms of slightly blurred vision, minimal acuity and field deficits, general salutary outcome, and no consistent correlation with the clinical control of hyperglycemia; diabetic retinopathy is usually of modest degree, and the prognosis for proliferative retinopathy is uncertain. Neurodiagnostic studies are not indicated and corticosteroid administration upsets diabetic control, without providing any known therapeutic effect. In the older insulin-dependent population, such diabetic papillopathy may be confused with common ION. While likely related to hypoxia of the prepapillary capillaries, 'diabetic papillopathy' enjoys a much better visual prognosis than most other forms of ischemic optic neuropathy.

Infrequently associated conditions

In 1973, Carroll originally called attention to a form of ischemic optic papillopathy occurring after uncomplicated *cataract extraction*, with sudden visual loss from four weeks to 15 months postoperatively[64]. In general, about half the patients with initial eye affected may anticipate visual loss following operation on the second eye. In Carroll's series, three patients were in their 50s and the disc infarction occurred with both retrobulbar or general anesthesia, and no patient experienced a loss of vision in a second eye, unless subjected to cataract extraction. Carroll also concluded that neither corticosteroids nor anticoagulants are effective therapies.

Peri-operative data are too incomplete to be able to incriminate a simple postoperative rise in ocular tension, although discs with marginal perfusion could be vulnerable. Hayreh's suggestion[65] of lowering ocular tension when second eyes are at risk seems reasonable. Optic neuropathy following cataract extraction represents a distinct variant characterized by a circumscribed time course and high incidence of bilaterality, to the point of predictability, when the second eye is operated on (even in the fifth and sixth decades)[66].

Acute disc edema or retrobulbar neuropathy causing visual loss in younger patients not yet included in the 'vasculopathic' age group, falls into categories where *collagen vascular or auto-immune arteritis* are suspected, or inflammatory neuritis may not be ruled out. This idiopathic ION of the 'young' tends to be bilateral and recurrent[67]. In a series of nine patients with vasculitis-induced optic neuropathy[68], there were seven women aged 31-62 years with systemic lupus erythematosus, rheumatic arthritis or Sjögren's syndrome. Serum ANA and double-strand DNA are valuable laboratory tests, and MRI images show enhancement with gadolinium contrast, involving mostly the intracanalicular and intracranial portions of one or both nerves and/or chiasm (Fig. 3). The question of retinal arterial vasospasm in ION is unanswered and, indeed, both uni- and sequential bilateral disc infarctions have been reported as a rare manifestation of *migraine*[69,70], and during cluster headache[71].

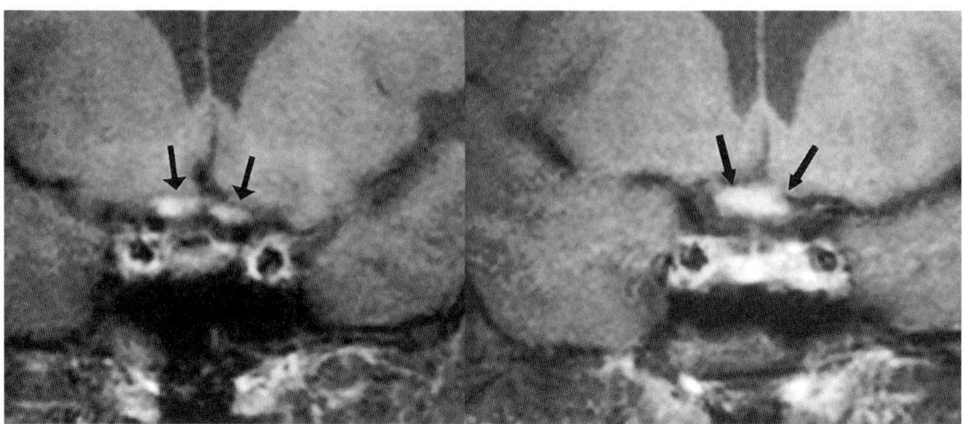

Fig. 3. Thirty-two-year-old women with systemic lupus erythematosus, bilateral visual loss. ANA 1:640, anti-double strand DNA 210 (normal <100). Coronal MRI (T-1 weighted) sections after gadolinium injection show (arrows) enhancement of (*left*) optic nerves and (*right*) optic chiasm.

Other varieties of ischemic disc swelling occur following marked or recurrent *blood loss*[72], most frequently from the gastrointestinal tract, but peculiarly delayed by days to weeks. This seems an infrequent complication of pulmonary bypass surgery[73], or other general surgical procedures where progressive postoperative red blood cell destruction drops hemoglobin levels[74]; visual loss has been reversed apparently by blood replacement. Bilateral retrobulbar infarcts with mild disc edema have been documented histologically[75]. The review by Katz *et al.*[76] catalogues instances of ION following surgical procedures which include: lumbar spine surgery (four cases), coronary artery bypass graft (19 cases), bilateral neck dissection (four cases), and miscellaneous procedures (seven cases). These authors suggest the common denominators of peri-operative anemia, intraoperative hypotension, and pre-existing arteriosclerotic risk factors. 'Blood loss', or hypoperfusion, ION is typically simultaneously bilateral, with moderate disc swelling, vision in the 20/200 range, and modest, if any, improvement.

Knox *et al.*[77] have reported a variety of *'uremic'* optic neuropathy characterized by bilateral visual loss with disc swelling in patients with severe renal disease manifested by uremia, anemia, and hypertension. Improvement followed hemodialysis, except in one case of actual cryptococcal meningitis. However, Hamed *et al.*[78] contend that 'uremic optic neuropathy' does not constitute a single pathophysiological entity, but includes complications of raised CSF pressure, severe consecutive anterior ischemic optic neuropathy, and adverse reaction to hemodialysis itself. Bilateral ION is reported in a young woman with optic disc drusen, chronic hypotension who was undergoing renal dialysis[79].

As noted above, *carotid artery disease* does not seem to play any regular role in ION; in fact, retinal arterial embolization and ION are mutually exclusive findings, except in the rarest of situations. Waybright *et al.*[80] documented three instances of typical ION with ipsilateral carotid occlusions, with retrograde filling of the ophthalmic artery by external carotid branches, perhaps indicating hypoperfusion of the nerve head, and Brown[81] reported a single case of abrupt visual loss at first with a normal disc, and then with pale edema, in an eye suffering chronic hypoxia from complete carotid occlusion. From a series of 612 patients with acute ischemic hemispheric strokes due to internal carotid occlusions with 'reversed flow in the ophthalmic artery', only three cases of simultaneous optic nerve infarction were uncovered[82]. Pulseless disease has also been complicated by ION[83].

In a patient with atrial fibrillation[84], emboli were found in the posterior ciliary arteries at autopsy, and Tomsak[85] recorded three patients with ION accompanied by retinal emboli, following coronary artery bypass surgery and cardiac catheterization. Acute disc swelling attributed to ION has been reported in eclampsia[86], porphyria[87], and pseudoxanthoma elasticum with platelet hyperaggregability[88].

Even as ION with disc swelling (*i.e., anterior*) does not constitute a single nosological disorder, so retrobulbar (*i.e., posterior*) optic nerve ischemia does not connote distinctive etiology, but represents a rare consequence of various diseases. This 'posterior' ION variant consists of abrupt unilateral, rarely bilateral, visual loss without disc edema. *Other compressive, inflammatory, toxic, traumatic or infiltrative causes should be rigorously excluded.* Hayreh[89] has included cases of lupus and cranial arteritis, and Isayama *et al.*[90] reported 14 cases, 20-73 years of age (six less than 54 years), with hypertension, diabetes, and infrequent carotid stenosis. Otherwise, polyarteritis nodosa[91], acute internal artery occlusion[92], blood loss[52] and intraoperative hypotension[93], are all rare causes of posterior ION. As noted above, MRI studies may prove to be exceedingly helpful in defining such cases of 'posterior' ION, and in avoiding misdiagnosis (Fig. 3). In those subsets of ischemic optic neuropathy where a degree of inflammation plays some role, the use of systemic corticosteroid therapy seems to be reasonable.

References

1. Boghen DR, Glaser JS: Ischaemic optic neuropathy: the clinical profile and natural history. Brain 98:689, 1975
2. Movsas T, Kelman SE, Elman MJ, Miller NR et al: The natural course of non-arteritic ischemic optic neuropathy [Abstract]. Invest Ophthalmol Vis Sci 42:951, 1991
3. Traustason OI, Feldon SE, Leemaster JE et al: Anterior ischemic optic neuropathy: classification of field defects by Octopus™ automated static perimetry. Graefe's Arch Clin Exp Ophthalmol 226:206, 1988
4. Kline LB: Progression of visual field defects in ischemic optic neuropathy. Am J Ophthalmol 106:199, 1988
5. Beck RW, Savino PJ, Schatz NJ et al: Anterior ischemic neuropathy: recurrent episodes in the same eye. Br J Ophthalmol 67:705, 1983
6. Borchert M, Lessell S: Progressive and recurrent nonarteritic anterior ischemic optic neuropathy. Am J Ophthalmol 106:443, 1988
7. Kao LY, Huang L, Chen TT: Anterior ischemic optic neuropathy: recurrent attacks in one eye in a bilateral case. Ann Ophthalmol 21:71, 1989
8. Optic Neuritis Study Group: The clinical profile of optic neuritis: experience of the Optic Neuritis Treatment Trial. Arch Ophthalmol 109:1673-1678, 1991
9. Hayreh SS, Zimmerman MB, Podhajsky P, Alward WL: Nocturnal arterial hypotension and its role in optic nerve head and ocular ischemic disorders. Am J Ophthalmol 117:603-624, 1994
10. Hayreh SS: Anterior ischemic optic neuropathy. V. Optic disc edema an early sign. Arch Ophthalmol 99:1030, 1981
11. Hayreh SS: Anterior ischemic optic neuropathy. I. Terminology and pathogenesis. Br J Ophthalmol 58:955, 1974
12. Olver JM, Spalton DJ, McCartney ACE: Microvascular study of the retrolaminar optic nerve in man: the possible significance in anterior ischemic optic neuropathy. Eye 4:7-24, 1990
13. Onda E, Cioffi GA, Bacon DR, Van Buskirk EM: Microvasculature of the optic nerve. Am J Ophthalmol 120:192-202, 1995
14. Katz B, Weinreb RN, Wheeler DT et al: Anterior ischemic optic neuropathy and intraocular pressure. Br J Ophthalmol 74:99-102, 1990
15. Kalenak JW, Kosmorsky GS, Rockwood EJ: Nonarteritic anterior ischemic optic neuropathy and intraocular pressure. Arch Ophthalmol 109:660-661, 1991

16. Barrett DA, Schatz NJ, Glaser JS et al: Progressive anterior ischemic optic neuropathy associated with transient increased intraocular pressure. (personal observation)
17. Trobe JD, Glaser JS, Cassady J et al: Nonglaucomatous excavation of the optic disc. Arch Ophthalmol 98:1046, 1980
18. Trobe JD, Glaser JS, Cassady JC: Optic atrophy: differential diagnosis by fundus observation alone. Arch Ophthalmol 98:1040, 1980
19. Frisen L, Claesson M: Narrowing of the retinal arterioles in descending optic atrophy: a quantitative clinical study. Ophthalmology 91:1342, 1984
20. Beri M, Klugman MR, Kohler JA et al: Anterior ischemic optic neuropathy. VII. Incidence of bilaterality and various influencing factors. Ophthalmology 94:1020, 1987
21. Lepore FE, Yarian DL: A mimic of the 'exact diagnostic sign' of Foster Kennedy. Ann Ophthalmol 17:411, 1985
22. The IONDT Study Group: Characteristics of patients with nonarteritic anterior ischemic optic neuropathy eligible for the ischemic optic neuropathy decompression trial. Arch Ophthalmol 114:1366, 1996
23. Guyer DR, Miller NR, Auer CL et al: The risk of cerebrovascular disease in patients with anterior ischemic optic neuropathy. Arch Ophthalmol 103:1136, 1985
24. Fry CL, Carter JE, Kanter MC et al: Anterior ischemic optic neuropathy is not associated with carotid artery atherosclerosis. Stroke 24:539-542, 1993
25. Jay WM, Williamson MR: Incidence of subcortical lesions not increased in nonarteritic ischemic optic neuropathy on magnetic resonance imaging. Am J Ophthalmol 104:398, 1987
26. Giuffre G: Hematologic risk factors for anterior ischemic optic neuropathy. Neuro-Ophthalmology 10:197-203, 1990
27. Watts MT, Greaves M, Rennie IG, Clearkin LG: Antiphospholipid antibodies in the aetiology of ischaemic optic neuropathy. Eye 5:75-79, 1991
28. Chung SM, Gay CA, McCrary JA: Nonarteritic ischemic optic neuropathy: the impact of tobacco use. Ophthalmology 101:779-782, 1994
29. Beck RW, Servais GE, Heyreh SS: Anterior ischemic optic neuropathy. IX. Cup-to-disc ratio and its role in pathogenesis. Ophthalmology 94:1503, 1987
30. Mansour AM, Shoch D, Logani S: Optic disk size in ischemic optic neuropathy. Am J Ophthalmol 106:587, 1988
31. Botelho PJ, Johnson LN, Arnold AC: The effect of aspirin on the visual outcome of nonarteritic anterior ischemic optic neuropathy. Am J Ophthalmol 121:450-451, 1996
32. Sergott RC, Cohen MS, Bosley TM, Savino PJ: Optic nerve decompression may improve the progressive form of nonarteritic ischemic optic neuropathy. Arch Ophthalmol 107:1743, 1989
33. Glaser JS, Teimory M, Schatz NJ: Optic nerve sheath fenestration for progressive ischemic optic neuropathy: results in a second series of 21 eyes. Arch Ophthalmol 112:1047-1050, 1994
34. The Ischemic Optic Neuropathy Decompression Trial Research Group: Optic nerve decompression surgery for nonarteritic anterior ischemic optic neuropathy (NAION) is not effective and may be harmful. JAMA 273:625-632, 1995
35. Wagner HP, Hollenhorst RW: The ocular lesions of temporal arteritis. Am J Ophthalmol 45:617, 1958
36. Biller J, Asconape J, Weinblatt ME et al: Temporal arteritis associated with a normal sedimentation rate. JAMA 247:486, 1982
37. Hauser WA, Ferguson RH, Holley KE et al: Temporal arteritis in Rochester, Minnesota, 1951 to 1967. Mayo Clin Proc 46:597, 1971
38. Bengstsson BA, Malmvall BE: The epidemiology of giant cell arteritis including temporal arteritis and polymyalgia rheumatica: incidences of different clinical presentations and eye complications. Arthritis Rheum 24:899, 1981
39. Hayreh SS, Podhajsky P: Visual field defects in anterior ischemic optic neuropathy. Doc Ophthalmol Proc Ser 19:53, 1979
40. Melberg NS, Grand MG, Diekert JP et al: Cotton-wool spots and the early diagnosis of giant cell arteritis. Ophthalmology 102:1611-1614, 1995
41. Sebag J, Thomas JV, Epstein EL et al: Optic disc cupping in arteritic anterior ischemic optic neuropathy resembles glaucomatous cupping. Ophthalmology 93:357, 1986
42. Barricks ME, Traviesa DB, Glaser JS, Levy IS: Ophthalmoplegia in cranial arteritis. Brain 100:209, 1977
43. Bienfang DC: Loss of the ocular pulse in the acute phase of temporal arteritis. Acta Ophthalmol (Kbh) 67(Suppl 191):35, 1989
44. Bosley TM, Savino PJ, Sergott RC et al: Ocular pneumoplethysmography can help in the diagnosis of giant-cell arteritis. Arch Ophthalmol 107:379-381, 1989

45. Siatkowski RM, Gass JDM, Glaser JS et al: Fluorescein angiography in the diagnosis of giant cell arteritis. Am J Ophthalmol 115:57-63, 1993
46. Model DG: Reversal of blindness in temporal arteritis with methylprednisolone. Lancet 1:340, 1978
47. Rosenfeld SI, Kosmorsky GS, Klingele TG et al: Treatment of temporal arteritis with ocular involvement. Am J Med 80:143-145, 1986
48. Diamond JP: Treatable blindness in temporal arteritis. Br J Ophthalmol 75:432, 1991
49. Hamilton CR, Shelley WM, Tumulty PA: Giant cell arteritis: including temporal arteritis and polymyalgia rheumatica. Medicine 50:1, 1971
50. Cullen JF: Ischemic optic neuropathy. Trans Ophthalmol Soc UK 87:759, 1967
51. Palm E: The ocular crisis of the temporal arteritis syndrome (Horton). Acta Ophthalmol (Kbh) 36:208, 1958
52. Hamrin B: Polymyalgia arteritica. Acta Med Scand (Suppl)533:2, 1972
53. Boyd RV, Hoffbrand BI: Erythrocyte sedimentation rate in elderly hospital in-patients. Br Med J 1:901, 1966
54. Milne JS, Williamson J: The ESR in older people. Gerontol Clin 14:36, 1972
55. Miller A, Green M: Simple rule for calculating normal erythrocyte sedimentation rate. Br Med J 260:Jan, 1983
56. Klein RG, Campbell RJ, Hunder GG, Carney JA: Skip lesions in temporal arteritis. Mayo Clin Proc 51:504, 1976
57. Coppeto JR, Monteiro M: Diagnosis of highly occult giant cell arteritis by repeat temporal artery biopsies. Neuro-Ophthalmology 10:217-218, 1990
58. Lipton RB, Solomon S, Wertenbaker C: Gradual loss and recovery of vision in temporal arteritis. Arch Intern Med 145:2252, 1985
59. Liu GT, Glaser JS, Schatz NJ, Smith JL: Visual morbidity in giant cellarteritis: clinical characteristics and prognosis for vision. Ophthalmology 101:1779-1785, 1994
60. Roche NE, Fulbright JW, Hunder GG et al: Correlation of interleukin-6 production and disease activity in polymyalgia rheumatica and giant cell arteritis. Arthritis Rheum 36:1286-1294, 1993
61. Skillern PG, Lockhart G: Optic neuritis and uncontrolled diabetes mellitus in 14 patients. Ann Intern Med 51:468, 1959
62. Lubow M, Makley TA: Pseudopapilledema of juvenile diabetes mellitus. Arch Ophthalmol 85:417, 1971
63. Barr CC, Glaser JS, Blankenship G: Acute disc swelling in juvenile diabetes: clinical profile and natural history of 12 cases. Arch Ophthalmol 98:2185, 1980
64. Carroll FD: Optic nerve complications of cataract extraction. Trans Am Acad Ophthalmol Otolaryngol 77:623, 1973
65. Hayreh SS: Anterior ischemic optic neuropathy. IV. Occurrence after cataract extraction. Arch Ophthalmol 98:1410, 1980
66. Serrano LA, Behrens MM, Carroll FD: Postcataract extraction ischemic optic neuropathy. Arch Ophthalmol 100:1177, 1982
67. Hamed LM, Purvin V, Rosenberg M: Recurrent anterior ischemic optic neuropathy in young adults. J Clin Neuro-Ophthalmol 8:239, 1988
68. Sklar EML, Schatz NJ, Glaser JS, Post JD, Ten Hove M: MR of vasculitis-induced optic neuropathy. AJNR 17:121-128, 1996
69. O'Hara M, O'Connor PS: Migrainous optic neuropathy. J Clin Neuro-Ophthalmol 4:85, 1984
70. Katz B: Bilateral sequential migrainous ischemic optic neuropathy. Am J Ophthalmol 99:489, 1985
71. Toshniwal P: Anterior ischemic optic neuropathy secondary to cluster headache. Acta Neurol Scand 73:213, 1986
72. Hayreh SS: Anterior ischemic optic neuropathy. VIII. Clinical features and pathogenesis of posthemorrhagic amaurosis. Ophthalmology 94:1488, 1987
73. Sweeney PJ, Breuer AC, Selhorst JB et al: Ischemic optic neuropathy: a complication of cardiopulmonary bypass surgery. Neurology 32:560, 1982
74. Jaben SL, Glaser JS, Daily M: Ischemic optic neuropathy following general surgical procedures. J Clin Neuro-Ophthalmol 3:239, 1983
75. Johnson MW, Kincaid MC, Trobe JD: Bilateral retrobulbar optic nerve infarctions after blood loss and hypotension: a clinicopathologic case study. Ophthalmology 94:1577, 1987
76. Katz DM, Trobe JD, Cornblath WT, Kline LB: Ischemic optic neuropathy after lumbar spine surgery. Arch Ophthalmol 112:925-931, 1994
77. Knox DL, Hanneken AM, Hollows FC et al: Uremic optic neuropathy. Arch Ophthalmol 106:50, 1988
78. Hamed LM, Winward KE, Glaser JS et al: Optic neuropathy in uremia. Am J Ophthalmol 108:30, 1989

79. Michaelson C, Behrens M, Odel J: Bilateral anterior ischemic optic neuropathy associated with optic disc drusen and systemic hypotension. Br J Ophthalmol 73:767, 1989
80. Waybright EA, Selhorst JB, Combs J: Anterior ischemic optic neuropathy with internal carotid artery occlusion. Am J Ophthalmol 93:42, 1982
81. Brown GC: Anterior ischemic optic neuropathy occurring in association with carotid artery obstruction. J Clin Neuro-Ophthalmol 6:39, 1986
82. Bogousslavsky J, Regli F, Zografos L et al: Optico-cerebral syndrome: simultaneous hemodynamic infarction of optic nerve and brian. Neurology 37:263, 1987
83. Leonard TJK, Sanders MD: Ischaemic optic neuropathy in pulseless disease. Br J Ophthalmol 67:389, 1983
84. Liebermann MF, Shahi A, Grenn WR: Embolic ischemic optic neuropathy. Am J Ophthalmol 86:206, 1978
85. Tomsak RL: Ischemic optic neuropathy associated with retinal embolism. Am J Ophthalmol 99:590, 1985
86. Beck RW, Gamel JW, Willcourt RJ et al: Acute ischemic optic neuropathy in severe preeclampsia. Am J Ophthalmol 90:342, 1980
87. DeFrancisco M, Savino PJ, Schatz NJ: Optic atrophy in acute intermittent porphyria. Am J Ophthalmol 87:221, 1979
88. Manor RS, Axer-Siegal R, Cohenn S et al: Bilateral anterior ischemic optic neuropathy, pseudoxanthoma elasticum, and platelet hyperaggregability. Neuro-Ophthalmology 6:173, 1986
89. Hayreh SS: Posterior ischaemic optic neuropathy. Ophthalmologica 182:29, 1981
90. Isayama Y, Takahashi T, Inoue M et al: Posterior ischemic optic neuropathy. III. Clinical diagnosis. Ophthalmologica 187:141, 1983
91. Hutchinson CH: Polyarteritis nodosa presenting as posterior ischemic optic neuropathy. J Roy Soc Med 77:1043, 1984
92. Sawle GV, Sarkies JNC: Posterior ischaemic optic neuropathy due to internal artery occlusion. Neuro-Ophthalmology 7:349, 1987
93. Rizzo JF, Lessell S: Posterior ischemic optic neuropathy during general surgery. Am J Ophthalmol 103:808, 1987

Visual loss in Graves' disease

Jonathan C. Calkwood and Ronald M. Burde

Department of Neurology/Neuro-Ophthalmology, Ochsner Clinic, New Orleans, LA, USA

Goiter in exophthalmos was first described in the literature somewhere around the 12th century. In 1825, Parry described a number of patients with diffuse goiter, tachycardia, without organic heart disease, one of whose eyes protruded from the socket[1]. Ten years later Robert Graves published three similar patients — "when the eyes were open the white of the sclera could be seen to be a breadth of several lines around the cornea"[2]. And about four years later in the German literature, Von Basedow also reported eye disease associated at that time with what was called non-organic heart failure or thyrotoxic heart failure[3]. Hyperthyroidism and exophthalmos were called Graves' disease until 1959 when Werner introduced the term 'euthyroid Graves' disease' for those patients with ophthalmic signs and symptoms of hyperthyroidism but without other manifestations of thyroid dysfunction[4]. The term Graves' disease may refer to hyperthyroidism with or without orbital changes. For the ophthalmologist the term implies orbital disease typical for thyroid dysfunction with or without systemic signs and symptoms. Graves' ophthalmopathy is a better term that may avoid confusion.

Ophthalmic signs are present in approximately 40% of dysthyroid patients[5]. The incidence of euthyroid Graves' disease has been described in 8% of dysthyroid ophthalmopathy patients but may be as high as 20% so the absence of clinical findings of systemic thyroid dysfunction does not exclude the diagnosis[6,7]. Graves' ophthalmopathy can often be diagnosed by the clinical signs alone. Lid retraction is the most common and specific sign in acquired proptosis due to Graves' disease. When this sign is present no further testing is required to establish the diagnosis[8]. Lid lag on downgaze is a common accompanying sign in Graves' disease that may be due to a mechanical restriction although some have suggested it is caused by increased sympathetic tone[9,10]. Other important clinical signs include conjunctival injection over the medial and lateral rectus muscle insertions and an inflammatory myositis typically affecting the muscle belies of the medial and inferior recti resulting in restrictive elevation and abduction deficits. The lateral rectus muscle and the insertions of the ocular muscles are rarely affected. Glaucoma in Graves' ophthalmopathy is uncommon but pseudo-elevation of intraocular pressure may occur in primary position and with gaze in the direction of a restricted muscle. This

Address for correspondence: Jonathan C. Calkwood, MD, Department of Neurology/Neuro-Ophthalmology, Ochsner Clinic, 1514 Jefferson Highway, New Orleans, LA 70121-2483, USA

Peril to the Nerve – Glaucoma and Clinical Neuro-Ophthalmology, pp. 249–252
Proceedings of the 45th Annual Symposium of the New Orleans Academy of
Ophthalmology, New Orleans, LA, USA, April 25-28, 1996
edited by Barry J. Leader and Jonathan C. Calkwood
© 1998 Kugler Publications, The Hague/The Netherlands

phenomenon may also be useful in clinical diagnosis since the intraocular pressure increases with upgaze.

There is considerable evidence that Graves' disease is an autoimmune disease. In 1956, Adams and Purvis reported on long-acting thyroid stimulator[11], Kriss *et al.* showed that long-acting thyroid stimulator was an IgG molecule[12], Smith and Hall further defined thyroid-stimulating immunoglobulins in Graves' disease[13]. Roitt *et al.* described autoantibodies in Hashimoto's disease[14] and in 1974, Volpe said that Hashimoto's disease and Graves' disease were separate but related[15]. Solomon *et al.* postulated a shared underlying immune dysfunction between Graves' ophthalmopathy, idiopathic hyperthyroidism, and Hashimoto's thyroiditis[16]. Autoimmune diseases tend to run together and approximately 0.6% of patients with Graves' will have myasthenia gravis. Conversely, about 5% of patients with myasthenia will also have thyroid ophthalmopathy[17]. A Tensilon test should be considered when ptosis is present with other clinical features of Graves' ophthalmopathy.

Neuroimaging findings of Graves' ophthalmopathy are characteristic, often showing bilateral findings with a predilection for involvement of the muscle bellies of the lateral and medial rectus muscles. The tendinous insertions are relatively spared and there may be a generalized increase in orbital fat content in the acute stages of the disease. Relative muscle size is best appreciated on coronal views of the orbit. Orbital fat content and muscle size decreases during the chronic stages associated with fibrosis of the muscles. Despite marked engorgement of the extraocular muscles no consistent signal abnormalities are demonstrated on magnetic resonance imaging[18]. In compressive optic neuropathy, CT and MRI show a markedly congested orbital apex due to the enlarged extraocular muscles.

The medical management of Graves' ophthalmopathy depends on the clinical features present. In mildly symptomatic disease no treatment may be necessary but all patients should be treated for any underlying thyroid dysfunction which may improve the ocular symptoms in some patients. The use of systemic steroids for proptosis and ductional deficits is controversial. Oral prednisone may be effective in some patients and response to steroids may relate to the type of underlying immune dysfunction[19]. Prednisone for ductional deficits is administered for two weeks. If no clinical improvement occurs treatment should be discontinued. Improvement of symptoms should prompt a slow taper titrating the dose by clinical signs. Steroid therapy should not last longer than three months[20]. Intraorbital corticosteroid injections are an alternative to systemic steroids that has been shown to be quite effective for ocular motility problems[21]. Radiotherapy has also shown efficacy in Graves' ophthalmopathy[22].

Optic neuropathy in Graves' disease may present insidiously or have a more fulminant course. Typical symptoms include acuity and color vision loss in the clinical setting of Graves' orbitopathy. Other ocular pathology in Graves' patients may obscure the diagnosis and cause delay in treatment. When optic neuropathy occurs it is believed to result from compression at the apex due to enlarged ocular muscles. Feldon *et al.* and Barrett *et al.* have separately shown optic neuropathy to be related to extraocular muscle volume[23,24].

A relative afferent pupillary defect (Marcus-Gunn pupil) may be present since the optic nerve involvement may be unilateral or asymmetric. The optic disc examination is not always helpful in diagnosis. The optic nerve may be normal, pale or edematous at presentation. Visual field testing is important in diagnosis and may reveal a classic compressive optic neuropathy pattern of cecocentral or central scotomata. Arcuate visual field defects and generalized depression may also occur. Serial perimetry is important for determining the patient's response to therapy[24].

Optic neuropathy in Graves' disease should be considered an ophthalmologic emergency and requires prompt treatment with systemic corticosteroids. Some studies have shown good results with oral prednisone up to 200 mg/day while others advocate intravenous methylprednisolone up to 1 g/day for three days[25,26]. Cyclosporin as monotherapy is less effective than steroids but in combination with steroids may be helpful in refractory patients[27]. Plasmapheresis is not as effective as systemic steroids and is not recommended as first line therapy[28]. A variety of surgical approaches for optic neuropathy have been used and are effective, especially if the medial and inferior walls are decompressed. Surgical decompression is generally reserved for cases refractory to medical management. Orbital radiation with fractionated doses of 1500–2000 cGy over ten days has been shown to be effective in the management of optic neuropathy due to Graves'[29].

In conclusion, acute vision loss in Graves' disease from optic neuropathy should be considered an ophthalmic emergency. Optic neuropathy may be difficult to diagnose or the vision loss attributed to other causes. Prompt and aggressive treatment may reverse or limit permanent visual loss.

References

1. Parry CH: Collections from Unpublished Medical Writings of the late Caleb Hillier Parry, Vol 2, p 211. London: Underwoods 1825
2. Graves RJ: Med Surg J 7(Part II):516, 1835
3. Von Basedow CA: Exophthalmos durch Hypertrophie des Zellgewebes in der Augenhöhle. Wochenschr Ges Heilk 6:197, 1840
4. Werner SC: Euthyroid patients with early eye signs of Graves' disease. Am J Med 18:608, 1959
5. Sridama V, DeGroot LJ: Treatment of Graves' disease and the course of ophthalmopathy. Am J Med 87:70-73, 1989
6. Wiersinga WM, Smit T, Van der Gaag R et al: Temporal relationship between onset of Graves' ophthalmopathy and onset of thyroidal Graves' disease. J Endocrinol Invest 11:615-619, 1988
7. Marcocci C, Bartalena L, Bogazzi F et al: Studies on the occurrence of ophthalmopathy in Graves' disease. Acta Endocrinol 120:473-478, 1989
8. Burde RM, Savino PJ, Trobe JD: Clinical Decisions in Neuro-Ophthalmology, p 257. St Louis, MO: CV Mosby Co 1985
9. Feldon SE, Levin L: Graves' ophthalmopathy. V. Aetiology of upper eyelid retraction in Graves' ophthalmopathy. Br J Ophthalmol 74:484-485, 1990
10. Miller NR: Walsh and Hoyt's Clinical Neuro-Ophthalmology, Vol 2, 4th Edn, p 953. Baltimore, MD: Williams & Wilkins 1985
11. Adams DD, Purvis HD: Abnormal responses in the assay of thyrotropin. Univ Otago Med Sch Proc 34-11, 1956
12. Kriss JP, Pleshakov V, Chien JR: Isolation and identification of the long-acting thyroid stimulator and its relationship to hyperthyroidism and circumscribed pretibial myxedema. J Clin Endocrinol Metabol 24:1005, 1964
13. Smith BR, Hall R: Thyroid stimulating immunoglobulins in Graves' disease. Lancet ii:427, 1974
14. Roitt IM, Doacch D, Campbell PN, Hudson RV: Auto-antibodies in Hashimoto's Disease (lymphadenoid goiter). Lancet ii:820, 1956
15. Volpe R, Farid WR, Von Westarp C, Row VV: The pathogenesis of Graves' disease and Hashimoto's thyroiditis. Clin Endocrinol 3:239, 1947
16. Solomon DH, Chopra IJ, Chopra U, Smith FJ: Identification of subgroups of euthyroid Graves' ophthalmopathy. New Engl J Med vol. 296, 181-186, 1977
17. Burde RM: Graves' ophthalmopathy and the special problem of concomitant ocular myasthenia gravis. Am Orthop J 40:37-49, 1990
18. Kucharczyk W (ed): MRI: Central Nervous System, p 414. New York, NY: Gower Medical Publishing 1990

19. Sergott RC, Felberg NT, Savino PJ et al: Graves' ophthalmopathy-immunologic parameters related to corticosteroid therapy. Invest Ophthalmol Vis Sci 20:173-182, 1981
20. Burde RM, Savino PJ, Trobe JD: Clinical Decisions in Neuro-Ophthalmology, p. 389. St Louis, MO: CV Mosby Co 1985
21. Thomas ID, Hart JK: Retrobulbar repository corticosteroid therapy in thyroid ophthalmopathy. Med J Aust 2:484-487, 1974
22. Kriss JP, Petersen IA, Donaldson SS et al: Supervoltage orbital radiotherapy for progressive Graves' ophthalmopathy: results of a twenty-year experience. Acta Endocrinol 121(Suppl 2):154-159, 1989
23. Feldon SE, Lee CP, Muramatsu SK et al: Quantitative computed tomography of Graves' ophthalmopathy: extraocular muscle and orbital fat in development of optic neuropathy. Arch Ophthalmol 103:213-215, 1985
24. Barrett L, Glatt HJ, Burde RM et al: Optic nerve dysfunction in thyroid eye disease: CT. Radiology 167:503-507, 1988
25. Klingele TG, Hart WM, Burde RM: Management of dysthyroid optic neuropathy. Ophthalmologica 174:327-335, 1977
26. Guy JR, Fagien S, Donovan JP et al: Methylprednisolone pulse therapy in severe dysthyroid optic neuropathy. Ophthalmology 96:1048-1053, 1989
27. Prummel MF, Mourits MP, Berghout A et al: Prednisone and cyclosporine in the treatment of severe Graves' ophthalmopathy. N Engl J Med 321:1353-1359, 1989
28. Burde RM, Savino PJ, Trobe JD: Clinical Decisions in Neuro-Ophthalmology, p 390. St Louis, MO: CV Mosby Co 1985
29. Donaldson SS, Bagshaw MA, Kriss JP: Supervoltage orbital radiotherapy for Graves' ophthalmopathy. J Clin Endocrinol Metabol 37:276-285, 1973

Idiopathic intracranial hypertension

Norman J. Schatz

University of Miami, Bascom Palmer Eye Institute, Miami, FL, USA

Idiopathic intracranial hypertension (IIH) is a syndrome of elevated intracranial pressure without known cause. Dandy set down the following criteria, which still should be fulfilled in order to establish an accurate diagnosis: signs and symptoms of increased intracranial pressure; absence of localizing findings on neurological examination; absence of displacement or obstruction of the ventricular system on neuro-imaging; otherwise normal neuro-diagnostic studies, except for increased intracranial pressure; an alert and oriented patient; no other specific causes of increased intracranial pressure present[1].

Symptoms of increased intracranial pressure include headaches, usually described as severe, daily, pulsatile, commonly increased with bending, and may last for hours. In a recent review of 50 patients with IIH[2], 94% of patients presented with headaches, 39 of the 50 patients described their headaches as pulsatile, and headaches predominantly lasted for more than an hour. The headache is often reported as different from previous headaches and, for the most part, described as the most severe headache they have ever experienced.

The next most frequent symptom encountered was that of transient visual obscurations, described variably as brief, less than a minute episodes of dimming of vision, usually lasting seconds. In Wall's series, changes in posture, such as rapidly assuming the standing position, lying down, bending over, or performing the Valsalva maneuver, were the predominantly precipitating events, although several patients reported obscurations provoked by glare or by changes in illumination from dark to bright. The mechanism of transient visual obscurations has remained speculative, but theoretically includes vascular compromise at the peripapillary capillary level, blockage of axoplasmic flow, and even vitreous traction. Obscurations are generally not believed to be correlated with the degree of intracranial pressure, or with the extent of disc edema. Transient visual obscurations are not necessarily associated with ultimate poor visual outcome, but are useful in establishing the diagnosis of increased intracranial pressure. They can be seen in almost any cause of disc elevation, including drusen, and in normal individuals[3].

Pulsatile tinnitus occurs in over half the patients with IIH. The noise is synchronous with the heartbeat and is usually attributed to either venous vascular compression with secondary venous turbulence, or hydrops and dilatation of the nerve sheath in the internal auditory canal. Diplopia is encountered in about one-third of

Address for correspondence: Norman J. Schatz, MD, Mercy Neuroscience Institute, Suite 209, 3661 South Miami Avenue, Miami, FL 33133, USA

Peril to the Nerve – Glaucoma and Clinical Neuro-Ophthalmology, pp. 253–256
Proceedings of the 45th Annual Symposium of the New Orleans Academy of
Ophthalmology, New Orleans, LA, USA, April 25-28, 1996
edited by Barry J. Leader and Jonathan C. Calkwood
© 1998 Kugler Publications, The Hague/The Netherlands

the patients, usually secondary to unilateral or bilateral VIth nerve paresis, this phenomenon may be secondary to downward displacement of the brain stem with stretching of the VIth nerve, tethered against the dural edge[4].

Visual loss is the main symptom to which treatment should be directed. A quarter of patients may suffer significant visual field loss, which takes the form of enlargement of the blind spot, isopter constriction, nasal, especially inferonasal field loss, arcuate scotomas, other nerve fiber bundle type defects and, more rarely, central visual loss and blindness. Field loss generally follows the distribution of the retinal nerve fiber bundles, and the pattern shows 'disc-related' (connected to the blind spot) defects similar to those found in glaucoma or drusen of the optic nerve head. In all series that analyze the frequency of field patterns, at least 80% of the visual defects are disc-related, only a small percentage of patients presenting with central or paracentral scotomatous field loss, which can usually be accounted for on the basis of retinal changes extending to the macula[5-7].

The mechanism of the visual loss is related to disc edema in IIH that results when raised intracranial pressure is transmitted to the subarachnoid space within the optic nerve sheath. At the level of the lamina cribrosa, visual axons angulate sharply and axoplasmic flow stasis occurs. Intracellular swelling of the nerve fibers manifests as optic nerve head swelling, involving disc tissue in front of the lamina cribrosa. These mechanisms presuppose the intact communication between the intracranial compartment and the anterior portion of each optic nerve. Anatomical differences in this potential space may act in preventing such transmission[8]. Hayreh[3,9,10] clearly summarizes the important concepts to be considered in the pathogenesis of visual field loss in IIH: *1.* all nerves that become edematous from IIH are presumed to have stasis of axoplasmic flow; *2.* the great majority of swollen optic nerves resulting from IIH do not exhibit optic nerve-related field loss; *3.* there does not seem to be a clear correlation between the degree of optic nerve edema and the risk of developing optic nerve-related field loss; *4.* when the optic disc-related field defects do occur, they may be permanent or reversible; *5.* when the field loss shows recovery after medical or surgical treatment, the rate of recovery is usually gradual, but can occur over a short period of time; *6.* systemic hypertension, ocular hypertension, and anemia may be significant risk factors for visual field loss; and *7.* when field loss occurs, the pattern corresponds to nerve fiber bundle loss similar to glaucoma. Although ischemia is likely to be the major factor, axoplasmic flow stasis plays a major factor in visual field loss. Some would argue that profound degrees of visual loss for significant periods of time may be reversed by lowering intracranial pressure or sheath pressure, suggesting that such recovery is at least functionally related to the restoration of axoplasmic flow.

With regard to management, the major goals of therapy are relief of the symptoms, especially headaches, and restoration or preservation of visual function. In that regard, visual loss remains the most feared complication of the disease. Therapy should also be directed towards weight reduction, although the relationship between body weight and management is unclear. Recent weight gain has been strongly associated with visual deterioration. In some patients, when placed on severe diets, or after stomach stapling procedures with significant weight loss, complete remission of their disease has occurred. Regardless, weight loss is strongly recommended.

Of oral agents, acetazolamide has been found effective in lowering intracranial pressure. It is a diuretic that also reduces cerebrospinal fluid production. The recommended dose of 500 mg b.i.d. is suggested. Furosemide has been effectively used as an alternative, both as a diuretic and to decrease cerebrospinal fluid production. A recent review of the subject by Goodwin *et al.*[11,12] suggested that digoxin can reduce cerebrospinal fluid production by its effect on the sodium potassium ATPase in the choroid plexus. This has not been in use at all, however, in clinical management.

The use of corticosteroids in the management of pseudotumor has generally been discouraged. This is a high complication risk group of obese females. Long-term steroids for chronic disease have little use or benefit. Corticosteroids do reduce interstitial brain edema, but influence cerebrospinal fluid production. Recently, Liu *et al.*[13] described the limited use of i.v. methylprednisolone in patients with IIH who have acute visual loss with macular exudates. This series demonstrated reduction of optic nerve swelling, and restoration of visual function even after 1 g a day of i.v. methylprednisolone for three to five days, followed by the rapid taper of oral steroids. This situation is probably the one exception in which steroids may be of benefit.

With regard to the management of visual loss, after the diagnosis has been established, the clinician must rely on visual fields to follow progress. It is impractical in this day and age to consider following patients in any other way than computerized automated perimetry, which is now so readily available and standardized. Visual fields should be repeated weekly after the diagnosis is established, until vision is stable or improved. If disc edema persists and there is evidence of significant progression in field loss, in spite of maximum medical management, then optic nerve sheath decompression on the worst involved eye is the suggested treatment. Optic nerve sheath decompression, although an effective method of reversing visual loss, is not without risk of loss of vision in the perioperative period[14].

Serial lumbar punctures have been recommended in the past in the management of pseudotumor cerebri. However, spinal fluid is replaced completely within a 24-hour period, in spite of the fact that 'spinal taps' may be associated with some potential shunting of cerebrospinal fluid to subcutaneous tissues. The punitive nature of repeated taps, failure of compliance and difficulties with having patients return, may be more hazardous than any benefits than can be derived. We would discourage this form of treatment. The role of lumboperitoneal shunt in the management of pseudotumor has been suggested for treatment of intractable headaches. However, because of the high rate of shunt failure[15] and other complications, the procedure should be limited to patients who have progressive visual field loss in spite of maximal medical management and optic nerve sheath decompression. Its use in the treatment of headaches *per se*, should be discouraged. With regard to the management of chronic headaches, in patients with pseudotumor cerebri without field loss, this becomes the only problem of chronic headache management and combinations of tricyclic medications in the therapeutic range varying from 150 to 200 mg daily of amitriptyline may be of benefit.

In summary, IIH is a disorder which can be a significant threat to visual function. Careful visual fields at frequent intervals determine the clinical direction in management. Documentation of fields, serial disc photographs, and prompt intervention, if visual function fails, on maximal medical management, would appear to be our major responsibility. The association of IIH with obesity demands that weight reduction also be a goal of treatment. *Other associations with hypervitaminosis A should be eliminated, as well as all probable associated causes.* Special caution should be taken in all patients who do not fit the clinical profile of disease and in all cases of IIH in males, or in slender females, and an index of suspicion of another evolving etiology should be kept in mind.

References

1. Wall M: Idiopathic intracranial hypertension. Neurol Clin 9:73-95, 1991
2. Wall M, George D: Idiopathic intracranial hypertension: a prospective study of 50 patients. Brain 114:155-180, 1991
3. Hayrey SS: Optic disc edema in raised intracranial pressure. VI. Associated visual disturbances and their pathogenesis. Arch Ophthalmol 95:1566-1579, 1977
4. Gluseffi V, Wall M, Siegel PZ, Rojas PB: Symptoms and disease associations in idiopathic intracranial hypertension (pseudo-tumor cerebri): a case control study. Neurology 41:239-244, 1991
5. Corbett JJ, Savino PJ, Thompson HS et al.: Visual loss in pseudotumor cerebri. Follow-up of 57 patients from five to 41 years and a profile of 14 patients with permanent severe visual loss. Arch Neurol 39:461-474, 1982
6. Lessell S, Rosman NP: Permanent visual impairment in childhood pseudotumor cerebri. Arch Neurol 43:801-804, 1988
7. Gittinger JW, Asdourian GK: Macular abnormalities in papilledema from pseudotumor cerebri. Ophthalmology 96:192-194, 1989
8. Hayreh SS: Optic disc edema in raised intracranial pressure. V. Pathogenesis. Arch Ophthalmol 95:1553-1565, 1977
9. Hayreh SS: Pathogenesis of oedema of the optic disc (papilloedema). Br J Ophthalmol 48:522-543, 1964
10. Hayreh SS: Pathogenesis of oedema of the optic disc. Doc Ophthalmol 24:289-411, 1968
11. Goodwin J: Medical Management of Idiopathic Intracranial Hypertension. NANOS Syllabus 1992
12. Neblett CR, McNeel DP, Waltz TA, Harrison GM: Effect of cardiac glycosides on human cerebral spinal fluid production. Lancet 2:1008-1009, 1992
13. Liu GT, Glaser JS, Schatz NJ: High-dose methylprednisolone treatment of acute, severe visual loss in pseudotumor cerebri [Abstract]. Neurology 43(Suppl 2):A226, 1993
14. Corbett JJ, Nerad JA, Tse DT, Anderson RL: Results of optic nerve sheath fenestration for pseudotumor cerebri. The lateral orbitotomy approach. Arch Ophthalmol 106:1391-1397, 1988
15. Sergott RC, Savino PJ, Bosley TM: Modified optic nerve sheath decompression provides long-term visual improvement for pseudotumor cerebri. Arch Ophthalmol 106:1384-1390, 1988

Round Table and Question and Answer Period

Undiagnosable progressive optic neuropathies – etiology, management and empiric treatment

Moderator: Jonathan Calkwood, MD

Round Table

Jonathan Calkwood, MD: Undiagnosable optic neuropathies are the bane of neuro-ophthalmologists. Often we find ourselves rounding up the usual suspects and still winding up without any clear diagnosis. It is most difficult when it is a progressive optic neuropathy and not a stable problem. I have assembled two cases from my practice and will use the expertise of our panel to answer several questions. Is there anything that I have missed; is there anything else that needs to be thought of; would Dr. Glaser or Dr. Schatz have done differently; or is there anything else we can try?

The first case is a 64-year-old lady who was in very good health, no history of hypertension or diabetes or other small vessel risk factors other than her age. She had a sudden onset of painless vision loss in her right eye, no other associated symptoms, no symptoms of giant cell arteritis. She was first seen in my clinic in June of 1994 for this problem. The only other important point in her ocular history is the presence of a previously diagnosed branch retinal artery occlusion in her left eye.

Joel S. Glaser, MD: Did you say you saw the occlusion?

Dr. Calkwood: No, the retinal artery occlusion happened nine years previously. At the time I initially saw her, her visual acuity was 20/30 in both eyes. She had a 0.9 log unit relative afferent pupillary defect measured in her right eye and optic disc edema in the eye. (The right eye again is the symptomatic eye. The left eye is the eye with the old apparent branch retinal artery occlusion.) *This is a visual field* of the symptomatic eye showing what I described in the slide as an altitudinal defect, but it would probably be better described as a broad arcuate defect. (Fig. 1b) The field in the fellow eye, which was the eye affected nine years ago from an apparent branch retinal artery occlusion, looked like this (this will become important later on because she developed changes in this eye as well.) (Fig. 1a) The right optic disc shows edema more prominently in the superior portion of the disc with some hemorrhage. (Fig. 2) The left optic nerve attention we see looks pretty normal and I want to draw your attention to the temporal portion of the neural rim because you are going to see some changes there on subsequent photographs. Her initial workup was negative and the diagnosis of non-arteritic anterior ischemic optic neuropathy was made (NAION). Her acuity and her visual fields were stable for a

Peril to the Nerve – Glaucoma and Clinical Neuro-Ophthalmology, pp. 257–269
Proceedings of the 45th Annual Symposium of the New Orleans Academy of
Ophthalmology, New Orleans, LA, USA, April 25-28, 1996
edited by Barry J. Leader and Jonathan C. Calkwood
© *1998 Kugler Publications, The Hague/The Netherlands*

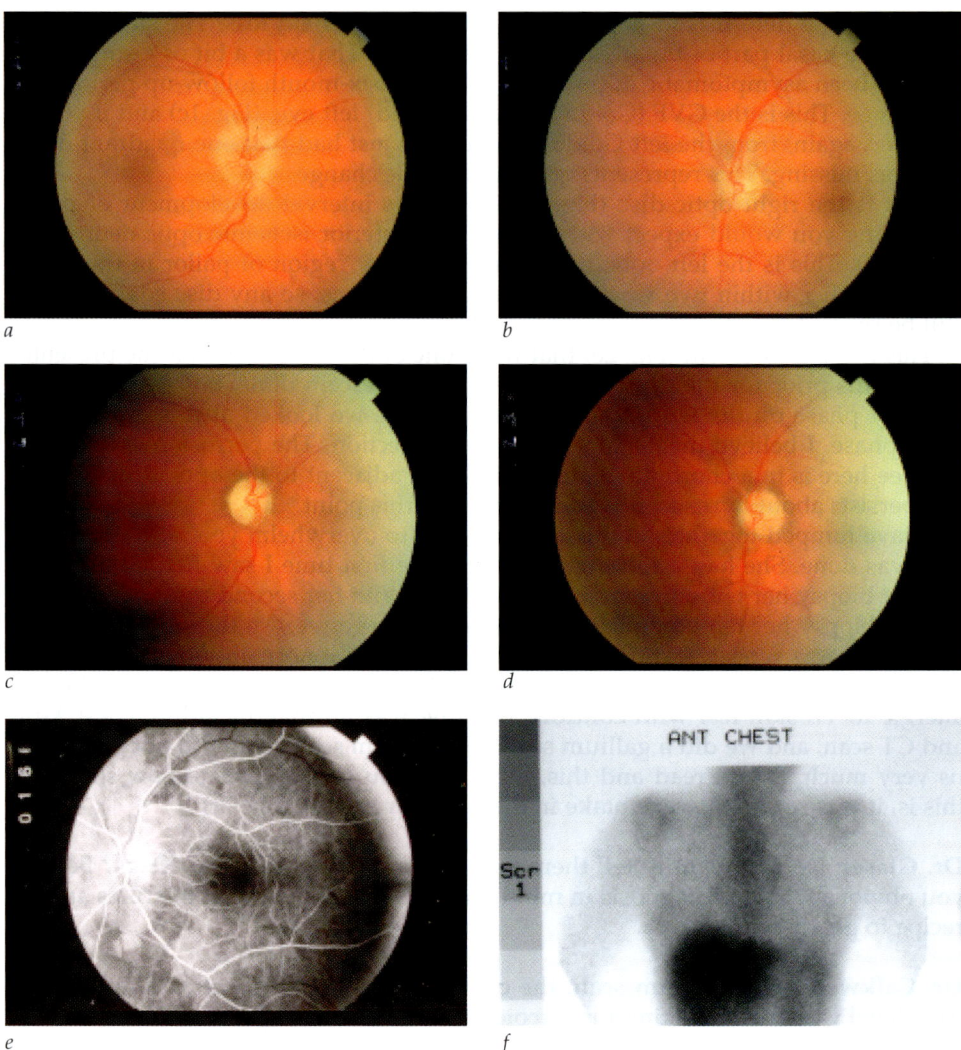

Fig. 2a-f. Fundus photographs on initial presentation showing disc edema with superficial hemorrhages in the right eye (a) and normal nerve with left eye (b). Six-month follow-up photos reveal resolution of edema in the right eye (c) with interval development of sectoral pallor in the superior temporal portion of the disc. The left optic nerve (d) shows interval development of pallor in the superior temporal neural rim. The IVFA shows early phase (16 second), chondial perfusion defect in a vertical watershed distribution in the left eye (e). Forty-eight hour tumor localization Study (Gallum Scan) shows abnormal tracer uptake in the perihiliar region(f).

are not too sure, and I took the thing around to two other radiologists, and they all said, well, we are not very impressed.

Dr. Glaser: We are not saying we know any more about the details of the scan than the nuclear radiologist, but you have kind of run out of things to diagnose that you can help this lady with. Obviously, it is not the garden variety ischemic optic neuropathy of any kind. It is not cranial arteritis: I did not think it was going to be because of the way it has progressed. Sarcoid can do very peculiar things in the optic nerve, including swelling the front end with no visual loss, or doing in the canalicular or intraorbital end without showing any change in the optic nerve. We have recently had a young girl from San Paulo, Brazil, who came with severe visual loss and a big fat chiasm, but a little bit rough and ragged in the chiasm, very slight elevation of protein on the LP that she came with from San Paulo, and also when we repeated our lumbar puncture, again an elevation of protein, but also serum ACE negative, CSF ACE positive for sarcoid.

Dr. Calkwood: The story gets better. We went on to do a lumbar puncture (LP). In her serum she had beta 2 microglobulins, which has been associated with sarcoid as well as with a whole lot of other diseases including lymphoma and leukemia, but in her CSF, the beta 2 microglobulins were negative. I also asked them to run an ACE on the CSF, and that was negative. I was not sure that this was sarcoid, but I gave her an empiric trial of steroids and her fields got a little better. Every time I tried to taper her down below about 40 mg per day, she would lose more vision and we would not always get it back. There is the field. Again, that is the right eye, (Fig. 1f) and the left eye, and you can appreciate that there has been a little bit of field recovered with corticosteroids in the left eye. (Fig. 1e) The right eye really did not improve much. So, this was a lady who ultimately failed two attempted tapers of oral corticosteroids. In fact, I did the initial treatment with IV corticosteroids. I started off with giving her 1 g methylprednisolone a day for three days. That was with the acute vision loss in her left eye, the second involved eye, and then put her on oral Prednisone and tried to taper her rapidly. She lost vision again with a rapid taper. I bumped her back up to around 60 mg and gave her a very long, protracted taper and as soon as she got below 40, almost every time she started to lose vision, and she never really tolerated getting below 20. So ultimately we wound up in consultation with a rheumatologist, putting her on methotrexate. Since she has been on the methotrexate, we have been able to taper the steroid dose down to 20 mg a day, which is where we are currently, and I have not gone any further.

Dr. Schatz: When you face the problem of slowly progressive optic neuropathy, of course this is what we were talking about when we said the atypical optic neuritis. An atypical optic neuritis means that you are dealing with vasculitis, sarcoid, or infiltrative disease, or contiguous disease of other structures, like neoplasms or sinus inflammatory disease. The difficulties, of course, are that occasionally you will find fungal disease, that when you put patients on steroids they have had an infiltrative optic neuropathy related to aspergilli or something, so your imaging really has to be very good. Everything has been done in this particular case to try to establish a diagnosis. But do not think that lymphoma is out of the picture yet, although when you look at the subtle clues, sarcoid seems at least a viable diagnosis, a patient who is anergic, who has some suggestive laboratory studies of sarcoid and a little bit of hilar uptake. The usual protocol for investigation short of transbronchial biopsy has been gone through rather completely in trying to establish the diagnosis of sarcoid. When you find steroid dependency in sarcoidosis, the use of methotrexate is well recognized as a successful way to lower the steroid dose. The other form of treatment is radiation therapy, that has been suggested in some patients with localized sarcoidosis to cut down the response. I feel much safer with the use of methotrexate in the immune response.

Sarcoid has three ways of presenting itself in the central nervous system: (1) a vasculitic form, so it will present as stroke, (2) a parenchymous form where it presents just as a globular mass or tumor, which you would expect to see, suprasellar

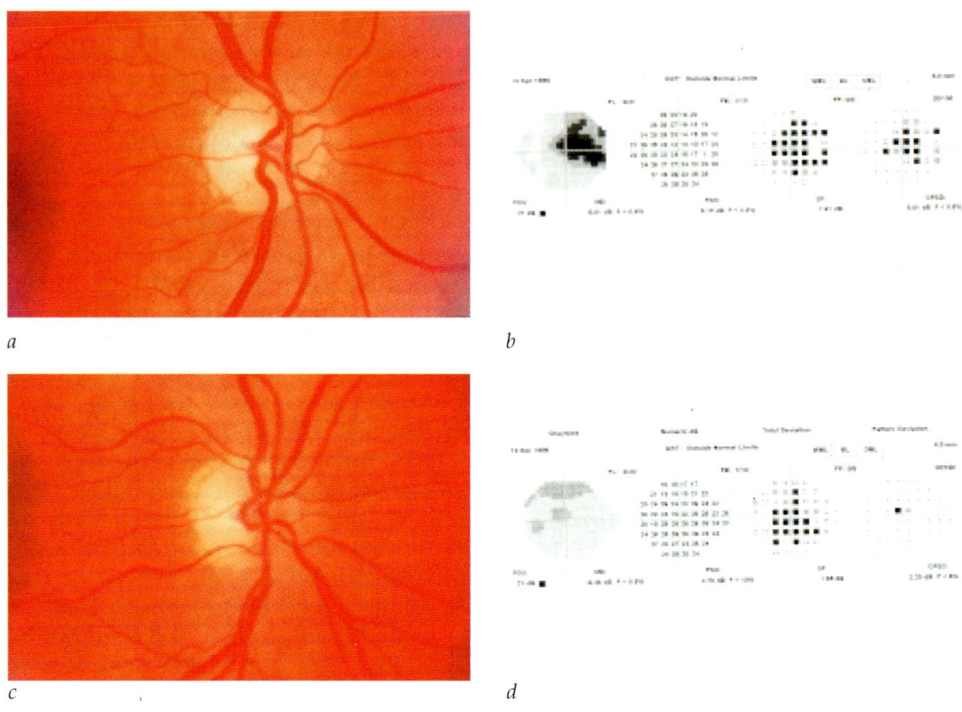

a

b

c

d

Fig. 3a-d. Fundus photography of the right optic nerve (a) shows temporal pallor with a ceco-central scotoma on Humphrey perimetry (b). Fundus photography of the left eye (c) shows temporal pallor and cecocentral scotometic on Humphrey perimetry (d).

tumor with diabetes insipidus and a chiasmal mass, and (3) the meningeal form, which is the form that infiltrates the nerves and goes down both nerves. We usu-ally see the nerves light up with gadolinium, but they do not have to. I do not know that we know what this disorder is, but steroid-sparing immunosuppression and minimizing the steroid dose seems the best thing to do.

Dr. Glaser: The quality of the MR scan is very important. And in patients where you are looking for some occult or atypical form of optic nerve disease, you have to be very specific in what you order, and if you order a brain MRI, it is insuffi-cient. The person who is doing the MRI needs to understand that you need thin sections, which are 3 mm. They need to know that you want to see exquisitely the picture of the intraorbital, the intracanalicular and intracranial optic nerves and chiasm. You do not get that particularly well on a standard brain MRI scan. So, if you are looking for lesions in the anterior visual pathway, you have to really de-sign the MRI, and of course, to do it without gadolinium is an incomplete scan. And then I suppose you yourself need to go to the radiologist with whatever your favorite weapon is in the parish, put it up against him and say to him, "Tell me those optic nerves are 100% normal. What is that little ragged, etc., on the side? That optic chiasm is not smooth." Unless you have that kind of cooperation, that kind of study, you will miss sarcoid, and sarcoid is not rare. I thought it was rare. It is not rare. And the reason we know it is not rare is because we are getting better and better MRI scans and are finding paradoxically enlarged nerves and enlarged nerves and chiasm that are not tumor, and then to complete the work-up, etc., and hopefully find something outside the head that you can biopsy and establish the diagnosis of sarcoidosis.

Dr. Schatz: There is one other problem that you have in this case. Ordinarily, vision gets bad enough to get tissue from one blind nerve, but this acuity stayed so good that this was not an option. Because you know, as these disorders of the swollen disc and progression occur, there is a time that, when a nerve is blind for a period of time, taking the nerve and looking for tissue can establish the diagnosis. That has been the way to establish the diagnosis in the lymphoma cases.

Dr. Glaser: Have you seen a case of sarcoid that will do one optic nerve and then continues to do them nine years later with no tissue that is available? That is a way of shouting, hey, come biopsy me!

Dr. Schatz: I do not know that disorder. The branch retinal artery occlusion presumed if that was first bout of optic neuritis, I do not know that disorder.

Dr. Calkwood: Well, she has had three MRIs now, at least two of them are axial and thin section coronal, all the way back as far as the field strength will go to the chiasm, and then I do a head on top of that, and go over them with the radiologist and go over them myself.

Dr. Glaser: I am not questioning...although you did not show them.

Dr. Calkwood: I did not show them. That is what I am telling you. I did not show them, but she has had three now and I still have yet to find any tissue, although doing a blind transbronchial biopsy probably would have been a good idea.

Dr. Glaser: A repeat LP for a CSF ACE I do not think is out of the question, and I do not know that I would hesitate to push her internist, or whoever is looking after her, to get on with a look at this hilar business. Because she is youngish and she is committed here already to methotrexate.

Dr. Schatz: Of course, the methotrexate may have reversed everything in the chest. It might be nice to see if her hilar business is clear.

Dr. Calkwood: Repeat a gallium scan and see if it resolves?

Dr. Schatz: I would get her off steroids as quickly as you can, keep her on the minimum methotrexate for a period of time, and then see in six months from now if you can get her off the methotrexate.

Dr. Calkwood: I have had trouble with other sarcoid patients getting them off steroids on just immune suppressants. Is that something..?

Dr. Schatz: That is if you are going to get them off immunosuppressants, at least you can get her to every other day of steroids.

Dr. Calkwood: How fast would you go at this point?

Dr. Schatz: Two-and-a-half mg a week on alternate days. So that you will end up with her at 20 every other day in about ten weeks.

Dr. Calkwood: Maybe this is sarcoid, maybe it is not. I guess I am perplexed by these undiagnosed optic neuropathies. Is there another group of disorders causing optic neuropathy as yet undefined?

Dr. Glaser: Why do you think there was such a huge difference between our pictures 21 years ago and today? It is perplexing, but you have to live with it in some cases.

Dr. Schatz: There have been a lot of reports on associations with progressive optic neuropathies in rheologic studies that show platelet abnormalities, that show thromboplastin abnormalities, that show other abnormalities which people have reported as being consecutive ischemic neuropathies in certain patients. That does not look quite like what this patient is. In fact, one nerve you distinctly showed was retrobulbar in its onset. So we have taken it away from the disorders that we would think of as progressive vascular occlusive disease or ischemic neuropathy, once you showed it was a retrobulbar event in the second eye. So, we are left with what sort of infiltrative disease this is. The next question was, is there a disorder that produces branch retinal artery occlusions and has optic neuropathy as part of it? So, there are all sorts of endotheliopathies, even associated with just plain ordinary hypercholesterolemia which we think produces vascular spasm, etc. But again, they present as disc swelling. So I think that what we are left with is this disorder as we know it, tumor infiltration or is it sarcoid or granulomatous disease that produces it? You have looked for Wegener's and you have done all the things that you should do. I do not know that we can answer what this disorder is, but for lack of knowing, hilar adenopathy, some changes in blood that suggests sarcoid, a clinical picture that we all accept as possible sarcoid, that seems acceptable. And you did Leber's titers on her.

Dr. Calkwood: As a matter of fact, I did not.

Dr. Glaser: Good for you.

Dr. Schatz: Thank goodness, because that is not the picture of Leber's.

Dr. Calkwood: I did do antiphospholipid antibodies, although I personally have never seen an ischemic optic neuropathy, or at least a picture of anterior ischemic optic neuropathy from that. And they were negative, they were normal, as everything else was.

I have one more case that sort of comes at the other end, another tough optic neuropathy without disc swelling. And this is a situation of a gentleman who, at the time I saw him, was 46 years old and who had been through multiple other neurologists, ophthalmologists, neuro-ophthalmologists. Age 20 is when he first noticed some color vision problems, present in both eyes. He did not notice any other visual problems until he was 23, at which time he had lost a little central vision in his right eye. No-one could ever find anything, and he had no diagnosis. He went along roughly stable visual-wise until he was 38, at which time he had a sudden loss of vision in his right eye. At age 25, he had an episode of meningitis, presumably viral meningitis, and has a long history of migraine headaches. His visual acuity when I saw him was 20/70 and 20/50. Color plates were down, again a little more so on the left than the right, and contrast sensitivity was abnormal, and he had an afferent pupillary defect of 0.9 log units in the right eye. His visual fields I will show you in a minute, but they basically show central scotomata consistent with his confrontation and cecocentral defects, and there was pallor in the temporal portion of the optic nerves. This bilateral cecocentral scotomata was seen on serial Humphrey visual fields. This has remained fairly stable since I have seen him, although going back, he has a stack of Humphrey summary sheets that probably measure an inch and a half in each eye, that show a fair amount of fluctuation, loss of field, recovery of field, loss of field, again, always in the central and cecocentral region. These are the optic nerve photos, shown next to the corresponding Humphrey visual field (Fig. 3). The same old story, pretty much negative laboratory evaluation performed on multiple occasions. In this gentleman we did, in fact, do a Leber's profile, which was negative, multiple negative MRI scans, some of which were good MRs, some were not, but the good ones are the most recent ones and are adequate studies. Abnormal visual evoked potential with diminished latencies and a relative sparing of the amplitudes. Fluorescein angiograms were normal. It is much more difficult in him really to quantitate his vision. He is a very reliable person, again, and he notices the visual change when it is confirmed by fields; sometimes it is not, but when it is confirmed by Humphreys, he tends to notice a visual change several weeks before you actually pick up on the perimetry. So I tend to believe him much more so. He is a professor at UNO and heavily relies on his vision in his work. Treated with a whole bunch of stuff, basically, including the kitchen sink, methylprednisolone, IV methylprednisolone protocol. Oral steroids have been the mainstay of his treatment for the last eight years. He has had pulsed cyclophosphamide which did not seem to cause any improvement in his vision. IgG therapy, in fact, was tried by a neurologist at LSU, and most recently he has been started on Imuran, which has allowed us to get the corticosteroids down to about the 15- to 17-mg range. The main positive response to the steroid sparing agent of the Imuran seems to be his subjective view of his vision, that whenever steroids get down below about 20 mg, his vision starts to go down.

Dr. Glaser: How bad does it get? Because you said that his vision wobbles all over the place.

Dr. Calkwood: He has been down to as much as 20/200 in his left eye.

Dr. Glaser: But you have him 20/70 and 20/50.

Dr. Calkwood: Which were his most recent acuities. And he has been fairly stable in that range. The big thing that bothers him is...

Dr. Glaser: Has he really documented an acute drop of a significant level?

Dr. Calkwood: Yes, and in fact I wanted to include a series of Humphreys done at Tulane by Mike Wall when he had an acute decline in his left eye and there clearly was a huge drop-off with a big cecocentral scotoma in that eye that resolved, again, on oral steroids for approximately six months, improved to roughly what you see in the left eye.

Dr. Glaser: In his left eye?

Dr. Calkwood: In his left eye. It was his right eye that was affected first at age 38.

Dr. Glaser: Did the pupillary response reflect that change? Did the afferent defect switch to the left, do you know?

Dr. Calkwood: That was not documented in the records.

Dr. Glaser: I will tell you why I am asking and maybe you have other evidence that I am way off base, but that is all right too. Could you go back to the fundus photographs and cut the lights back a little bit. I want to show you something about these discs, and also his history is a little bit peculiar. Let us set aside the very acute phase for just a second. This disc has a peculiar, very focal amount of temporal pallor and again it is two dimensional and I am kind of shooting from the hip, but it seems to me that it is really quite focal in this temporal aspect. I cannot comment on whether there is also some excavation in the temporal aspect of this disc.

Dr. Calkwood: It is shallow, scooped cupping.

Dr. Glaser: Shallow, scooped on the edge and the rest of it looks very good, does it not? Rosy pink, red, yes?

Dr. Schatz: Yes.

Dr. Glaser: Thank you. Let us look at the other. It is just facing the wrong way, but we still understand that this is the temporal aspect of the disc, right? And again, we have here a nice pink, rosy color of all the disc, except precisely that temporal aspect, and what I am proposing is that he is a dominant optic atrophy. The problem I am having is the fluctuations in vision. He is a college professor, but what does he teach? I am just kidding. These discs with focal atrophy in the papillomacular bundle, levels of vision which seem to fluctuate anywhere from 20/30 to 20/70 occasionally lower, but they seem to come back, precisely the visual acuity range of the dominant optic atrophies. He has got precisely the area of disc that shows this principal defect and, in one of the fields, this is really great and why I am jumping on the discs, there seems to be just next to the fixational area, if anything it is in temporal field, and a number of the dominant optic atrophies have chiasmal type field defects in the temporal field and most of the time almost hemianopic. So what I would do with him is to re-record his color vision. I would use the Farnsworth-Monsel 85 or D15, I would look for a tritan axis, because the only acquired optic nerve disease with a tritan axis is dominant optic atrophy. He may have a diffuse dyschromatopsia which does not disprove it. If he has a tritan axis, it is dominant optic atrophy and you can also look at his brothers, sisters, father, mother, if he has children, and if you can find another member in the family, then that is what this is. My only problem is these acute changes that I cannot shake. But anyhow, you have a discussion of dominant optic atrophy out of it.

Dr. Calkwood: The fluctuation has been his hallmark of his vision, up and then down and then up and down, but within a range, and certainly part of that is due to the location of his visual field defects that they are central..

Dr. Glaser: We know that acquired optic neuropathies, especially inflammatory ones, can become steroid-dependent. We also know that patients can become medicine-dependent, and they feel a lot better when you give them something, and when you take it away, they do not feel quite as good, whatever way their symptoms, etc., express themselves. So I am not trying to be pushy, I am just saying that that is the direction I would look in this fellow, and as you say, you have rounded up all the usual suspects, and you are certainly treating him with some very severe, if not punitive, medications, and if he has got a tritan axis and another family member...

Dr. Calkwood: This is a gentleman who did a literature review and suggested azathioprine, among a few others. He has also seen various other neurologists and neuro-ophthalmologists who have suggested.....

Dr. Schatz: I would send him to someone else also.

Dr. Glaser: But you do not have an answer. You may not get an answer, but pursue this business of the tritanopia in other family members.

Dr. Calkwood: Okay. In dominant optic atrophy, that typically occurs at a younger age, though, usually?

Dr. Glaser: Sure. But the level of vision can be quite progressive. I am not saying sudden, that is peculiar. I think that would be rare, and I must say I think I have also seen it once but without a return of vision, a drop from something like 20/50 to 20/70, and the patient was quite sure and we had already seen her before personally in my own records, and pushed hard. Every patient goes through an iron maiden visual acuity. So you have to be very careful that you do not explain changes in visual acuity because a high school drop out in somebody's office did a visual acuity and got 20/200. They got to Calkwood's office and he put a thumbscrew on and refracted them and would not let the patient go until they were 20/30, and you know that is the way some patients are. Do you have an answer?

Dr. Calkwood: No, I have no answer to that whatsoever. No, I think that certainly is a reasonable thing to do. Your point is taken about the disc appearance that looks very dramatic. I did not really see the nerve fiber layer drop-out as I have seen in some of the others, although usually the other dominant optic atrophies I have seen are much younger, and so you have a more stark contrast between their healthy nerve fiber layer and the nerve fiber layer that is gone. So perhaps that is why it is not so prominent in him. Who knows what the years and years of steroids have done too. One other interesting note, just to throw this out. This man is about 6'7" tall, very slender. Does that do anything for you? I have been thinking about it for years trying to associate...

Dr. Schatz: The air is too rare up there, I think.

Question and Answer Period

Dr. Glaser: Could I answer a question that somebody asked? Actually, two questions that one person asked. In the post-cataract procedure, ischemic optic neuropathy, and you have got to do the second eye, what do you do in terms of the surgical preparation? And I tell you, I really do not know. But obviously there are two good general rules. One is to wait as long as possible before having to do the second eye, so that when the patient comes crawling across the floor to the surgeon, and the surgeon has been holding him off for whatever years, then of course the time has come because the patient cannot function. I guess the thing you need to do is just to make sure as best you can that at no time after the procedure is there a rise in pressure, and just be prepared to look after that. Any other precaution, I do not know.

Dr. Schatz: And is the data in on second eye involvement? That is, if you do the second eye, the likelihood of an ischemic event.

Dr. Glaser: In Caroll's original description, no patient in his series has yet had a second eye with ischemic neuropathy, unless they had been subjected to a cataract procedure. And this was even true in the age group into the 40s, the rare ones who have cataracts done then, so I think there may be something that tips over a disc at risk.

Dr. Calkwood: Now this is in the cataract associated AION? Now, do you distinguish that from, let us say, someone who has had AION in one eye and a disc at risk in the other, and you are thinking of doing the cataract in the unaffected eye?

Dr. Glaser: I do not know that the same precaution applies to the one that followed hard on the heels of a cataract procedure with regard to monitoring the intraocular tension.

Dr. Schatz: But you suspect it is so, do you not?

Dr. Glaser: No, do I?

Dr. Schatz: Yes, I think so.

Dr. Glaser: The other question somebody wanted to know about. They really wanted to know what to do with the patient with ischemic optic neuropathy, no signs or symptoms of cranial arteritis, polymyalgia rheumatica, but a sed rate of 70. Nothing particular in the fundus that suggests cranial arteritis, but now you have got the tail wagging the dog, what do you do with a 70? And I must admit that I treat the patient until the dust clears and I can figure out what is going on, including during that time arranging for a temporal artery biopsy. But I think if there is any question in your mind, and maybe if its based on the sed rate, then you do need to 'protect that patient's second eye' over the period of time that you are trying to decide whether it is cranial arteritis. Of course, the biopsy comes back negative, you still have the sedimentation rate of 70. If you start them on steroids and the sed rate is cut in half in 48 or 72 hours, then that is presumptive evidence of arteritis, that you have dropped the sed rate.

Dr. Schatz: And, at that stage, you have two choices. If your biopsy is negative and your sed rate does not move, you can consider getting the patient off steroids. If the biopsy is negative and the sed rate drops down to 15, then you should titrate the patient according to sed rate and then, finally, if the biopsy is positive, you know the answer.

Dr. Glaser: An important point in protecting the second eye in giant cell arteritis, the great weight of evidence is if the eyes are not involved bilaterally or within 48 to 72 hours one versus the other, the longer you go in days, weeks, or months, and the second eye has not become involved, the likelihood is very very small. And so you can kind of play your steroid dosage and whether the steroids that the patient is taking are eating up the patient, and you can back off fairly quickly, even by let us say the four-month or six-month mark, if what you are doing is protecting the second eye. Giant cell arteritis involves other vessels in the body, and it is very difficult to come up with information which indicates that, even if you treat giant cell arteritis without ocular involvement, it makes any difference to the patient. Most of them are already in the 80 age group, and so that the actuarial tables are already not much in their favor. It is very difficult to see that steroids do anything for that in the long haul. For the eye, you are probably off the hook by about six months, if not four.

Dr. Calkwood: Do either of you find a role for using C-reactive protein and perhaps the serum protein electrophoresis, as well as looking at whether they are anemic or not? Because the people with anemia seem to have a higher incidence of sed rate negative giant cell arteritis.

Dr. Glaser: Right. I have seen a poster go by on C-reactive protein and I have tried to find the evidence that it is a useful test over and above the sed rate. And either I cannot find it or it is not, but I did try to look.

Dr. Schatz: But the anemia is a rather important one. You know that fits into the category of another sign of chronic disease, just like fatigue and muscle aches and other signs and symptoms. So the anemia is of some help.

Dr. Calkwood: Okay, I guess we are under directives to wrap it up for today so they can prepare the room for this evening.

you want the 24 versus the 30, I use the 24 without a fast pack as a screening field. I use a 30-2 or a 32, depending on what system you are using for looking at chiasmal lesions because the two separates. There is nothing right on the midline. It is on each side of the midline. If you use a 31 or 30-1, that gives you something that goes straight down the center. I cannot answer the questions in specifics because each question you have asked, and the questions are excellent, are really patient-specific.

Norman J. Schatz, MD: Yes, I will disagree with Ron. We did a study at Bascom using the Humphrey screening field on all the neuro patients and glaucoma patients. We then did 30-2s on the same patients and, using double-blinded observers, we classified all our fields into non-diagnostic, hemianoptic, nasal contraction, etc. The observers did just as well with the five-minute screening field from the standpoint of picking up a field deficit.

For the past six months, I have been doing all my own automated fields. It takes about five minutes with the patient to educate them and for you to know whether or not you can leave them in a room alone and get a reliable field, but you certainly do have to have an education curve between you and your patient. If you are following a neurodiagnostic patient, that is, if what you are doing is not trying to make a diagnosis, but trying to see whether the nature of the disease is better, worse, or the same, then you had better use the same parameter that is reproducible each time; and we use a 30-2 for that particular job. There is no doubt that you can get all the information you need from fast screening, and in the patients that you need Goldmann, all the Goldmann machines will be made into salad bowls very shortly, they will not be there any more; because there is a kinetics program on all the new Humphreys. It is a fairly good kinetic test and, in your patients in whom you cannot get information another way, putting in a kinetic test is not a bad one. Remember, when in doubt, after you have gotten this black picture with no information, you had better have written down what the confrontation fields show, "how many fingers is that?", "how many is this?", can they compare them, and do they recognize colors in the quadrant. And if your confrontation does not agree with your Humphrey field, throw the damn thing out.

Dr. Burde: I think it is also important to remember that an Amsler grid is a half-penny Humphrey static perimeter. When you use your Amsler grid, you are doing a super-threshold static field, no more, no less. And if you have a cooperative patient, they will give you a tremendous amount of information. But again, it is patient specific. You cannot rely on it. But, in fact, these are sorts of static fields that are very helpful.

Question: "Is it true that over 90% of neurological deficits can be found within the central 30 degrees of field?" and "How often should you perform fields to follow a neurological deficit?"

Dr. Schatz: If we consider where neurological deficit starts and say it is optic nerve, everything in the optic nerve is a 90% central conducting organ. So that anything past the center 30 degrees to the brain is stupid. The optic nerve does not have a great investment in anything outside 20 degrees. Because we are a super conducting highway. The only exception is the monocular temporal crescent which starts at 60 degrees and goes to 90 degrees in one eye and that you find by confrontation. The only case I have ever seen of the monocular crescent being knocked out was a man who had a catheterization for coronary artery disease and, during the catheterization, he had an embolus. He saw flashing lights, sparkles, zigzag, had a homonymous hemianopia, and when things cleared, all he had was 30 degrees of field loss in his temporal crescent. And in his anterior lip of calcarine cortex at the splenium he had an infarct. We had missed that on all our field techniques short of static 90-degree full field. There is a full field program, even on the static programs on the Humphrey. You do not need it! Yes, almost all neurological fields can be detected in the central 30 degrees. They all come to the midline.

Dr. Calkwood: Dr. Burde is going to present a case for discussion.

Dr. Burde: This is a 45-year-old man who came to Jacobi, which is the Bronx Municipal Hospital, with a week's history of blurred vision and left-sided headache. The headache was said to be frontoparietal. It was about 4/10, if 10 is a very severe headache. It was alleviated by the use of acetaminophen, and he complained about double vision that was worse in right gaze.

Dr. Schatz: So he had a left VIth nerve palsy.

Dr. Burde: I will just make the comment that it was difficult to communicate with the patient. The past medical history, he had hypercholesterolemia and everything else was really non-contributory. On examination, his vision was 20/20 OU; color and brightness were equal. Look at his pupil. The pupil was 4.5 on the right side, briskly reactive to 2.5. On the left side, the side of the pain, he had a pupil that was a half millimeter larger, but briskly reactive, that was in the light, and similarly, briskly reactive but anisocoric in dim light. If one looked at ductions, there was a marked limitation in the field of the left inferior rectus, a mild reduction of action in the field of the left inferior oblique.

Dr. Schatz: But Ronnie, you said that he was worse in right gaze?

Dr. Burde: That is correct.

Dr. Schatz: So there is some symptomatic paradox?

Dr. Burde: Correct. And he measured what we thought were 15 diopters of left hypertropia and about 6 diopters of left exotropia in the primary position. The resident said, "Is this a partial IIIrd nerve palsy, and if it is, is it a pupillary sparing palsy?" And the remainder of the examination was normal with the exception of the flattening of the right side of his face with some residual from an old VIIth nerve palsy.

Dr. Schatz: So he had a history of an old VIIth?

Dr. Burde: Right. So the residents now called and said, "How shall we go about taking care of this patient? Does this fit the definition of a partial IIIrd? Is this what they mean when they talk about pupillary sparing?

Dr. Schatz: It is a very interesting question. This is a pupillary involving IIIrd. That is, if you look at what is contained in inferior division and what it requires to... when we say pupillary sparing IIIrd, we mean the lids droop completely, the eye will not adduct, the eye will not elevate, and the eye will not depress, and the pupil is a little bigger, but it still works. So that is pupillary sparing. But when you say there is a little inferior rectus and a little bit of pupil enlargement, and a little bit of inferior oblique, and everything else is spared, then the pupil is likely just as involved as all of the rest of IIIrd nerve function and from my standpoint, 45-year-old patients are not allowed to have vasculopathic IIIrd's to begin with, so now once you have established that the distribution of motility is in a IIIrd nerve pattern and the pupil is involved although it still works, your obligation is a simple one: find the cause of his partial IIIrd nerve palsy.

Dr. Burde: Jonathan, do you want to add something?

Dr. Calkwood: I think the pain also is important and would tip me off and warn me to investigate this further with neuroimaging.

Dr. Burde: So we have pain, painful partial IIIrd nerve palsy, and I think that whether this pupil is involved or not... Norm, what about the briskness? In other words, if this were a neurogenic IIIrd, would you not expect to see some difference in the reactivity of one pupil versus the other?

Dr. Schatz: So far you have shown us a patient with a motility disturbance and an essential anisocoria, and nothing about the pupil gives us any clue about it at all. And yes, this could be orbital myositis...we do not have one clue that the pupil is a motor pupil. You did not tell me when the lights were on they were even more unequal? You said they were the same. You did not say when they were dark they became more equal like we see in motor pupil. So whatever information we are getting about the pupil, it is not useful in solving the problem.

Dr. Burde: That is one of the critical points we would like you to take home with you. That pupil may look abnormal. There may be nothing but an essential anisocoria and, unless you have information to tell you that this is definitively pupillary sparing, you have an obligation to work this patient up and to evaluate the patient.
They could not get an MR, but they could get an angiogram. So my next question to you is, under any circumstances would you have gotten an angiogram immediately just because you could get it, versus waiting for an MR or CT?

Dr. Schatz: If the pupil was involved, I would have gone straight to the angiogram and not requested an MR. In this circumstance, I am still a little bit teased by the fact that orbital ultrasound might have been a nice way, if you could not get an MR, get orbital ultrasound and see if there was a fat muscle or dirty fat or something that suggested orbital pseudotumor. We have not established the anatomy yet as to where this lesion is located. It is nice to have the angiogram out of the way in a 45-year-old with what we thought might have been an incipient IIIrd.

Dr. Burde: The day after the angiogram, the inferior oblique was working a little less than before. There is a question now about how brisk that pupil was, but we are past the angiogram. The inferior rectus is still not working. At this time, we were able to get some imaging.

Dr. Schatz: So here we see the left orbit and that is the one of concern. Now let us follow structures backward and we will see. The lateral rectus looks okay, medial rectus is okay. He may be a little myopic. This is an unequal cut so you can see that we are at the bottom of one orbit, at the top of the other. So that makes looking at symmetry a little bit difficult. Let us go into cavernous sinus and see what there is there. We see two clinoids. They are okay. The pituitary fossa is all right. There is some question about whether this carotid is a little bit bigger. Here is the junction of where: this is the posterior clinoid, clivus, and then here is the interpeduncular space. So here is the IIIrd coming out here and the only thing that I see is that I cannot tell about that carotid.

Dr. Burde: What do you think this stuff intramedullary is?

Dr. Schatz: I am sorry, I missed a little bit of the something that is in the brainstem. So here on the T2, now we are at the little of the IIIrd nerve nucleus; here is the collicular plate; and you see that in the area of the periaqueductal gray, following the fasciculus of the IIIrd is this right T2 image. Then you see back over here a second.

Dr. Burde: What do you think that is?

Dr. Schatz: It looks like a met to me, but it has increased fluid content. I have to see it on T1 and on gad. I guess multiple lesions suggest the possibility of toxoplasmosis. Here is a periventricular lump that corresponds and here is that area that turned bright on T2 in the middle of the pons, and middle of the mesencephalon that was actually loosened as if it were cystic, so it is loosened on T1 and there it is ring-enhancing. So now we go through the ring-enhancing multiple lesions and toxo gets high on our list. So now we want to know his HIV status, lymphoma less likely.

Dr. Burde: Normal.

Dr. Schatz: Normal.

Dr. Calkwood: Any travel to Central America?

Dr. Burde: He is from Mexico. So what is this?

Dr. Schatz: It looks like cysticercosis.

Dr. Burde: Exactly.

Dr. Schatz: So this is just a case of cysticercosis. It is interesting that cysticercosis happens to like to be in the posterior IIIrd ventricle. It is one of the areas where deposition and trapping of cysticerci occur. This is sitting right in that posterior end of the IIIrd ventricle and then it has this lucency sitting anterior to it. It has partial hydrocephalus, so he is partially obstructed at the aqueductal level.

Dr. Burde: This is so-called *Taenia solium* or cysticercosis. Pig is the intermediate host. The only true host completing the life cycle is in man. The drug we use now is praziquantel. Some people go back to albendazole, and using it along with corticosteroids and anti-seizure medication. When we went back in his history, we found that he had had a grand mal seizure one year prior to being seen and a partial seizure two months prior to being seen. So here is somebody who presented with this multitude of lesions within the CNS who had a partial IIIrd nerve palsy that was likely to be probably not pupillary sparing, but only partially involved. Do we have any more questions from the audience?

Dr. Calkwood: We have a stack of questions from the audience, literally. I am just going to take them one at a time.

Are there as many cases of optic atrophy following topical retrobulbar anesthesia?

Dr. Schatz: You mean in the post-cataract extraction ischemic optic neuropathy, does anesthesia make a difference? We looked at this in our series and it certainly did not make any difference at all. The stay suture did not make a difference. The site of the incision did not. The technique did not make a difference. It would appear that the risk at disc and the pressure spike may be the major factors, but again, we do not have a full handle on it. There are those cases, as you know, where you know you have an orbital hemorrhage and the patient wakes up blind; that is a different disease. Those cases when you image them and you find a sheath hemorrhage with blood in the sheath itself or orbital blood, that is a different disorder.

Dr. Calkwood: Question directed for Dr. Schatz. What doses of Diamox do you use in idiopathic intracranial hypertension, and how often do you follow stable patients with papilledema?

Dr. Schatz: The starting dose is 500 mg a day just to see if they will tolerate it, and they usually do tolerate it. Patients do get tingling and paresthesias and all the rest, but you can usually manage that. The headaches you can manage with amitriptyline. Most patients end up within two weeks on 500 mg twice a day. That is what I would consider maximal medical management, and we treat their headaches with nortriptyline, amitriptyline, something that you know has both 5-hydroxy... an anti-pain, anti-nociceptive which improves the sleep pattern and helps them handle chronic illness. How often do you follow fields? We follow our pseudotumor patients weekly until fields are stable or improving; monthly until we see that their patterns have improved; and then every four months when their stable patterns have been shown to be improved, unless they call and say that there has been a change.

Dr. Burde: I hate to disagree with Norm. The fact is there is only one good paper on Diamox and that was in the *Journal of Neurosurgery* and they were using Diamox to lower pressure in people who had brain tumors. And that is the only good work. It showed that you required a minimum of 4 g of Diamox a day to be effective in lowering the pressure. I find that most people will not tolerate that much, but you can, if they do not tolerate that much, try methazolamide which is a Neptazane. Neptazane passes through the blood-brain barrier much better than acetazolamide and, therefore, you can get away with lower doses. The trade-off is that Diamox makes people sleepy and Neptazane makes them more sleepy, obviously because it is the amount getting in. But we have had patients who have tolerated 3 and 4 g of Diamox a day, whom we managed to hold until we got past whatever we had to get past.

Dr. Calkwood: Do you find that titrating the dose up slowly over a few days at a time lessens the side-effects?

Dr. Burde: I have not been aware of lessening of the side-effects by taking people up slowly. Diamox is a wonderful drug for people who get headaches in the mountains. So if you are a skier and you get skier's headaches, go on 250-500 mg of Diamox.

Dr. Schatz: You can go up to 2-3 g a day of Diamox if patients have a very difficult time tolerating it and, for the most part, you can manage your patients with 500 mg b.i.d. There is no doubt that if you are losing visual function, you should increase the dose and I do not disagree with Ron about that.

Dr. Calkwood: What would you use in someone who is allergic to sulpha?

Dr. Schatz: You are in trouble. Lasix has sulpha in it. You really have to know what the allergy is to sulpha. Stevens-Johnson syndrome, first time it happens, you know how much trouble you are in.

Dr. Burde: That is the patient in whom you might consider steroids.

Dr. Calkwood: Another question, shifting gears here a little bit, have the advantages of intravenous corticosteroids over oral therapy been conclusively demonstrated in the treatment of giant cell arteritis/ischemic optic neuropathy?

Dr. Burde: No, nobody has ever done this study to make a definitive statement. What we do know is that there are a number of cases of giant cell arteritis in which people are being treated with relatively high doses of steroids, who either reactivate or break through the steroids, lose vision in the other eye, and develop an ischemic retinopathy on top of it. And when you give them i.v. steroids by pulse, that in fact they respond within 24 hours and then you can slowly take them off it. There are no definitive tapers. Everything is really clinical opinion that is being offered.

Dr. Schatz: But at least in Grant Liu's review of the use of i.v. methylprednisolone, it was surprising to see that there was about 15% of improvement of visual function in a group of patients, so that when you suspect giant cell arteritis in this day and age in a patient of 70 years or above with a unilateral ischemic neuropathy, that patient should be hospitalized, placed on i.v. methylprednisolone, put on bed rest because, by the time ischemic neuropathy occurs, they are on the end of a perfusion system that already has their external carotid compromised, their internal carotid compromised, and their perfusion to the whole base of their skull compromised. They need plasma expanders without throwing them into failure, and they need urgent care. So, that is a group of patients. Now, even then, some of them develop the second eye, even with that therapy; but at least there is a group of those patients who recover visual function.

Dr. Burde: As many of you know, I have been a champion of large doses of steroids and have been using anywhere from 500 mg to 1 g four times a day. When I see these particular types of patients, what I do is go to a spinal cord steroid dose over 24 hours. You are getting the pulse in, and all that methylprednisolone is gone within 24 hours and what you have done is you have it in the right concentration to stabilize the membranes. Then I keep them on something like 60 a day and I slowly taper them down. Is there any evidence that that works? The answer is no.

The fact is that we need to set up a number of studies, but they are not even in the works yet.

Dr. Calkwood: A follow-up to that steroid question regarding multiple sclerosis in optic neuritis. "Barring any contraindications, should all patients with optic neuritis be offered i.v. steroids to delay the risk of MS, or perhaps just those at higher risk?"

Dr. Schatz: I addressed the issue yesterday and that is a pretty direct question about it. You are still in the area where clinical judgment is the best choice. Here is what we do not know. We know that if you have done your study and found a female with a single attack of optic neuritis and you find grade i.v. MR scan, the likelihood of that patient having MS over the next two years is something like 70%. We do know that if you gave i.v. methylprednisolone, the statistical number of new white matter lesions over that two years would be about 23% less than if you had never given i.v. steroids. And I think that really has changed our attitudes. That does not mean you need them hospitalized. Right now, i.v. steroids with a visiting nurse or outpatient delivery can be done very easily, but I think that is our obligation. Given the patient with good acuity, single attack, no lesions in central nervous system, our predictability of attacks over two years is much less, and that patient needs a rescan in six months. But those are the kind of protocols we are going to start working out to see what formula is the best, that patient does not need i.v. steroids. Their likelihood of returning to 20/20 vision is excellent. Their likelihood of having MS over the next two years is less. And the risks of imposing that aggressive a treatment on them are a little too much, we are not in the safety code now.

Dr. Calkwood: Another question along the same lines is, "Should i.v. methylprednisolone followed by oral steroids be given for repeat attacks of optic neuritis?"

Dr. Burde: I think there is so little evidence that, unless you are really backed up against the wall, the use of i.v. steroids is not going to do anything or p.o. steroids are not going to do anything but maybe shorten an attack by a couple of days, and so I do not think it is worth the difference. In fact, now we have the blessing that in chronic progressive disease where we used to use corticosteroids, we now have β-interferon available. We have other interferon products that are coming out and being looked at that are already in Phase III studies. So, no, unless the patient were severely impaired, I would probably choose not to treat the patient.

Dr. Schatz: I think we have all decided that one of our markers of activity of disease is going to be new gadolinium-enhancing lesions that may tell us something about active disease without clinical manifestations. And remember, it is the addition of more and more confluent lesions that leads to the euphoria, dementia, and things that begin to sneak up on what we call chronic relapsing, and add to the debility. So, we are at this science fiction of the answers. Science fiction of today is the truth of tomorrow. We are almost there with myelin basic protein, betaseron with the new form, even the i.v. methylprednisolone role in delaying new lesions of the central nervous system. On our way, I do not think we can get over-reactive. If you see an optic neuritis patient for the first time and they have four or more ovoid or periventricular and they show active gadolinium enhancement, that is active disease and that calls for looking at what you can do to make it inactive and what you can do to prevent the next attack. We have some things that suggest we can do both. Betaseron is not without complications of fever, pyrexia, fatigue, etc., but it is getting better and more refined, and the new protocols are looking even better. I think what you will see around the country is the proliferation of multiple sclerosis total care clinics in which MR will become part of the assessment as we have new protocols to evaluate patients.

Dr. Calkwood: This is a question addressed to Dr. Burde. "Are there any theories regarding the male predominance of Leber's optic neuropathy?"

Dr. Burde: Simply, that when you look at the gametes as there is cell division to form the egg and the sperm, the sperm has no room to have mitochondria in it. And we know that it is the mitochondrial DNA that leads to.. the particular mutation is occurring in the mitochondrial DNA. Therefore, it is only the ovum that can carry that particular genetic species, and therefore, when you have the sperm come in, it does not add anything to it. So that if the mother has it, the likelihood is that it will be maintained and passed; whereas, why you get a 1:1 ratio in Japan is a much more difficult question to address.

Dr. Schatz: The question was if maternal DNA has the mitochondrial all the time, why do they not get the disease?

Dr. Burde: Women do get the disease in a ratio of 1:4. The fact is that there is a dilution in the number of mitochondria.

Dr. Calkwood: The next question is really a case. A 40-year-old with a closed head injury presents six months after a motor vehicle accident. No loss of conscious occurred. Complaints are blurred vision, intermittent headaches, no refractive error with presbyopia, what studies would you do, and would you follow this patient, and if so, for how long?

Dr. Schatz: You have not given us one objective sign of visual disturbance. We need an acuity, an afferent pupillary defect, a field that shows something is wrong, and if not, he has a post-traumatic syndrome and we will treat him accordingly.

Dr. Burde: The truth, though, is that there is a post-traumatic syndrome that is real in a small percentage of patients. And those people often get overlooked because everybody said this is occurring six months down the road. Obviously, we do not have enough information to go on further, but indeed, every patient has the right when coming to us to have a total evaluation and not to be predetermined that he has his lawyer in hand.

Dr. Schatz: The post-traumatic syndrome of headaches, myalgias, sleep disturbance, etc., may really in fact have as their base a secondary gain, but many times the patients are trapped in that and they have to be treated as any unconscious conflict would be treated with appropriate neurotransmitters and taking away secondary gain. The syndromes of post-traumatic migraine have just been recently reviewed again in the *Green Journal on Neurology* and this post-traumatic syndrome, by a rather cynical approach. I have never had that approach. I think these patients respond well to medical management, sometimes requiring Prozac and other drugs to get their sleep pattern back to normal, to get their circadians back to normal, and to have them reassured. The post-traumatic syndrome does in fact build on itself.

Dr. Burde: And I think that over the next few years our responsibilities as ophthalmologists are going to grow and that we will be responsible for knowing how to use certain drugs that we have talked about, for example, the tricyclic antidepressants in the treatment of headaches. We will have to learn to use Prozac or Zoloft, and where it is appropriate and where it is not. I think that, in the past, we could askew that to other people, but I think that the way things are going now and what will be required of us in terms of being a general ophthalmologist will be to know how to use these drugs appropriately.

Dr. Schatz: And I think what Dr. Burde meant was to use it ourselves as we get more and more depressed.

Dr. Calkwood: Here is a more open-ended question. "How do you differentiate optic neuritis from ischemic optic neuropathy?"

Dr. Schatz: We can first talk about the overlaps. You have seen that the fields can be the same; you have seen that the discs can be swollen in both; you have seen that there is a difference in age group. We have said that optic neuritis has a mean onset of 33 years and we have said that ischemic optic neuropathy has a mean of 68 years. That means that, at any given case, there are cases you will not be able to distinguish. We have said that streak hemorrhages on the disc are almost unheard of in optic neuritis. They are the rule in ischemic optic neuropathy. We have said altitudinal field defects, arcuates are the rule, but they occur in optic neuritis. So the answer to the question is, sometimes you cannot, but for the most part, if you go through your checklist of age, morphology of disc, nature and character of field disturbance, predisposing factors, you can come up with an educated guess as to which it is.

Dr. Calkwood: A question for Dr. Burde. "If a patient presents with hyperthyroidism and exophthalmos, do you recommend surgical thyroidectomy as opposed to radiation therapy?"

Dr. Burde: I think the best way to treat these people is with medications such as propylthiouracil. In those people, about 4.2%, so it is said, will go on to develop the ophthalmopathy or dysthyroid ophthalmopathy. About 5.2% develop ophthalmopathy after surgery and 6.8% or so after radioactive iodine, so I prefer to treat these patients using medical therapy if at all possible, and the majority of patients will respond to the medical therapy.

Dr. Schatz: But Ron, that is somewhat in contrast to what endocrinologists like to do for the long-term management of Graves' disease of the thyrotoxicosis, and do you think there is a place anticipating orbitopathy, the patient with early orbitopathy that you or the endocrinologist wants to give radioactive iodine, to give steroids through the period of treatment?

Dr. Burde: There is one paper in the *Lancet* which says, if you pretreat patients with prednisone in a dose of between 60 and 80 mg per day before you give the radioactive iodide, that the incidence of dysthyroid orbitopathy will be reduced to nil. The problem is that that paper is about eight years old and I have never seen it repeated. I have never seen any confirmatory data.

Dr. Schatz: We are trying to repeat it now and the data look pretty good, but I cannot tell you for sure. Our numbers are too small.

Dr. Burde: I really think that, if you can treat these patients medically, you can actually reverse the autoimmune phenomenology that exists, that is, the T4, T8 helper cell/suppressor cell ratio on medical therapy will revert to normal. I think if you can do that and get rid of the autoimmune component, the patient is going to be better off in the long run.

Index of authors